Preface

This is the sixth edition of the handbook for doctors that the International Planned Parenthood Federation has published. The first three were called simply the *IPPF Medical Handbook*. From the fourth edition in 1974 the title has been *Family Planning Handbook for Doctors*.

Information on the methods of family planning continues to increase, as does that on subjects surrounding contraception. Because of this, the book has been expanded substantially, with five new chapters. The great majority of the chapters that appeared in the fifth edition have been completely re-written and brought up to date. In addition, an important and, we hope, useful innovation has been the inclusion of the authoritative policy statements of the IPPF International Medical Advisory Panel (IMAP).

This Panel, which was constituted in 1979, is made up of members of the medical profession who are acknowledged by the international medical community as experts in the family planning field. Since 1980 the Panel has produced statements on all the main methods of family planning, on infertility and on the acquired immune deficiency syndrome (AIDS). Many of the statements put out in the early 1980s have been brought up to date when new knowledge has been forthcoming. These statements are now incorporated in this *Handbook* at the ends of the chapters to which they refer.

Of the five new chapters in the *Handbook*, one discusses breast feeding as it is related to fertility and contraception. Lactation is still playing an important role in birth spacing in many parts of the world, and its practical aspects in connection with fertility are gone into in some detail. There is also a useful chapter explaining some of the statistical terms used in family planning work; terms which may puzzle some of those working in this field. Adolescents, as well as older women in the decade before the menopause, pose problems in the choice of contraception, and a new chapter addresses the particular difficulties both these groups, and those advising them, may come across when choosing a suitable method of contraception.

7

Long-acting hormonal contraceptives now occupy a special chapter. In the previous edition of this book, these forms of contraception were incorporated in the chapter on systemic contraception. Now they are on their own, and oral contraception occupies a substantial chapter by itself. Post-coital contraception, which was mentioned briefly in 1980, now merits a chapter of its own as well.

In the previous edition, a chapter dealt with community based distribution of contraceptives. This has been expanded to cover non-clinic service delivery, which incorporates a section on the rapidly growing delivery system of social marketing.

As with previous editions of the *Handbook*, although it is primarily addressed to doctors, the information in it will be useful to all members of the family planning team: doctors, midwives, nurses, and para-medical workers. It will be useful in clinics and doctors' surgeries and offices, as a book of reference to remind members of the family planning health team of the latest information in 1988 about all forms of contraception, and allied subjects such as infertility. Much stress has been laid throughout the book on counselling potential users of contraceptive services. The separate counselling chapter has been re-written and enlarged, and where applicable throughout the book, many separate chapters contain useful and important counselling advice.

Once again we hope the 1988 *Family Planning Handbook for Doctors* will be as useful as previous editions have proved to be. It should play an important role in the day-to-day work of all family planning doctors and many health workers, whether in the IPPF system or outside it, giving, as it does, up-to-date information on a range of family planning methods and allied subjects.

Acknowledgements

The various chapters in the *Family Planning Handbook for Doctors* were drafted by experts in their fields. They include: Prof. Michael Adler, Dr Leonard Barron, Dr John Cleland, Prof. Elizabeth Connell, Dr Nicholas Dennis, Dr Harold Francis, Prof. Ian Fraser, Dr John Guillebaud, Dr Geraldine Howard, Prof. Peter Howie, Dr Douglas Huber, Dr Ali Kubba, Prof. John Marshall, Dr John McEwan, Dr John Paxman, Mr John Pike, Dr Malcolm Potts, Dr Madan Singh, Dr Robert Snowden, Dr M R van Santen, Dr Catherine Vaughan Williams, Dr Elspeth Williamson and Dr Robert Yule.

Additional material for some chapters was supplied by:

W. Roger March '89.

IPPF
MEDICAL
PUBLICATIONS

Family Planning
Handbook
for Doctors

Edited for the IPPF by
Ronald L. Kleinman
M.B., Ch.B., D.(Obst.)R.C.O.G.

6th edition
1988

INTERNATIONAL PLANNED PARENTHOOD FEDERATION

International Office
PO Box 759, Inner Circle, Regent's Park, London NW1 4LQ, England
Telephone: 01-486 0741   Fax: 01-487 7950
Cables: IPEPEE LONDON   Telex: 919573 IPEPEE G

AIMS OF THE
INTERNATIONAL PLANNED
PARENTHOOD FEDERATION

IPPF, believing that knowledge of planned parenthood is a fundamental human right, and that a balance between the population of the world and its natural resources and productivity is a necessary condition of human happiness, prosperity and peace, has as its aims:

(*a*) *to advance the education of the countries of the world in family planning and responsible parenthood in the interest of family welfare, community well-being and international goodwill;*

(*b*) *to increase the understanding by people and governments of the demographic problems of their own communities and of the world;*

(*c*) *to promote population education, sex education and marriage counselling;*

(*d*) *to stimulate appropriate research in the following subjects: the biological, demographic, economic, eugenic, psychological and social implications of human fertility and its regulation; methods of contraception, fertility, subfertility and sterility; and to collect and make known the findings of such research;*

(*e*) *to stimulate and assist the formation of family planning associations in all countries;*

(*f*) *to stimulate and promote family planning in all countries through other appropriate organizations;*

(*g*) *to encourage and organize the training of all appropriate professional workers such as medical and health personnel, educationalists, social and community development workers in the implementation of the objectives of IPPF;*

(*h*) *to organize regional or international workshops, seminars and conferences;*

(*i*) *to take all appropriate measures to further the above objectives.*

Contents

Ms Caroline Clayton, Prof. Rebecca Cook, Prof. Bernard Dickens, Mr Sev Fluss, Dr Nicholas Ford, Prof. Stephen Isaacs and Dr Iqbal Shah.

Review of the chapters was divided among members of the IPPF International Medical Advisory Panel (IMAP) and of the IPPF Medical Editorial Advisory Board, as well as a number of acknowledged experts outside the IPPF system. Members of the IPPF Secretariat gave invaluable help as well, in particular Dr Pramilla Senanayake, Assistant Secretary General, Technical Services, and Dr Carlos Huezo, Head of Medical Programmes.

Current members of IMAP are: Prof. Mahmoud Fathalla (Chairman), Dr Phil Corfman, Dr Soledad Diaz, Dr Kerstin Hagenfeldt, Prof. Shan Ratnam, Prof. Allan Rosenfield, Prof. Fred Sai and Dr Badri Saxena. Former members of IMAP (Profs. Lidja Andolsek, Ulf Borell and Rodney Shearman) also reviewed the book.

Current members of the IPPF Medical Editorial Advisory Board are: Prof. Max Elstein (Chairman), Dr John Cleland, Miss Ann Cowper, Prof. Robert Edwards, Dr Harold Francis, Dr Ros Goddard, Dr Jan Karbaat, Prof. David Morley, Dr Madan Singh and Dr Robert Snowden.

Chapter 1

The Doctor's Role in Family Planning

Doctors have been at the forefront of family planning programmes for many years. They have promoted the health rationale for family planning and have been able to explain and put into perspective some of the more controversial issues related to family planning.

It is recognized that in many countries there are very few doctors per head of population. In some countries the ratio can be as low as one doctor to 100,000 people. This must be borne in mind when deciding on the role a doctor can play in a family planning programme. In addition, it has been felt even in countries where doctors are more freely available that their role need not necessarily be in the day-to-day delivery of routine family planning services.

The doctor, however, has very many functions to perform in the organization, administration and delivery of family planning services. These will be discussed below.

Service delivery

It is now accepted by many that counselling and delivery in relation to oral contraception and barrier methods of contraception, such as condoms and diaphragms, can be effectively delegated by doctors to other trained health professionals, such as nurses and midwives or paramedical workers. In many countries, community-based family planning services use trained lay personnel for the delivery of some of these services (see Chapter 20, page 311).

A doctor, however, should always be available for referral of clients who are unable to use these methods of contraception or who have side-effects or problems associated with their use. In addition, the doctor should play an important role in the training of health workers and lay personnel in counselling and delivery of services.

The doctor does play an important part in delivering surgical methods of contraception. For example, in some countries it may be necessary for the doctor to be the team leader in the provision of male and female sterilization. In other countries, doctors have effectively trained other health personnel in these surgical techniques. In either situation the doctor has to be responsible overall for the client and for the services provided. The fitting of intrauterine devices has also been effectively delegated to other trained health personnel in many countries.

In all these situations, the doctor should be responsible for providing the training and acting as a referral point for problem or complicated cases.

When new methods of contraception become available, it has usually been the doctor's responsibility to carry out the necessary training and be engaged in the delivery of these methods. For example, the insertion of Norplant, when it first reached the stage of clinical trials, was confined to doctors, but now, with wider use and availability, many health professionals other than doctors have been trained in the delivery of this method.

Helping infertile couples is an important aspect of all family planning programmes. The doctor has a major role to play in this area. Some of the investigations and treatment required for helping these couples may have to be carried out by the doctor. In other cases, these could be delegated, under supervision, to trained health personnel. Doctors will be the ones to refer infertile couples to specialist hospitals if more complicated methods of treatment are required.

Research

The doctor has an important part to play in designing and carrying out research, both at the basic laboratory level and also at the field level. The design of clinical trials and epidemiological surveys can also be organized by the medical profession. Clients who are part of a clinical research programme need special attention. These clients are usually followed up by a doctor.

Advocacy

The doctor has a crucial role to play in advocating family planning at various levels. In providing counselling to the couple or to an individual, the doctor is in an ideal position to provide information on the benefits of delaying the first pregnancy, spacing births, reducing the total number of children to four or less and in ending child bearing once a woman has reached the age of 30 to 35.

In addition, the doctor, as a community leader, has an important part to play in educating the community about the benefits of family planning. He will also be in a position to allay any anxieties and concerns that the individual, the couple or the public at large may have in relation to family planning programmes in general, or to a particular method of contraception.

At the national level, the doctor has a role in convincing policy makers about the importance of family planning and the need for decentralized and well-organized service outlets. Often the doctor is called upon to discuss controversial aspects of family planning programmes and methods of birth control with the media. He should put forward positive facts abou the value of family planning and not simply react to adverse criticism. On occasion, he may indeed have to react to adverse publicity from the media, but he should use every opportunity to be forthright and positive and disseminate information on the health and social benefits of family planning.

Administration

The doctor is usually at the top of the pyramid in relation to both administration and service provision in family planning. Those in charge of the organization of a family planning clinic will have to supervise the work there, which includes such matters as budgeting, record keeping and liaison with health authorities and other government departments. The doctor will have to help to train the staff of a clinic, for example, in the correct way to keep records and statistics of the clients attending. This is a most important way of finding out what is happening with regard to the uptake of family planning in a particular area.

At the government level some doctors may be involved in the actual administration of family planning programmes in a particular country, and there they can bring their medical knowledge to bear on the problems involved in instituting national or local programmes. They would also have to make sure that doctors and other health personnel working in such programmes are adequately trained in the tasks they have to perform.

Chapter 2

Factors Affecting Human Fertility

Introduction

The ultimate constraints on human fertility — the production of live-born offspring — are biological in nature. In reality, however, many social, cultural and economic influences operate to depress fertility well below the biological maximum. Biological variations in the capacity to conceive and bear children are extremely important at the level of the individual couple, but play a relatively minor role in determining the differences in the level of fertility between societies, except in a few exceptional circumstances.

At the outset a fundamental distinction can be drawn between two types of reproductive regime: *natural* fertility, where no conscious attempt is made by couples to regulate the spacing and number of children; and *controlled* fertility, where couples deliberately influence the timing and limit the number of births. The contents of this *Handbook* are largely devoted to a discussion of the various ways in which individuals may regulate their fertility in a conscious and purposive manner. However, this chapter starts by considering fertility in the absence of deliberate control.

Biological limits to fertility

In an imaginary healthy population, where all women marry at the age of 15 years and remain married until at least age 50, and where no birth control or breast feeding is practised, the average woman will bear about 15 children over her life-time. In this hypothetical situation, the level of fertility is constrained by biological factors which determine the onset and end of reproductive life and the spacing between births.

Virtually all child bearing occurs between the ages of 15 and 45. Within this span, fecundity, or reproductive capacity, is relatively low in adolescence, reaches a peak in the early twenties, remains high until age 35, and thereafter declines sharply to reach zero by age 50. In non-contracepting populations, the average maternal age at the time of the last birth is close to 40 years.

A total of 15 births within this age span implies a rate of one child about every 18 months to two years. This interval between births is composed of four main parts: a delay of 1.5 to 2.0 months following each birth before ovulation is resumed (in the absence of breast feeding); an average waiting time, or delay, of six to seven months before a recognizable conception occurs (i.e. a conception which results in a delay of the first menses after fertilization); a further short average delay caused by embryo and fetal wastage after the first four weeks; and finally nine months gestation.

The short span of an ovulation following childbirth and the length of gestation are relatively fixed. The waiting time to conception is more variable between individuals and populations, because it is related to the frequency of sexual intercourse. At a coital frequency of 10 times per menstrual cycle (thought to be the average in most populations, though reliable evidence is fragmentary) the probability of conception in a cycle is estimated to be 0.28. This rises to an estimated probability of 0.43 at a frequency of 20 coital acts per month and falls to 0.04 at a frequency of once per month.

The other main determinants of the waiting time to a recognizable conception are failure of the fertilized ovum to implant or the occurrence of a spontaneous abortion before the first missed menses. Such early embryo wastage may be as high as 50% of all fertilizations, although evidence is again meagre.

The length of the average interval between live births is further increased by embryo and fetal wastage after the first four weeks. The overall risk of such intrauterine death after the fourth gestational week is probably about 20%, with the great majority of losses occurring at early gestational ages.

Fertility in the absence of conscious regulation

Even in the absence of contraception, fertility never reaches the average biological maximum of 15 births per woman. Rather, the average level in a population is usually confined to a range of four to nine births per woman. Thus all societies possess a powerful array of customs and practices which depress human fertility well below its biological maximum.

The factors which directly affect fertility are known as proximate determinants. These include nuptiality (the marriage condition), contraception, infertility and breast feeding. These proximate determinants are discussed throughout the rest of this chapter.

Social restrictions on sexual intercourse constitute a major fertility check through the institution of marriage. Child bearing outside recognized marital unions is usually discouraged with varying degrees of severity. Thus the proportion of women who marry and the age at which they do so are crucial determinants of the fertility level. The diversity of marriage customs is truly immense. At one extreme, many Asian societies have traditions of universal marriage for women as soon as puberty is reached, with betrothal arranged long in advance of puberty. At the other extreme, much of Western Europe before the 20th century was characterized by a high level of celibacy (with up to one-third of women unmarried at age 50) and late ages of marriage. Even today in China there is a high rate of celibacy among unmarried people and a later age of marriage.

The reasons for this fascinating diversity lie deep in social and economic structures. One major set of influences is social expectations concerning the economic independence of the newly wed couple. In Western Europe, marriage was discouraged until the couple could be self-supporting in their own household. The need for a man to be economically secure before seeking marriage acted as a major barrier, particularly at times of low national prosperity. In many Asian societies, this economic impediment to marriage does not operate; the newly married customarily reside with the husband's family, and there is no expectation that they will be self-supporting. These traditional arrangements have changed considerably over the last generation, particularly among the more educated persons, with the result that marriage ages have risen sharply in many Asian countries.

Customs concerning the dissolution of marriages and re-marriage are equally diverse, though, in general, societies characterized by unstable marriages tolerate re-marriage readily, and thus dilute the negative effect of instability on fertility.

Within marriage, rather little is known about cultural variations in the frequency of sexual intercourse. There is undoubtedly immense individual variability and a pervasive decline with the lengthening of marriage, which leads to longer birth intervals as the marriage progresses. Avoidance of sexual relations on religious festivals and the permanent cessation of a sexually active life when the eldest children in the family themselves start reproduction are reported for a number of societies, but the overall effect on fertility may not be great. Of far greater significance is the delayed resumption of sexual intercourse following childbirth. Prolonged post-natal abstinence may have been a common feature of traditional hunter-gatherers and other populations. Today, the custom persists most strongly in sub-Saharan Africa, where delays of one to two years are still common in many countries. Even in this region, however, there is evidence of a decline in this once powerful birth-spacing mechanism; younger, urban and educated couples typically abstain for an appreciably shorter duration than older, rural and uneducated couples.

Of equal importance to marriage and sexual customs in its influence on 'natural' fertility is breast feeding. It is now known that breast feeding inhibits ovulation through a complex hormonal path, triggered by the infant's stimulation of the nipple (see page 194). Suckling has to be maintained at a certain intensity to inhibit ovulation. Full breast feeding without appreciable supplementation is usually sufficient to protect the mother against the risk of conception. As supplementation is introduced and the frequency of suckling declines, ovulation and menstruation return.

In general terms, it is thought that each month of breast feeding provides a little over half a month of protection against conception. Thus 18 months of breast feeding are associated with nine months of post-partum anovulation. But the relationship varies considerably between individuals and populations, because of differences in the intensity of suckling. This variation, and the small but nevertheless appreciable risk that a breast-feeding woman will conceive before she is aware of her return to reproductive capacity through the occurrence of her first menses, limits the reliability of lactation as a method of birth spacing for an individual couple. It remains true, however, that lactation is a powerful check on fertility, perhaps preventing as many births as contraception.

Prolonged breast feeding of two years or more was probably the norm in traditional societies, and is very common among the rural populations of China, the Indian sub-continent and sub-Saharan Africa. It tends to decline in response to urbanization and modernization, which engender incompatible life styles. This tendency may lead to an increase in fertility unless counterbalanced by the use of contraception.

In comparison with marriage and breast-feeding customs, other checks on natural fertility, while often important for the individual couple, are much less powerful determinants of societal fertility. Reproductive capacity is not closely linked to nutritional levels.

Under-nutrition has to be extremely severe before ovulation ceases. Disease, of course, occasionally exerts a major influence on fertility. The level of primary infertility in some tropical African countries, in the 1960s, was as high as 20-30%, largely because of sexually transmitted diseases. This contrasts with a level of about 5% in the majority of populations. Some diseases, notably malaria, are known to increase the risk of fetal loss, though the relatively high level of natural fertility in regions of the world where malaria is endemic suggests that this effect is not a major restraint.

The advent of controlled fertility

The traditional restraints on human fertility, discussed in the last section, take the form of social customs, which are not consciously varied by individual couples to control family size. For instance, it appears that women who want no more children do not deliberately prolong breast feeding to achieve this goal. The advent of contraception represents a shift in reproductive control from social customs to decision-making by the individual couple. This increase in the ability of individuals to take charge of their own destiny is perhaps the most fundamental characteristic of contraception.

The link between sexual intercourse and child bearing and fetal development in the uterus is almost universally recognized. Knowledge of some methods of birth control — abstinence, withdrawal, and induced abortion — therefore must have been present for thousands of years. Undoubtedly, birth control and infanticide, in extreme situations, have been used throughout human history. However, the first recorded instance of widespread use of birth control to limit family size is provided by France in the 18th century. Between 1880 and 1930, the use of birth control spread throughout Europe and overseas European settlements. Over the last 30 years, the practice has been widely adopted in most Asian and South American populations, and there are signs of change in Africa and the Arab world.

The shift from natural to controlled fertility is truly a revolution. The breaking of the link between sexual intercourse and reproduction represents a new freedom in human relations. The effect on the lives of women has been especially profound. Under conditions of 'natural' fertility, a woman typically spends 20 years of her life in the delivery and rearing of six or so children. Under conditions of controlled fertility, family size can be restricted to much smaller numbers of children and the process of family formation may be accomplished in a mere five to 10 years.

In view of its importance, it is not surprising that the family planning revolution has attracted much attention and research. The commonest explanation for the change is that the modernization of societies changes the economics of child bearing in such a way that a large number of children become a disadvantage to parents. Fertility decline is thus seen as a rational response to changes in external economic circumstances. In traditional societies, it is argued, children are beneficial to parents from an early age as a source of labour; they are an investment for support in old age, act as an insurance against risk in a hazardous environment, and enhance the physical security and political influence of the family unit.

Modernization erodes these benefits either directly or by providing more attractive alternatives. The shift from family-based to larger-scale modes of production reduces the labour usefulness of children, and the advent of mass education further decreases their availability for work. New forms of investment and insurance arise and, increasingly, political and legal functions are taken over by specialized non-familial institutions. At the same time, growth of a cash economy may heighten awareness of the cost of children in terms of food and clothes. These costs are increased directly by educational expenses and, indirectly, by the lost opportunity for mothers to exploit the rising employment opportunities outside the home.

The factors set out above are basic in society and thus change at a relatively slow pace. Economic development and the growth of communication media, however, also bring new opportunities, goods, and services, which may affect what people buy and what they aspire to more rapidly. The desire for consumer goods may compete with the desire for children. Similarly, the increased opportunities, represented in particular by the educational system, for investing resources in children may act to raise parental hopes on their behalf. This introduces a conflict between 'quantity' and 'quality' of offspring.

A further powerful set of arguments about the causes of fertility reduction through family planning concerns mortality. Until recent times, human populations have suffered high death rates, in proportion to their smaller numbers, particularly at the hands of occasional but catastrophic famines, epidemics and warfare. There has been high maternal and infant mortality because of disease. Faced with this risk of decimation, social rules evolved that encouraged high fertility and discouraged birth control. When mortality falls, these rules are no longer necessary and birth control can flourish.

There is surprisingly little firm evidence to support either the arguments concerning the economic value of children or the role of mortality decline. Numerous social surveys have shown that poor rural couples in developing countries do not actively seek large numbers of children. Only in sub-Saharan Africa are large families desired. In other regions, there is overwhelming evidence that high numbers of conceptions are unwelcome. Economists may well have exaggerated the extent to which large numbers of offspring are needed in pre-modern societies.

The provision of family planning services

Even in settings where parents desire no more than two to four children, there may be considerable initial resistance towards the idea of family planning and suspicions about particular methods. Sympathetic understanding at this stage can make a vital difference to individual couples and to the general spread of contraception within a community.

It is commonly believed that the major source of initial opposition to family planning comes from husbands rather than from wives. It is true that the burden of child bearing and rearing falls disproportionately on the wife. However, there is little evidence that husbands universally want larger families or that they are hostile to contraception.

In many societies, contraception has first been established among more educated couples in their late twenties or early thirties, who already have as many children as they want. Limitation, rather than spacing, has been the prime motive, and the practice has spread at varying speeds from urban to rural areas and from the more educated to the less educated. One of the greatest contributions of family planning services is to hasten this diffusion and thus ensure that all sectors of society are equally free from the burden of unwelcome conceptions.

In view of the serious effects of inadequate birth spacing on the health of mother and child, it is regrettable that the provision of family planning contraception for limitation has sometimes overshadowed provision for spacing. It remains true that couples in many cultures will wish to prove their fertility as soon as possible after marriage and therefore be uninterested in postponing the first birth.

19

But once this milestone is achieved, the medical case is strong for routine advocacy of reversible contraception to ensure a reasonable interval of at least two years before the second child is born. The value of contraceptive use early in family building is underscored by the research finding that such early use leads to more efficient use at later stages.

The provision of contraception for birth spacing should be sensitive to the natural birth-spacing mechanisms discussed in the previous section. In cultures where prolonged and intensive breast feeding is the custom or where (as in many African countries) the resumption of sexual intercourse is delayed for 12 months or more, it is unnecessary, or even counter-productive, to advocate early post-partum adoption of contraception. Advice must be carefully attuned to the circumstances and needs of particular couples.

The diversity of experience over the last 100 years is so great that few confident generalizations can be made about the relative acceptability of particular contraceptive methods and the relative effectiveness of different ways of promoting contraception. In Western Europe between 1880 and 1930, for instance, the spread of birth control was dominated by withdrawal, with little involvement of the medical profession, and this method is still the most commonly practised form of contraception in certain Eastern European countries. The large decrease in fertility over this period is a warning against denigration of methods that are intrinsically less effective than more modern methods. More important than the theoretical effectiveness of a method is the willingness of couples to sustain its use, and the efficacy with which they actually deploy the method (use effectiveness). Discontinuation rates of 50% within 12 months of starting a method are commoly reported.

In striking contrast to historical Europe, the contraception revolution of the last 30 years has been dominated by effective modern methods, notably oral contraception, intrauterine devices and sterilization. There are very few instances where the practice of withdrawal or periodic abstinence has increased appreciably. The sharp variations between countries in the apparent popularity of different methods may reflect ill-understood cultural factors. Even more important, however, are differences in the availability and promotion of particular methods.

In societies where the principle of reproductive control is not still fully accepted, methods which do not require constant motivation (notably sterilization, injectables, intrauterine devices and implants) have an obvious appeal. In rural areas where sources of contraceptive advice and supplies are thinly dispersed, such methods have an additional advantage of avoiding re-supply problems. But there is a danger in this line of reasoning. Mass promotion of such methods as the intrauterine device without adequate provision of follow-up services has sometimes proved to be detrimental to the woman's health or to some family planning programmes. Genuine side-effects can be inflated by rumours and lead to steep declines in subsequent acceptability of the method. This is not to argue against such methods; the huge growth in the popularity of sterilization in Europe and North America, for instance, attests to the demand for permanent methods even in societies where alternatives are widely available. Adequate after-care, however, is essential.

Government attitudes to the provision of family planning services also vary widely. Much depends on the prevalent level of fertility and the perceived link between demographic trends and economic and national development. At one extreme are governments who perceive low birth rates as undesirable and who, on occasion, have withdrawn family planning services in an attempt to raise the level of child bearing. At the other end of the spectrum there are many more governments which regard high birth rates, and resulting rapid population growth, as an economic threat. In these circumstances, official family planning programmes are usually launched with the object of reducing birth rates. A wide range of strategies has been harnessed to popularize family planning. In some countries, mass media campaigns have been used and active involvement of communities has been sought. Such a high social prominence for the ideas of small families and family planning has played an important role in breaking the crust of conservative opposition and suspicion and has eased the rapid spread of contraception. In other settings, however, the advent of modern contraception has not been accompanied by strong publicity. The successful experience of one country cannot be transferred automatically to another.

In conclusion, the role of health personnel in the provision of contraceptive services is bound to vary according to local circumstances. At its heart, however, lie the basic rules of good clinical practice: sensitivity and patience in allaying the fears of individuals about novel practices; the tailoring of recommendations to suit individual circumstances; and a willingness to provide sustained after-care.

Chapter 3

Counselling and Contraceptive Choice

Counselling someone who comes for advice on family planning matters implies more than simply offering information and an expert professional opinion on what an appropriate course of action should be. While that person will quite properly expect expert advice, counselling also entails *listening* to her or his special, individual needs and circumstances. It allows the person concerned to take an active rather than a passive role in the decision-making process. In particular, it goes beyond mere questions of 'fact', and includes a discussion and exploration of feelings and relationships. All counsellors require adequate training in what is a complicated and often subtle two-way relationship.

The counsellor may be a doctor, or a midwife, nurse or paramedical member of the family planning team. It is often an advantage if the counsellor is of the same sex as the person being counselled, and, in certain situations, of the same ethnic or cultural group.

When community-based distribution of contraceptives takes place (see page 311), the distributor (often a satisfied user herself) may make an ideal counsellor.

Counselling allows clients to explore vague anxieties and uncertainties which may only be partially formulated in their own minds, and to work towards a satisfactory personal resolution of these feelings. Of course, this takes time, much more time than straightforward one-sided instruction or direction. But it allows a real 'consultation' between provider and client, and confers the overwhelming advantage of gaining the active and willing participation of the client in the course of action which is eventually decided. A well-informed client, who has taken a well-considered decision after the counselling, is much more likely to continue as a contented and successful family planning user.

Contraceptive choice

The use of any method of contraception is not always enjoyable; taking a hormone preparation regularly in order to inhibit fertility, fitting a cap or a condom, the insertion of an IUD, having a long-acting injection, testing the consistency of cervical mucus, or the prospect of a sterilization operation, all these have their drawbacks and difficulties, and are not experiences to which individuals look forward with any sense of pleasurable anticipation. Indeed, the reverse is nearer the truth. The methods of fertility regulation from which most couples choose represent a choice of the least unpleasant among the available alternatives. This choice is not so much a positive discrimination but a negative one, in that the methods *not* chosen are even more disliked than the method that *is* chosen. Nevertheless, it is also true that couples who come seeking contraceptive advice have decided that a choice from the available range of methods is better than no method at all. Their motivation to plan their family or to avoid pregnancy is the over-riding one.

To plan one's family successfully is no easy matter, and if a couple is to do so effectively, a variety of hurdles and obstacles has to be negotiated, often in a spirit of determination and tenacity. Perhaps the first hurdle to be faced relates to the actual *idea* of family planning. For some, the very thought of regulating fertility through the use of birth control is repugnant. The decision whether or not to take part in sexual activity which may lead to pregnancy is more complex than is often supposed. The approach that suggests 'doing nothing is the easiest way out' as far as taking precautions against pregnancy is concerned, does not necessarily imply a lazy and irresponsible attitude. It can also be a recognition that the necessary precautions are seen as so much of an intrusion that this outweighs the perceived risk of an unwanted pregnancy.

Provision of methods

Having overcome this first hurdle by accepting that to prevent undesired pregnancy is to behave responsibly, the next challenge relates to the *provision* of family planning methods. Individuals or couples wishing to make sure that their sexual activity does not lead to an unplanned pregnancy must obtain supplies from somewhere. Supplies can be obtained from a range of outlets: from mail order catalogues and slot machines to family planning clinics and general practice surgeries. Obtaining supplies of a contraceptive method can be a daunting task. Although some people are able to purchase supplies from a pharmacist confidently and without any shyness, other people may find the situation so embarrassing that they are quite unable to contemplate it. To consult a doctor about contraception may well be seen as even more daunting.

Sexual behaviour is perhaps the most private and sensitive area of personal life, and to discuss such behaviour with a comparative stranger (however professionally qualified) takes considerable courage and self-control. The difficulties associated with the accessibility of the provider (which can be measured in geographical, social or personal terms) lead many couples to choose methods of contraception which do not require medical provision but which can be bought over the counter, by mail order or from a slot machine, even though these methods may be considered less effective in preventing pregnancy.

Choosing a method

Having steeled oneself to pass the second barrier and to approach a particular family planning service, the third obstacle becomes apparent. This relates to the specific *method* to be chosen. Assessing benefits and risks, or the balance between the reported effectiveness of a particular method in preventing pregnancy and the knowledge that side-effects are also present, is not always easy. The morbidity (and even occasional mortality) among those using some of the modern methods of family planning, which is often publicized, adds to the uncertainty that many people experience.

In making a choice of contraceptive method the provider's interpretation of the needs of the user may, at one level, be obvious and often medically determined; a woman with a history of high blood pressure or thrombophlebitis is unlikely to be prescribed oral contraception. But at another level this interpretation of need may be far more subtle. Studies have shown that some methods are differentially favoured by providers because it is believed they require only a low level of motivation in their use.

For example, in an early USA study, proportionately more black than white women were fitted with intrauterine devices (IUDs), even when controlling for educational level. In the UK, in at least one area, proportionately greater numbers of council house tenants attending family planning clinics were fitted with IUDs than were women who were either renting private accommodation or were in the process of buying their own homes. Examples such as these indicate that the provider's choice of a particular method for a particular family planning user is being influenced by more than just a medical consideration. This, in itself, can be a positive characteristic of an efficient service, but if that choice is interpreted by the consumer as an attempt to impose a method based on a judgement which describes the consumer as 'irresponsible' in some way, the efficient use of the service is likely to be reduced. What the provider prescribes will also be influenced by his or her training, experience and personal preference.

The provider is most likely to be concerned with the ability of a method to prevent pregnancy, with its safety in use, and with its feasibility in terms of provision. The user of the prescribed method will, of course, also be concerned with its efficiency and safety. In addition she or he will be inclined to take into consideration the ways in which use of the method is likely to affect their personal and social *behaviour*. For example, a woman may decide against using a barrier method, not because she is concerned about the failure rate of the cap, but because she is put off by the thought of having to smear it with spermicide cream and insert it within her own body. Similarly, a man may decide against condom use because he is reluctant to interrupt an act of lovemaking to put it on.

Attributes of methods and users

One helpful way of making an appropriate choice of method easier is to determine the characteristics or *attributes* of that method. These characteristics or attributes describe a contraceptive method in terms of what behaviour is required for the use of the method to be effective.

They include answers to such questions as:
1. Who uses it?
2. When is it used?
   - before sexual intercourse?
   - during intercourse?
   - after intercourse?
   - independent of intercourse?
3. How is it used?
4. How does it act?
5. What part of the body does it affect?

25

6. What is involved in obtaining it?
7. What equipment goes with it?
8. How is it stored when not in use?
9. Where is it obtained?
10. How much does it cost?
11. How effective is it in preventing pregnancy?
12. What side-effects are associated with it?
13. How long do supplies last?

Similarly the characteristics of the user can be listed. These can also be presented as a series of questions, some of which may be of a highly personal kind, for example:

1. How old are you?
2. Have you already had a baby?
3. Is it your intention to have a baby in the future?
4. Have you a history of medical problems associated with pregnancy?
5. Have you ever had medical problems of a gynaecological nature?
6. Do you have one sexual partner, or more?
7. Are your sexual relationships of a stable kind?
8. How frequently do you have sexual intercourse?
9. Would you find it difficult to discuss contraceptive methods with your partner?
10. Do you smoke?

This approach identifies attributes which may at first sight seem trivial and of only tangential significance, but which can exert a considerable influence over the decision made about the choice, and continued use, of a particular family planning method. By looking both at the characteristics of the available methods of contraception, and at the characteristics and circumstances of the user, there is a better chance of choosing a suitable and appropriate method. For example, an older woman, particularly one who smokes, may not be well advised to use oral contraception. A woman who has more than one sexual partner is likely to be at greater risk of developing pelvic inflammatory infection and therefore may not be well advised to choose an IUD. A very young student, who sees her boyfriend only on the occasional weekend and so has sexual intercourse infrequently, may not be a candidate for taking the Pill continuously at this young age; it may be more appropriate that she or her boyfriend should consider a barrier method — a condom or diaphragm.

The reproductive life-cycle

Another important factor is that users will be at different stages in their reproductive life-cycle, and their future intentions regarding pregnancy will differ. For example, some may be *delaying* the birth of their first child; others may be in the process of family building and may be *spacing* the births of their children; while yet others may have achieved their desired family size and are now *stopping* having children (*limiting* their family). The needs of these three groups — delayers, spacers, and stoppers — are very different. For example, 'spacers' may be more willing to accept a method which has a slightly higher failure risk, while 'delayers' and 'stoppers' may feel a greater need to use a highly effective method. 'Delayers' will also wish to choose a method which is unlikely to impair their future fertility, while this factor will not be of so much concern to 'stoppers'.

Advice on using a method

Once a specific fertility-regulating method has been chosen, it is important that the user fully understands the correct procedures for using that particular method. A clear and accurate knowledge of what is entailed is likely to lead to a much more efficient use of the method. In addition it is important that the possibility and likelihood of side-effects is honestly discussed. A woman who is forewarned about likely side-effects of a particular method and informed of their significance and usual duration is much more likely to continue and persevere with its use. Known failure rates should also be discussed with the client.

Research has shown that the heightened level of anxiety which is often experienced by a client during a consultation with a doctor or other provider may reduce her or his ability to take in and absorb information in the usual way. Being preoccupied with such things as overcoming embarrassment and shyness about discussing sexual matters, the client may emerge from the consultation realizing that she or he cannot remember some of the fundamental points of the discussion. (Most people have suffered the similar experience of being so intent on presenting a favourable image of themselves to the person to whom they are being newly introduced, that the name of the new acquaintance completely fails to register.) It is therefore important to have some written material, such as information leaflets, available so that the client can go over the explanations and instructions again in a less stressful atmosphere. The client should also have clear instructions (preferably written where this is possible) about how and where to obtain further advice should she or he have any worries or uncertainties about the use of the chosen method.

Conclusion

To summarize, perhaps the most important element in counselling is skill in listening. The good counsellor spends more time listening than talking. This allows an atmosphere of trust and understanding to develop, and so the client is able to formulate, and to articulate, her or his needs more accurately and confidently. Secondly, consideration of the behavioural attributes of contraceptive methods, and of the individual characteristics and life-style of the potential contraceptive user, allows the provider to counsel on methods that suit the individual needs of the user more closely and to explain the reason behind the suggestions. Finally, counselling allows the contraceptive user to make an informed decision rather than to take a passive role in a matter that means so much to her or him. This approach will have the practical value of increasing the rate of continued contraceptive use; but much more importantly, it recognizes and acknowledges the human dignity and worth of each individual person and so treats that individual with the respect which is her or his due.

Chapter 4

Oral Contraception

Definition of oral contraception

A substance or a combination of substances (usually steroids) administered orally which prevent pregnancy. The main forms of oral contraception include the combined oral contraceptive containing both oestrogen and progestagen (COC), the progestagen-only Pill (POP) and hormonal post-coital contraception (PCC). The latter is used in emergencies.

The history of oral contraception

In the late 19th century scientists observed that ovarian follicles do not develop during pregnancy. Ludwig Haberlandt, a physiologist at the University of Innsbruck, Austria, first proposed the term 'hormonal sterilization' in 1921. He suggested that extracts from ovaries might be used as oral contraceptives. The idea attracted little interest for 20 years. Meanwhile, the molecular structure of the sex hormones was determined, and much knowledge accumulated on the endocrine control of reproduction. Oestrogens were identified in 1929, and progesterone in 1934.

In 1941 Marker used diosgenin from the Mexican yam as raw material for sex steroids. This led to the synthesis of norethisterone (norethindrone) by Carl Djerassi in 1950. At the same time, Frank B. Colton independently produced norethynodrel. These two compounds had progesterone-like activity and were called progestagens or progestins. By 1956, the animal effects of these progestagens had been investigated by Francis J. Saunders, Gregory Pincus and their associates. John Rock, an obstetrician, conducted clinical trials in Puerto Rico, using norethynodrel, and in 1956 Rock, Pincus and Garcia demonstrated that it suppressed ovulation. A larger clinical trial followed in Puerto Rico with the help of Edris Rice-Wray. This trial used a combination of 10 mg of norethynodrel and 0.15 mg of

mestranol (the first combined oral contraceptive). In 1959 this formulation became the first oral contraceptive marketed. Since 1960 many
different steroidal contraceptives have been developed, progressively
containing lower doses of both oestrogen and progestagen. There are
an estimated 60 million current users of oral contraceptives
throughout the world.

Usage of oral contraceptives

Pill use in the different countries of the world varies enormously, and
estimates may not reflect the true picture. Usage is affected by
biological factors such as age and family size, medical politics, the
effect of the media, religion, and the availability of outlets for
provision of oral contraceptives. Therefore rates of usage are seen
which vary from under 1% in Japan to over 40% in the Netherlands.

Types of oral contraceptives

Since the early 1960s female hormonal contraceptives have been used
increasingly in many countries. Steroidal contraception for men is still
in the research phase, and a number of biological difficulties have to
be resolved before a male steroidal contraceptive becomes available.

Combined oral contraceptives (COCs)

The most widely used hormonal contraceptives are oral preparations
of oestrogen and progestagen taken in constant amounts for 20, 21 or
22 days, followed by an interval without steroids during which uterine
bleeding occurs. The commonest regimen is a 21-day course, followed
by an interval of seven days, when no tablet is taken, or placebo, iron
and/or vitamin tablets are substituted. The tendency in recent years
has been to reduce the dose of both progestagen and oestrogen, with
some currently available preparations containing the minimum effective dose. Phasic preparations, with a changing dose of progestagen,
allow the use of smaller amounts of steroids while still maintaining
good cycle control. The pharmacological differences between preparations are still uncertain. In spite of this, the widening choice in oral
contraception means that theoretically the following preparations
may be needed in a family planning programme:
    1. Low-dose preparations (those containing a small amount of

oestrogen/progestagen in a fair 'balance' of oestrogenic and progestational effects).

2. Those with a relatively high progestagen content (one with a primary progestational effect, and another with a strong anti-oestrogenic action).

3. A more oestrogenic combined formulation.

Factors influencing the choice of preparation will include the cost, method of packaging (and hence ease of administration), and availability of supplies. However, a family planning programme using only a few preparations of these three categories will combine choice, economy and the advantages of bulk buying.

When large quantities of oral contraceptive tablets of the same brand are manufactured they can be produced and exported at a low cost (less than 30 USA cents per cycle).

Sequential oral contraceptives

In sequentials, oestrogen is given alone for 14-16 days, followed by a tablet containing an oestrogen and a progestagen for five to seven days. This is followed by an interval of seven days when no tablet or a placebo is taken, and during these treatment-free days uterine bleeding occurs. These preparations ought not to be used for contraception and have been withdrawn from the market in many (but not all) countries. Their serious disadvantage is the high initial dose of unopposed oestrogen required, which has been shown to increase the risk of endometrial carcinoma. They are also, surprisingly, less effective, probably because the oestrogenic first phase of the sequential regimen removes the added protection progestagen gives by altering cervical mucus and reducing sperm penetration.

Phasic oral contraceptives

While the fixed-dose oral contraceptive maintains the same concentration of oestrogen and progestagen in all the tablets in the cycle, phasic Pills aim to vary the concentration mainly of progestagens to allow the use of less total progestagen per cycle. Phasic preparations, therefore, try to mimic the normal cycle, with initial oestrogen dominance. There is as yet no proof that this has health benefits, except for allowing low doses of each hormone to be used, since like all COCs the phasic types eliminate spontaneous ovarian/menstrual cyclicity. There are now various triphasic and biphasic preparations using ethinyl oestradiol, and either levonorgestrel or norethisterone.

Continuous oral progestagens (progestagen-only preparations — POPs)

A microdose of progestagen used on a daily basis without breaks has a contraceptive effect without always inhibiting ovulation. There are no tablet-free days, and menstruation may be irregular.

POPs are useful for women who experience side-effects with oestrogen-containing preparations. Certain side-effects of the COC such as weight gain, headaches and chloasma are less likely with the POP. Women with a history of thromboembolic complications on a combined preparation can use the POP.

Efficacy of the POP is age related. Therefore it is an especially attractive choice for the older woman. It is also definitely the hormonal method of choice for those who are breast feeding. Lactation is not altered in any significant way.

Progestagen-only oral contraceptives will be discussed in more detail later.

Post-coital preparations

These are discussed in Chapter 6 (page 97).

Ovarian hormone actions

Actions of oestrogens

Generally oestrogens have the following effects:

- development of female sexual characteristics at puberty;
- increase in the rate of proliferation of the epithelia of the reproductive system, including regeneration and growth of the endometrium in the first half of the menstrual cycle;
- stimulation of the production of low-viscosity, readily penetrable, cervical mucus, which facilitates sperm penetration about the time of ovulation;
- hypertrophy and increased motility of the smooth muscle of the genital tract;

• approximation of the fimbria of the uterine tubes to the ovulating follicle, helping them to receive the ovum;
• modification of electrolyte, protein and fat metabolism;
• an influence on their own rate of production by their action on the hypothalamic-pituitary axis, both by positive and negative feedback.

Actions of progesterone

Progesterone is produced in significant amounts only at certain times in the reproductive cycle; primarily by the corpus luteum and, during pregnancy, by the placenta. Some of the actions of progesterone, mainly directed to preparing the genital tract for pregnancy, are:

• transformation of the regenerating and growing endometrium to a secretory pattern;
• production of a thick, viscid, impenetrable cervical mucus, which impedes sperm penetration and probably bacterial invasion;
• modification of various oestrogen-induced cellular and secretory responses, helping implantation and maintaining pregnancy by a variety of mechanisms;
• a slight increase in body temperature as manifested by the biphasic temperature chart;
• an influence on the hypothalamic-pituitary mechanism as part of the feedback system;
• a number of effects on both protein and carbohydrate metabolism.

Rhythmic bleeding

The overt manifestation of the primate menstrual cycle is the rhythmic occurrence of monthly vaginal bleeding, which is the result of a decrease in the circulating levels of the ovarian steroids, oestrogens and progesterone, when fertilization and implantation has not occurred in the cycle.

Pharmacology and mode of action of the contraceptive steroids

The molecular structures of steroidal contraceptives are related to those of oestrogen and progesterone, but are modified to render them effective in low dosage by mouth. A representation of the basic steroid nucleus is shown in Fig. 1.

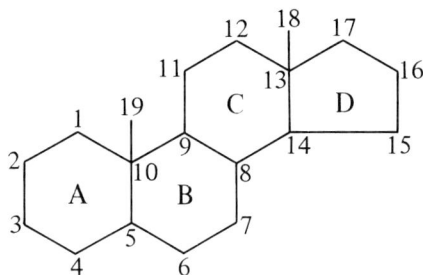

Fig. 1. *Schematic representation of the steroid nucleus, showing the numbering of the carbon atoms from 1 to 19.*

Oestrogens

A great number of chemical substances have oestrogenic activity, including steroidal oestrogens, non-steroidal synthetic oestrogens like stilboestrol, and many phenols.

Ethinyl oestradiol and mestranol (which is metabolically converted to ethinyl oestradiol with high efficiency) are synthetic oestrogens, effective for 24-36 hours when taken orally. They resemble natural oestrogen in their actions on the reproductive tract and hypothalamus, affecting luteinizing hormone production. They also cause changes in lipid metabolism and blood coagulation, similar to those found in pregnancy.

Progestagens

The synthetic progesterone-like substances, or progestagens (progestins), are structurally related to four parent compounds: testosterone, 19-nortestosterone, 17α-hydroxyprogesterone and progesterone itself.

19-norsteroids

The most widely used progestagens in oral contraceptives are 19-nortestosterone derivatives: levonorgestrel, norethisterone (norethindrone), norethynodrel, ethynodiol diacetate and lynestrenol. Newer, more discriminating progestagens include desogestrel, gestodene and norgestimate. Contraceptive efficacy is maintained with less metabolic impact, especially on the lipoproteins. In addition, cycle control is very good.

Oral 19-norsteroids remain active for 24-36 hours. They resemble progesterone, inducing secretory changes in the oestrogen-primed endometrium, producing viscous cervical mucus, affecting luteinizing hormone production, and inhibiting ovulation. In contrast they will not maintain pregnancy in oöphorectomized animals, do not increase basal body temperature, and are not metabolized to pregnanediol.

The 19-norsteroids also exhibit anti-oestrogenic properties to varying degrees. After five or six days of administration the secretory changes in the endometrial glands regress and relative atrophy of the glands occurs, while the stroma appears oedematous but of relatively low vascularity.

They do not virilize women at normal dosage levels, but their chemical relationship to testosterone may be why they have occasionally resulted in virilization of the female fetus *in utero* when high doses have been given in early pregnancy for reasons other than contraception. In high dosage they are mildly anabolic and may aggravate acne and slightly coarsen existing body hair. Unlike testosterone, they do not appear to increase libido in either women or men.

17α-hydroxyprogestagens

17α-hydroxyprogesterone occurs naturally. When given by mouth it has no contraceptive action. Synthetic derivatives (mainly chlormadinone, megestrol and medroxyprogesterone acetate) inhibit ovulation without androgenic, anabolic or oestrogenic effects. However, the oral contraceptives containing 17-acetoxy progestagens have been mainly withdrawn from use, because of animal work showing adverse effects of debatable human relevance, particularly the development of breast nodules in the beagle dog, and disturbances of carbohydrate metabolism. Indeed, medroxyprogesterone acetate, a widely used and highly effective injectable progestagen, has not yet been approved as a contraceptive by the US Food & Drug Administration. The Toxicology Panel of WHO and the IPPF International Medical Advisory Panel (IMAP), among many other national and international scientific advisory bodies, however, have approved the use of depot medroxyprogesterone acetate (see page 80).

Progesterone

Natural progesterone is inactivated by gastric digestion. Alternative routes of administration have been used, including vaginal pessaries and an IUD. A contraceptive role in lactating women is being explored.

Mechanisms of contraceptive action of the combined Pill

All steroidal methods of contraception operate by a combination of direct and indirect effects at ovarian, endometrial, and cervical levels. The primary action of the COC in most women is cessation of ovulation brought about by inhibition of pituitary follicle-stimulating hormone, thus inhibiting follicular maturation in the ovary and by the abolition of oestrogen-mediated positive feedback, which is the physiological trigger for the ovulatory surge of luteinizing hormone. Cervical mucus is affected, mainly by progestagen, and rendered inhospitable to sperm. The receptivity of the endometrium to the blastocyst is also reduced. These latter two mechanisms act as a backup to the main ovarian effect. The relevance to contraception of alterations in tubal function is unknown.

There is very little link between the COC cycle (and the withdrawal bleed) and the menstrual cycle (and menstruation). The normal menstrual cycle controlled by the hypothalamic-pituitary-ovarian axis is abolished during the use of the COC. Withdrawal bleeding is an end-organ response to withdrawal of the artificial hormones and is irrelevant to events elsewhere in the body. Abolition of the withdrawal bleed by taking COC continuously may be used in certain situations such as:

1. Simply to avoid the bleeding whether for aesthetic, social or medical reasons.

2. To avoid symptoms associated with withdrawal of steroidal hormones, such as headaches.

3. Where reduced bioavailability of the COC hormones is anticipated (e.g. in those with a history of a breakthrough pregnancy, and in those taking interacting drugs).

4. Using a progestagen-dominant combined Pill continuously for the treatment of endometriosis. A 'tricycle' regimen allowing a withdrawal bleed every three months is usually used (four packets consecutively followed by a seven-day break).

Absorption of steroidal hormones

After absorption of oestrogen and progestagen in the upper small bowel they are carried to the liver. Liver metabolism creates metabolites of both hormones in the form of sulphates and glucuronides. These re-enter the bowel with bile. Bacterial flora of the gut remove the sulphate and glucuronide groups from ethinyl oestradiol and allow re-absorption of the active agent, helping to maintain blood levels. All synthetic progestagens in current use, however, remain biologically inactive, even after re-absorption. The practical significance of this so-called entero-hepatic circulation is that drugs that inhibit bacteria in the gut may reduce the levels of ethinyl oestradiol. In an unknown minority of users this could reduce the efficacy of the COC. Such drugs include broad-spectrum antibiotics.

There is great individual variation in both the absorption and the metabolism of steroidal hormones. Absorption, of course, is affected by local conditions in the bowel, and therefore diarrhoea and/or vomiting would reduce the availability of both oestrogen and progestagen. Liver metabolism is increased by drugs that induce liver enzymes.

Efficacy of the combined oral contraceptive

Failures (pregnancies) range from 0.2 to 1 per 100 woman-years. Non-compliance is the cause for the majority of failures, but individual variation in absorption and metabolism would account for a minority. It seems that the modern low-dose combination may fail in those women where the bioavailability of steroidal hormones is reduced. In these cases minor errors of compliance may have an adverse effect on efficacy. The weight of the woman probably does not influence efficacy, i.e. overweight women are not at a high risk of pregnancy when using a low-dose oral contraceptive, although some data do suggest the reverse.

Missing Pills in such a way as to lengthen the Pill-free interval, i.e. by not finishing the previous packet to the last Pill or by starting the new packet late, may lead in some women to breakthrough ovulation and result in pregnancy. After any type of Pill omission, advice should therefore be to return to regular Pill taking, but to use extra precautions for seven days. If these seven days continue to beyond the end of the current 21-day packet, then the next packet should be started without the normal break (since the woman has already made her own 'break' by missing pills). This is preferable to the old 'end-of-packet rule'. Vomiting and/or diarrhoea imply the same potential loss of efficacy, during and for seven days after the attack.

Drug interaction

While the number of reported drug interactions with oral contraceptives is small, the increasing use of lower dose products make this problem particularly relevant. Oral contraceptive users who take other drugs concurrently may be affected in a number of ways. The contraceptive steroid may interact with other drugs and interfere with their action, or other drugs may reduce the efficacy of oral contraceptives, resulting in breakthrough bleeding and occasionally unwanted pregnancies.

Broad-spectrum antibiotics (especially ampicillin and tetracyclines) may alter bacteria in the bowel, as mentioned above, and could reduce the rate of production of deconjugated ethinyl oestradiol. The importance of this interaction has yet to be fully assessed, but caution when using broad-spectrum antibiotics, especially in short-term high-dose courses, is prudent: e.g. recommending extra contraceptive precautions during treatment and thereafter for seven days. Longer courses of low-dose antibiotics, such as in the treatment of acne, do not influence the bacteria in the bowel.

A more important category of drugs is liver enzyme inducers. An increase in the activity of liver enzymes increases the production of metabolites of contraceptive steroids and therefore reduces their efficacy. Top of the list is the antituberculosis drug rifampicin, where the use of an alternative contraceptive is recommended. Anticonvulsants, especially barbiturates, ethosuximide, primidone, carbamazepine and phenytoin (but not sodium valproate or clonazepam) are also implicated. Some hypnotics such as chloral hydrate, dichloralphenazone and glutethimide also induce liver enzymes. Other drugs such as chlorpromazine, meprobamate, phenylbutazone, griseofulvin and spironolactone are also implicated.

In all these cases an additional contraceptive has to be used, if the course of treatment with these drugs is short (as is the rule for antibiotics). For longer term therapy (except for antibiotics) an alternative method has to be considered, or a combined oral contraceptive with at least 50 µg of oestrogen has to be used. A shortening of the Pill-free interval may be advisable. The rules apply up to four weeks after stopping the drug in question.

On the other hand, oral contraceptives can alter the effectiveness of other drugs. Some antidepressants and anxiolytic drugs such as chlordiazepoxide, diazepam and tricyclic antidepressants either have an altered effect or a slightly increased chance of toxic effects, though this is not believed to be of clinical importance. The control of blood pressure and diabetes by the relevant drugs or anti-coagulation by warfarin will become more difficult if the combined Pill is used at the same time. These are areas where combined oral contraceptives should normally not be used in the first place.

The systemic effects of oral contraception

General aspects

The steroidal contraceptive agents, especially in the combined oral form, are highly predictable in preventing pregnancy but, inevitably, have certain side-effects. These effects may be due either to the direct actions of the synthetic steroids or to their indirect actions through the woman's own endocrine system.

The intensive investigation of a small group of women can provide much information about the metabolic effects of contraceptive steroids, though not necessarily about the pathological significance of these effects. However, the objective assessment of minor symptoms and of rare adverse effects requires large groups of women. Double-blind cross-over trials, i.e. where the same group of women is exposed to two or more preparations in sequence for a number of cycles each, can provide exceptionally useful information and need to be much more widely used.

It is always necessary to remember that women who choose to use oral contraceptives tend to differ from those who choose the intrauterine device or barrier methods in various ways. These include their past experience of fertility, frequency of sexual intercourse, standards of sexual hygiene, smoking, and age. Therefore simple comparisons between oral contraceptive users and those using other methods of contraception are rarely valid, and symptoms apparently more frequent in oral contraceptive users may reflect some other factor in their lives. Large groups of women (up to 100,000) are needed in so-called cohort studies, if the incidence of rare adverse side-effects is to be measured prospectively. In retrospective case-control studies, the frequency of oral contraceptive use in women who have a suspected adverse reaction is compared with the frequency of their use in matched controls without that reaction (see page 321). These studies require much smaller groups, sometimes only about 100 cases and their controls. Other information is derived from individual clinical case reports communicated to medical journals or to drug-monitoring agencies. However, such data alone provide inconclusive evidence for an association between drug exposure and the development of disease.

The difficulties involved in the study of the effects of steroidal contraception must be borne in mind when considering the data on adverse effects. It is even more difficult to study the beneficial effects of COCs, since protective and potentially life-saving effects of the Pill are far more difficult to recognize than morbidity and mortality associated with COC use. However, we can recognize both contraceptive and non-contraceptive beneficial effects of COCs.

Contraceptive beneficial effects

1. Highly effective in preventing pregnancy, with regular withdrawal bleeds giving regular reassurance of that fact.
2. Highly convenient, non-intercourse-related.
3. Reversible.

Non-contraceptive benefits

1. Most disorders associated with the menstrual cycle are reduced; so menorrhagia is less, causing less anaemia. Dysmenorrhoea and the pre-menstrual syndrome are less likely to be present and there are no ovulation-related symptoms such as pain or mid-cycle bleeding.

2. A reduction in the risk of pelvic inflammatory disease has been found in users of OCs when compared with users of other methods of contraception or with non-users.

3. Extra-uterine pregnancies are reduced since ovulation is inhibited.

4. Functional ovarian cysts are less common; so is endometriosis.

5. A reduction in endometrial and ovarian cancers (see page 46).

6. A reduction in benign breast disease, probably related to the progestagen component.

7. Possibly less thyroid disease (both over-active and under-active syndromes), although the protection is rather modest.

8. Some studies show a reduced incidence of mainly sero-positive rheumatoid arthritis in COC users. Other workers have failed to demonstrate this effect.

9. Less sebaceous disorders (if oestrogen-dominant COCs are used).

10. Possibly less duodenal ulcers.

Major adverse effects of COCs

Three areas of concern exist These are circulatory disease, both venous and arterial; liver disease; and possible adverse effects on some cancers.

Circulatory system disease

Overall, diseases of the circulatory system constitute the most important deleterious effects of combined OC use. The available data are from the developed countries of Europe and North America; there is little information from the developing countries.

From 1961 onwards reports have been published of venous thrombosis, pulmonary embolism, cerebral artery thrombosis, and coronary artery disease among women from developed countries taking oral contraceptives. Contraceptive steroids, especially oestrogen, affect blood clotting factors and the process of fibrinolysis in the blood and vessel wall. Most clotting factors are increased. The anti-clotting factor, antithrombin III, is reduced and the tendency for platelet aggregation is also increased. Fibrinolysis is enhanced in the blood, but reduced in the vessel walls.

Case-control and cohort studies undertaken in the UK, USA, and Scandinavia show evidence of a relationship between the use of oral contraceptives and thromboembolic complications, both venous and arterial. The risk of arterial disease increases with advancing age. However, in 1981 two major British prospective studies demonstrated the profound effect that cigarette smoking has on increasing the risks of circulatory disorders. The duration of use of OCs may play a part. The overall mortality risk ratio (see page 328) from the prospective study of the Royal College of General Practitioners in the UK was 4 for all vascular diseases. Epidemiological estimates of the risk ratio for the individual conditions vary between 1.5 and 6. Very few deaths or incidence of disease have been described under the age of 35, and in these few cases smoking seems to play a very important predisposing role.

Since the early 1970s, data have been accumulating on the relationship between both the oestrogen and progestagen components in the combined oral contraceptive and the occurrence of circulatory disease. Reports of thromboembolic disease attributed to different oral contraceptives monitored by the national drug registration authorities in the UK, Sweden and Denmark revealed an excess of cases in women using preparations containing more than 75 µg of oestrogen. In the UK it was therefore recommended that, wherever possible, COC formulations containing not more than 50 µg of oestrogen should be used. The main currently used preparations contain 30 to 35 µg of oestrogen and are likely to have a much less pronounced effect on circulation dynamics.

The incidence of thromboembolic disease, in the absence of steroidal contraception, shows marked geographical variation. It is not known if this is due to ethnic or environmental differences, but it is the impression of many observers that thromboembolic disease is especially rare in most developing countries. The frequency of post-operative, post-partum and other types of thrombosis in women (whether they are using oral contraceptives or not) needs to be established in developing countries. This may enable a more precise estimate of the risks of oral contraception to be made in different ethnic groups. Studies are now in progress to help clear up these points.

If women with sustained hypertension are identified and their COC use discontinued, the risk of both arterial and venous disease does not appear to increase with the length of past use of COCs. The key factor seems to be the age of the woman, not the number of years she has been on COCs. Ex-use of COCs may have an effect on cerebro-vascular disease, according to a UK prospective study. A USA study in 1981 suggested an ex-use effect on myocardial infarction, but no further evidence to confirm the association has emerged since, and most of the data related to smokers over the age of 35 taking high-dose oestrogen/progestagen Pills.

Risks of oral contraceptives have to be balanced against their contraceptive and non-contraceptive benefits as well as the risks and efficacy of alternative methods and the morbidity and mortality rate associated with accidental pregnancy. In countries with higher maternal mortality and especially where the evidence suggests that the women have a lower incidence of thromboembolic diseases, the equation is very much in favour of oral contraceptives. This is especially so in younger women. In older women with added risk factors, especially smokers, the risks have to be weighed very carefully.

In some countries manufacturers are obliged to insert information in packages of oral contraceptives concerning possible predisposing conditions to thrombosis and other rare adverse side-effects. Such package inserts may be aimed at providers and/or users of oral contraceptives.

Whenever a woman has a relative contra-indication to the use of COCs, the risks to her health of taking the Pill should be carefully considered against the risks of an unplanned pregnancy or of using other less effective forms of contraception.

Venous thromboembolism

The association between COC use and venous thromboembolism is strongest when the diagnosis is certain or probable. The risk is limited to current users and unrelated to duration of use.

COC users have a slightly higher mortality than non-users from this cause. These deaths are mainly from pulmonary embolism. The oestrogen component of OCs is the main associated factor. Therefore COC formulations containing under 50 µg of oestrogen are preferred. Whenever major elective surgery is contemplated, the woman should be advised to stop using COCs four weeks before the operation. Alternative effective contraception should be advised. This could be an oral or injectable progestagen. COCs may be restarted at the first menstrual period, or two weeks after full mobilization following surgery, whichever is later. In the meantime, other effective contraception should be continued. In emergency procedures the surgeon may consider prophylactic anti-coagulant measures around the time of the operation.

Hypertension

In almost all COC users there is a slight increase in both systolic and diastolic blood pressure within the normotensive range. Only about 2.5% of women become clinically hypertensive. Several reports suggest that the progestagen component of COCs plays a part in determining the blood pressure effects, but only when given with oestrogens. The use of low oestrogen/low progestagen formulations is therefore advisable. Hypertension remains a most important risk factor in Pill users, especially since it is a risk factor for other arterial disease.

Pregnancy-induced hypertension is not now considered a contra-indication to COC use provided the blood pressure continues to be monitored.

Myocardial infarction

Present data relating to myocardial infarction and use of OCs are conflicting. However, there is no doubt that women who use OCs and smoke and/or are hypertensive show an excess death rate from this condition. As well as intra-arterial thrombosis, it is probable that arterial wall damage caused by changes in plasma lipids is involved. The latter is much more obvious with high-dose COCs, and the relationship, if any, between currently used low-dose COCs, plasma lipids, and myocardial infarction requires further study.

Cerebrovascular accidents

Thrombotic stroke is increased six-fold in COC users compared to non-users. The data on haemorrhagic stroke, including subarachnoid haemorrhage, are much less convincing. Some cases of the latter are in reality caused by cerebral venous thrombosis. Hypertension with or without steroidal contraception is an important cause of subarachnoid haemorrhage.

Liver disease

Recurrent idiopathic cholestatic jaundice and recurrent generalized pruritus of pregnancy are thought to be a response to a change in hormonal environment. Steroids, and in particular the 17-alkyl-substituted steroids, are known to cause alterations in liver function and cholestasis. Clinical reports of jaundice in women using oral contraceptives have appeared in the UK, the USA, and especially in Scandinavia and Chile. A past history of cholestatic jaundice of pregnancy or jaundice associated with COC use contra-indicates the use of steroid contraception.

COC users have a higher risk of developing hepatocellular adenomas of the liver, especially after prolonged use of COCs (in excess of three years). The magnitude of the risk increases with the dose of steroid, duration of use, and age of the user. New data (1986) also suggest a possible causative association with primary hepatocellular carcinoma. The background prevalence of these conditions is extremely low (of the order of 2-3 in a million, overall, though somewhat higher in areas where hepatitis B infection is frequent). Hence the increase in risk is acceptable for the overwhelming majority of COC users. It is likely that the new lower-dose preparations carry less risk of hepatocellular adenomas and carcinoma.

Combined oral contraceptives also change the composition of bile, making cholesterol less soluble and therefore increasing the risk of cholelithiasis. The bile changes are totally reversible on stopping COC. It is suggested that OCs may accelerate the clinical presentation of gallstones in those who are predisposed. This will therefore occur in the first few years of COC use. There is no evidence linking COC use to a total increase in the incidence of gallbladder disease. However, past or present gallstones are a relative contra-indication to prescribing oral contraceptives.

Other liver conditions where oral contraceptives should be withheld include those producing a history of chronic idiopathic jaundice (Dubin-Johnson and Rotor syndromes). Women sensitive to steroidal contraceptives will usually develop pruritus or severe discoloration of the urine about 10 to 15 days after beginning the use of oral contraceptives. Women suffering from jaundice should not be given the Pill, and if they are on COCs these should be stopped and be replaced by another effective form of contraception. If infective hepatitis is diagnosed, liver functions have to be checked and be shown to have returned to normal before restarting COCs. Other forms of contraception have to be provided, remembering that pregnancy might be more of a stress on the liver.

COC and neoplasia (*benign and malignant*)

Cancer is a multi-factorial disease characterized by a latent period of varying duration. Biological behaviour and exposure to environmental agents throughout life can lead to the appearance of cancer with a latent period often lasting 20-30 years. As long as we remain ignorant of the cause or causes of malignant disease, the effect of exogenous steroids on the incidence of cancer remains unquantifiable. Hormones affect the risk of cancer in both directions (i.e. reducing the incidence of some and increasing the incidence of others). Some benign neoplastic conditions are benefited by OC use (e.g. benign breast disease). Some are promoted (e.g. the very rare liver adenomas). Malignant tumours are affected in the same way. Carcinoma of the ovary and endometrium are less frequent in COC users while cervical neoplasia in its pre-cancerous and cancerous stage may be slightly increased in long-term COC users, especially those with other risk factors, such as sexually transmitted disease and multiple partners. The picture is still confused and more evidence needs to be collected.

Animal research conducted to clarify the association between steroids and neoplasia is not conclusive. High-dose oestrogens given over a relatively long period of time have been associated with the development of cancer in rats, mice, hamsters, rabbits and dogs, but not in guinea-pigs, cows, pigs or monkeys. Much animal work cannot be extrapolated to man because of differences in reproductive cycles and steroid metabolic pathways.

Other influences on carcinogenicity include the time of life at which the individual is exposed to the agent in question, and the interaction with other factors (e.g. in breast cancer, a family history of this condition increases the risk). There is also the largely unknown but important influence of the types and doses of steroid hormones incorporated in various formulations of oral contraceptives.

Benign neoplasms

The Pill has a definite protective effect against benign breast disease. This is probably related to the progestagen component of the COCs and increases with the duration of use of COCs. As discussed, hepatocellular adenomas occur 10 to 20 times more frequently in COC users than in other women, but these tumours remain extremely rare. Other benign tumours, including pituitary adenomas, show no association with COCs. A modest protective effect of COCs on uterine fibroids was recently demonstrated, and is likely to be due to the progestagen component of COCs.

Malignant neoplasms

Several case-control studies have shown a protective effect of COCs on carcinoma of the ovary, reducing the risk by about 40%. Protection is highest with increased duration of use, and continues for 10-15 years after stopping COCs. A similar protection against carcinoma of the endometrium has been demonstrated. The frequency of trophoblastic disease is not increased in COC users. However, because of an apparent increase in the risk of chorio-carcinoma if OCs are started before all traces of a hydatidiform mole have gone, some workers in the UK recommend withholding them until human chorionic gonadotrophin becomes undetectable in urine and blood.

Carcinoma of the cervix: Patterns of sexual activity, the choice of the male partner, the association with some viral genital tract infections and smoking have all been linked to cervical neoplasia. By 1986 there had been eight case-control and six prospective studies, the majority of which showed an association between cervical dysplasia or carcinoma and COC use. In a 1983 UK cohort study there was a positive effect of duration of COC use among about 7,000 parous COC users who were compared to a group of IUD users. The incidence of all forms of cervical neoplasia rose from 0.9 per 1,000 woman-years in those with up to two years' COC use to 2.2 per 1,000 woman-years after eight years. In 1985, a World Health Organization case-control study (WHO Collaborative Study of Neoplasia and Steroidal Contraceptives) reported more than a 50% increase in the risk of invasive cancer of the cervix in women who had used the COC for more than five years. The latter study did not control for the effect of tobacco smoking or the sexual activity of the male partner; and the earlier study had limited data on the sexual background of the cases. Both of these confounding variables and other sources of bias may explain the excess risk in the user group, as was shown previously in the Walnut Creek prospective study. COCs may prove to be a co-factor in the aetiology of cervical neoplasia, possibly accelerating the changes, but not the prime carcinogen.

Clinically, the regular taking of Papanicolaou smears is sound preventive medicine. This test should be offered, if available, to those sexually active women requesting the COC. The test is not necessarily a prerequisite for prescribing or making available oral contraceptives. The places where a comprehensive cytology service cannot as yet be made available are also the places where maternal and infant mortality are very high. In such areas the efficacy of the method in reducing maternal mortality from pregnancy and infant mortality by increasing child-spacing more than compensates for any (unproven) increased risk of cervical cancer caused by COCs.

47

The COC and breast cancer: The evidence about this common form of female cancer is copious, complex and at times confusing. On the whole the data are still reassuring for the generality of women. Certain groups of women may have an increased risk of developing breast cancer; they include those with a history of benign breast disease or a family history of breast cancer and those who delay their first full-term pregnancy.

In 1983 a study conducted in the USA reported an increased risk of breast cancer in women who used COCs containing 'high potency' progestagens before the age of 25 for at least four years. Other studies from the UK and Sweden were confirmatory, but the largest USA study, the 'cancer and sex hormone' or CASH study, failed to show an association even with early Pill use at a young age. Other studies have shown that those women who had never used oral contraceptives had appreciably more advanced tumours at presentation than those who had been using oral contraceptives during the year before the breast lump appeared. Past users occupied a middle position. Oral contraceptives may therefore have a protective effect on tumour growth.

The possibility of a long latent period between exposure to a carcinogen and development of malignancy exists, and COCs have been in use for a relatively short time. Definite conclusions have to await further evidence. A good practice in preventive medicine is to encourage women to carry out breast self-examination and to make use of local screening facilities where available.

Endocrine effects

Endogenous ovarian activity is depressed in COC users. The exogenous artificial hormones replace ovarian function. The release of gonadotrophins from the pituitary is suppressed, though it partially recovers during the Pill-free interval. The production of insulin, growth hormone, adrenal steroids, thyroid hormones and prolactin is increased. Globulins binding to hormones in the blood are also increased, but the effective blood levels of the latter are usually not much altered. The changes in thyroid function mimic the changes in pregnancy, with an increase in thyroxin-binding globulin and protein-bound iodine.

The relationship between COC use and *future fertility* has been investigated by several workers. In 1986 a UK study demonstrated a delayed return of fertility in nulliparous COC users aged 30 to 34 compared to non-users. Most women would accept a delay of two to three months in the time taken to conceive after stopping COC use. This may occur naturally, but in any case it is good medical practice to recommend such a delay so that normal periods will have resumed before conception occurs. There is no evidence that COCs can cause permanent sterility. There is no link between duration of use of COCs and impairment of future fertility.

There are no valid data to justify 'breaks' — interruption of the use of oral contraceptives at arbitrary intervals — in order to determine if ovulation will occur. Any presumed benefits are small if they exist, and are more than outweighed by the unplanned pregnancies which will probably result.

The term 'post-Pill amenorrhoea' is used to describe cases of secondary amenorrhoea of more than six months' duration, following discontinuation of oral contraceptives. In a recent Swedish study 1.8% of the population reported amenorrhoea of more than six months' duration. This is especially common in the extremes of reproductive life.

The use of COCs does not appear to increase the risk, but would camouflage a tendency to amenorrhoea by the occurrence of regular withdrawal bleeds in response to the contraceptive hormones. Post-Pill amenorrhoea of more than six months' duration happens in about 1% of cases, and is not different from non-OC related amenorrhoea in its causation and its excellent response to treatment.

Women giving a past history of secondary amenorrhoea may request oral contraception after the return of their periods. If the periods are regular and no current disorder is suspected, OCs may be allowed. If the woman has four periods or less per year, the COC should be withheld until conditions such as pituitary adenoma have been excluded. Women have to be warned that fertility cannot be proved in advance of becoming pregnant.

Metabolic changes

Most metabolic changes thought to be associated with the use of oral contraceptives have not been shown to have any pathological significance. *Glucose tolerance* is reduced with the use of oral contraceptives as it is in pregnancy; it also alters with the phases of the menstrual cycle. There are now fairly extensive studies to indicate a contra-insulin effect in the majority of both normal and diabetic subjects. The physiological significance, if any, of this change is not fully understood, and women quickly revert to normal when the oral contraceptive is discontinued. In truly non-diabetic subjects, the long-term use of oestrogen-containing hormonal contraceptives does not appear to cause overt diabetes. Women known to have had previously abnormal glucose-tolerance tests should be regarded as an at-risk group and should be watched more carefully, since in them overt diabetes may be induced. Oral contraceptives can be given short-term to young women with established diabetes, provided they are free of arteriopathy/retinopathy and of all other risk factors (see page 53) including smoking. Extra care in observation is then essential and minor modifications in diabetic therapy during the first few months may be needed. The progestagen-only preparations also affect carbohydrate tolerance, but to a much lesser degree than those containing oestrogen as well. They are the hormonal contraceptives of choice for diabetics.

Women using steroidal contraception sometimes complain of *weight gain*. Not all OC-associated weight gain is caused by OC use. Pre-menstrual weight gain is oestrogen-linked and is spontaneously reversible. An increase in appetite is to blame in the majority of cases of weight gain, but sometimes changes in cortisol metabolism producing an 'anabolic' effect may contribute. Giving appropriate dietary advice and prescribing lower-dose brands is adequate in most cases in preventing or controlling this problem.

Some changes in *blood biochemical indicators of vitamin status* take place during OC use. These changes are sub-clinical and their significance is unknown. There are no data to suggest the need for routine vitamin supplementation in OC users. Blood levels of iron are increased, which is beneficial in those suffering from iron deficiency.

Lipid metabolism is affected, both by oestrogens and progestagens in COCs. Progestagens, especially derivatives of 19-nortestosterone, increase low-density lipoprotein cholesterol and decrease high-density lipoprotein (HDL) cholesterol. This possibly atherogenic effect is counterbalanced by that of oestrogen. These data are from developed countries, where factors such as obesity, smoking and consumption of alcohol have a part to play, and most of the studies were done on higher-dose combined Pills. The changes with the currently available low-dose Pills may be much less. The new generation progestagens (desogestrel, gestodene and norgestimate) have either no effect on or raise the HDL cholesterol.

Choice of contraceptive

The alternatives available to a couple choosing a contraceptive are many. The choice depends on a delicate balance of risks and benefits of the different methods compared to the risks and gains of pregnancy. The role of the personnel supervising distribution is to provide the information to allow the couple concerned to make an informed personal decision. The information provided has to be given in such a way as to accommodate the social and educational background of the people concerned. The contraceptive needs of a particular couple may undergo several changes during their fertile lifetime. In the early days of their sexual relationship, the couple may require maximum effectiveness and therefore often elect to use a combined oestrogen-progestagen preparation; this is of particular value when they have no previous sexual experience. Oral contraception permits them fully spontaneous sexual expression at all times.

Efficacy of COCs depends on the woman's reliability in ensuring their regular use as part of a daily routine. Pills should be taken at the same time every day, and if any are forgotten beyond 12 hours they should be taken as soon as possible with extra precautions (see page 37). Careful Pill-taking also reduces the risk of spotting and breakthrough bleeding, especially with the low-dose preparations.

It is essential that a woman takes the tablets which have been prescribed for her and that she does not exchange these with her friend or neighbour who may have another formulation. Oral contraceptives should be stored out of reach of children. If a child eats oral contraceptives, no treatment is necessary and no serious harm will result. A pre-pubertal girl may experience a brief episode of uterine bleeding a few days afterwards, without major consequence.

Communities appear to benefit by having access to all methods of family planning, and there is no evidence that the available methods compete with one another. Most reported differences in initial method selection are mainly due to clinic staff bias. Those supervising oral contraceptive distribution should keep in mind the possible value of alternative methods, just as they should remember that systemic contraceptives can be a useful change from intrauterine devices or mechanical or chemical contraceptives. It should be recognized that when pregnancies do occur during contraceptive use, women may resort to abortion, depending on the facilities and the legal situation in the particular country.

The IPPF *Directory of Hormonal Contraceptives* contains useful information about which oral contraceptives are available in countries throughout the world. It also indicates which oral contraceptives, with different brand or trade names, have the same or similar formulation.

COCs may sometimes be prescribed on medical grounds to treat certain gynaecological problems. These include the relief of dysmenorrhoea, regulating the menstrual cycle, relieving premenstrual tension, controlling menorrhagia, preventing functional ovarian cysts and controlling endometriosis. If prescribed in this way, it may be permissible to use higher-dose preparations or to give the COC to women who have what would be contra-indications in the context solely of contraception.

Absolute contra-indications to COC use

1. Past or present circulatory disease, including any arterial or venous thrombosis in the past, current ischaemic heart disease and severe essential hypertension or past Pill-induced hypertension. Varicose veins are only a contra-indication if there has been an association with venous thrombosis.

2. Conditions where the risk of thrombosis is higher, such as atherogenic lipid profile; or a known pre-coagulatory abnormality of clotting or fibrinolysis.

3. Any condition favouring cerebral ischaemia, including severe migraine, focal migraine (migraine with focal cerebral ischaemic symptoms), ergot-treated migraine, or transient ischaemic attacks without headaches.

4. Valvular heart disease, especially with pulmonary hypertension (though COCs may be permitted in certain situations after expert advice).

5. Sickle-cell anaemia may not be an absolute contra-indication (see page 53).

6. Liver diseases, such as a history of cholestatic jaundice of pregnancy, disorders of hepatic excretion (e.g. Dubin-Johnson syndrome), infective hepatitis (until liver function returns to normal), porphyria, and liver adenomas.

7. History of any serious condition affected by sex steroids, such as conditions occurring or worsening in a previous pregnancy (e.g. herpes gestationis, haemolytic uraemic syndrome, chorea, and otosclerosis).

8. Steroid-dependent cancer (e.g. breast cancer), unless permitted by the oncologist after discussion, or pre-cancer (hydatidiform mole).

9. Undiagnosed genital tract bleeding.

10. Actual or possible pregnancy.

11. Allergy to either steroid in the Pill.

12. Recent trophoblastic disease (until hCG is undetectable in blood and urine).

13. The woman's unrelieved anxiety about using the method even after full counselling.

It is important to note that some of these contra-indications may not be permanent.

Relative contra-indications to COC use

1. Multiple risk factors for arterial disease. These include:

(*a*) cigarette smoking

(*b*) treated hypertension

(*c*) increasing age (especially if combined with cigarette smoking)

(*d*) obesity

(*e*) diabetes mellitus

(*f*) family history of arterial disease such as ischaemic heart disease and ischaemic cerebrovascular accidents.

A combination of some of these may be considered an absolute contra-indication.

2. Hyperprolactinaemia.

3. Oligo-menorrhoea. This should be investigated first.

4. Severe depression.

5. Pre-surgery, at least four weeks before and, starting at the first period, at least two weeks after major surgery or immobilization.

6. Chronic systemic diseases (e.g. Crohn's disease, diabetes, malabsorption syndromes and chronic renal disease). In the three latter conditions high density lipoprotein cholesterol is reduced.

Carriers of the sickle-cell trait are allowed the use of COCs. The situation is uncertain in relation to homozygous sickle-cell disease (SS and SC genes). In theory there is an increased risk of thrombosis with this condition. Research has shown that injectable progestagens extend the interval between sickle-cell crises, so in the West Indies and

West Africa the COC is now considered to be only relatively contra-indicated in sickle-cell disease, especially when balanced against the greater risk of pregnancy. However, further direct evidence is required and studies are in progress in this field.

Choice of COC formulations

The general principle is to choose a formulation containing the minimum effective dose of both oestrogen and progestagen. Efficacy is not reduced among compliant users by using lower dosage, but the main drawback may be the occurrence of breakthrough bleeding. Ideally, COC users should be maintained on the lowest dose of both hormones which each individual's uterus will permit, i.e. just above her own bleeding threshold.

For less compliant women and those who cannot tolerate or will be confused by breakthrough bleeding or the absence of withdrawal bleeds, a preparation which is unlikely to cause breakthrough bleeding rather than one which gives the lowest possible metabolic impact should be chosen. If women are warned and counselled about breakthrough bleeding, they tend to accept it if it is mild and disappears after a few cycles. Persistent and troublesome breakthrough bleeding necessitates a change of formulation, and the use of a phasic Pill or one with a higher dose first of progestagen and then of oestrogen.

Preparations containing more than 30 to 35 µg of oestrogen should normally be selected for special categories, especially women on long-term interacting drugs and those who have had a previous contraceptive failure with COCs. Breakthrough bleeding rarely signifies a reduction in the effectiveness of the COC used; conversely, the regular occurrence of a withdrawal bleed is not a guarantee that no pregnancy will occur.

Women should be instructed to start the first cycle of oral contraceptives on either the first or the fifth day of established menstruation, depending on what is acceptable in a particular country. If the first packet is started on day 1 of menstruation, there is no need for additional contraceptive precautions. Where oral contraceptives are started later than day 3 in the first cycle, additional contraceptive precautions have been advised during the first 14 days of that cycle. The British Family Planning Association now recommends that this precautionary time be reduced to seven days.

Monitoring and supervision

Depending on the local resources and availability of health personnel to deal with inquiries and to check users, regular follow-up has to be organized. Ideally, someone starting the use of oral contraceptives should be seen three months later, and then at least every six months. At each visit the health personnel dealing with the woman should endeavour to identify any new risk factors developing, should discuss any side-effect, be it minor or major, and be especially vigilant for warning signs of circulatory problems. These are, most importantly: rise in systolic and/or diastolic blood pressure; the occurrence of migraine in someone who has never experienced migraine previously; or the onset of focal migraine with transient neurological deficit. Any major changes in weight have to be discussed with the woman. When available, cervical cytology should be carried out, and breast self-examination should be encouraged.

The emergence of any new factors or the discovery of serious warning signs, such as a systolic blood pressure over 160 mm Hg, and a diastolic blood pressure over 100 mm Hg, have to be considered as indications for reviewing the choice of contraception for the woman.

Below are some of the side-effects and conditions that need special attention in COC users.

Side-effects and complications

If a COC user has any of the following symptoms then she should be advised to seek urgent medical advice:

1. Severe pain in the calf of one leg, since this may be an indication of deep-vein thrombosis.

2. Severe central chest pain or pain on either side of the chest aggravated by breathing. The former can be a symptom of myocardial infarction and the latter of pulmonary embolism.

3. Unexplained shortness of breath with or without the coughing up of blood-stained sputum.

4. Severe abdominal pain.

5. Any unexplained neurological symptom explicable in terms of transient cerebral ischaemia, such as weakness affecting one side of the body, a marked sudden disturbance of vision, inability to speak, or focal epilepsy.

6. The onset of jaundice.

Depression

Short-term changes of mood in women of fertile age can often be correlated with phases of the menstrual cycle, and the use of steroidal contraceptives usually relieves pre-menstrual tension, irritability and depression in many women. A UK study did show a slight increase in depressive illness in COC users. The progestagen in COCs is blamed for mood changes and, in a proportion of users, altered tryptophane metabolism leading to low pyridoxine levels does occur. In these cases, pyridoxine (vitamin B6) can be tried or an oral contraceptive containing a different progestagen may be used. In extreme cases a change of method is advisable. In 1985 a cohort study in the UK ruled out any association between COC use and serious psychiatric illness.

Changes in libido

Sexual behaviour in mammals is partly dependent on the level of circulating steroids. There is some evidence in humans that frequency of sexual intercourse varies with the menstrual cycle and with pregnancy, but psychogenic factors probably override hormonal changes in most women. It has been reported that the use of steroidal contraceptives alters libido in many women, but the changes may be in either direction. A double-blind study has shown the presence of a post-ovulatory drop in the frequency of sexual intercourse in normal cycles. This is abolished by oral contraceptives. Frequency of intercourse may increase owing to freedom from the fear of unwanted pregnancy. But the anti-oestrogenic effect of some formulations in some susceptible women may result in impairment of vaginal lubrication during sexual intercourse and thereby cause coital difficulties.

There is no test to identify those women whose libido may decrease. If loss of libido becomes a genuine drawback to the use of combined oral contraceptives in particular women, attempting to modify these effects by altering the progestagen and its dosage might first be tried before changing to alternative methods of contraception.

Teratogenicity

Sex steroids can be teratogenic. Confounding factors such as smoking, or use of alcohol and other drugs confuse the picture. The type of steroid, the time of exposure, and the duration of exposure are important considerations. Diethylstilboestrol (DES), a non-steroidal oestrogen, can harm the human fetus with effects that show later in life. Some studies on hormone use in early pregnancy suggest an increased incidence of rare congenital abnormalities, but the existing epidemiological evidence is still reassuring. The two main UK studies showed no excess of congenital abnormalities among COC users as compared to non-users. A major US study confirmed these data, and studies from some European countries are also reassuring. However, in these studies multiple births were commoner among breakthrough pregnancies in COC users, though maternal age may contribute to this increased risk.

Women should be clearly advised not to continue using oral contraceptives if they think they are pregnant. In their first cycle on OCs, they should be careful to start taking the Pill at the beginning of menstruation. They should be warned against the pointless practice of using large doses of oral contraceptives as a supposed abortifacient.

Having been given these instructions and warnings, a woman who inadvertently continues the use of COCs in early pregnancy should be counselled on the lines that at least 2% of all births are complicated by a major abnormality and that a normal outcome of pregnancy can never be guaranteed. The Population Council estimates that seven out of every 10,000 COC-exposed pregnancies might have a possibly attributable abnormality. This is a risk that many women will accept. Ex-COC use carries no proven risk of teratogenicity, though some concern about vitamin/mineral changes has prompted a few authorities to recommend delaying conception for two to three months after discontinuing COCs.

A WHO Scientific Group (1981) concluded that OC use before the conception cycle carries no proven adverse effects on the fetus. With regard to OC use after conception, "the evidence for an increased risk of congenital malformations is not clear. If such risks exist, they are very small".

Lactation

Breast milk is the main source of nutrition for many infants, particularly in developing countries. It also protects the infant against some diseases. Therefore, it is important not to interfere with breast feeding by inappropriate use of certain forms of contraception. Combined OCs do appear to have an adverse effect on the quantity of milk produced and on the duration of lactation, although data on currently used low-dose OCs are not available. Therefore, progestagen-only OCs (POPs) are the hormonal method of choice in lactation, usually commenced within seven days of delivery. Some authorities have shown that delaying the start of the POPs to the beginning of the fourth week after the birth, reduces the incidence of persistent lochia, with no reduction in efficacy. Combined OCs should ideally be withheld until the infant is weaned.

Tropical diseases

Because oral contraceptives are widely used in developing countries their interaction with conditions and diseases common in those countries is particularly significant. One common disease found in the tropics is schistosomiasis (bilharziasis). The results of liver function tests remain the same in OC users whether they have uncomplicated schistosomiasis or not. The same applies to the common Asian parasitic disease caused by the liver fluke (*Opisthorchis viverrini*).

The eye

If acute loss of vision, even if only temporary, occurs, the Pill should be stopped and the cause investigated. It may be caused by thrombosis or haemorrhage of a retinal artery or vein or by transient cerebral ischaemia, in which case COCs are contra-indicated. Visual disturbances can accompany diffuse migraine and if the relevant history (i.e. no field defects) and investigations are negative, COCs are still allowed. COCs do not aggravate glaucoma.

A few contact-lens wearers may experience discomfort when they start COCs owing to corneal oedema and a resultant change in the corneal surface. If this happens the woman should remove the lens to avoid corneal damage. She should see her optician in case the lens needs refitting. Nowadays this side-effect is rare with the use of low-oestrogen COCs and the introduction of soft lenses.

Nausea or vomiting

Nausea may occur when COCs are started, but vomiting is not usual. If persistent vomiting happens then it will interfere with steroid absorption and therefore efficacy. Taking OCs at bed-time reduces the risk of nausea. It may recur to a slight degree at the beginning of each cycle but tends to decrease with continued use of the preparation.

Nausea should be viewed with suspicion if it occurs later on; then the woman should be examined to exclude pregnancy and other causes. Lowering the dose of oestrogen may relieve the condition. If a woman vomits within three hours of taking her Pill another one should be taken.

Headaches

These are very variable. Sometimes the complaint of headache is really related to the woman's anxiety over taking oral contraceptives. Some women notice headaches on the tablet-free days, and these may be similar to pre-menstrual headaches. This may be an indication for the tricycle regimen described earlier (see page 36). Migraines may be improved or worsened by the use of oral contraceptives and their significance was discussed on page 55.

Urinary tract infection

Several studies have shown that urinary tract infections are commoner in COC users than in controls. In some cases this may be due to an increase in frequency of sexual intercourse, so-called 'honeymoon cystitis', but since bacteriuria does occur, recurrent symptoms necessitate a change of method.

Alterations in the menstrual pattern

The significance of *breakthrough bleeding* to the first and subsequent choice of COCs has been discussed (see page 54). However, it is important to examine the cervix, since local pathology may be responsible. The possibility of a drug interaction or erratic Pill-taking must also be considered and appropriate action taken. Absence of withdrawal bleeds may occur separately or in association with breakthrough bleeding. If this withdrawal amenorrhoea persists over several cycles the woman should be examined and a pregnancy excluded. A change in the formulation (initially to a phasic brand) may solve this problem. Absence of withdrawal bleeds is not a reflection of poor fertility.

A minority of COC users complain of a pre-menstrual type of syndrome at the end of each Pill cycle, with fluid retention, breast tenderness, and possible changes in mood. These symptoms may be commoner with oestrogen-dominated phasic Pills, and usually clear following a change of formulation.

Vaginal discharge

Excessive vaginal discharge may be caused by cervical ectropion (wrongly called cervical erosion), which is more common in Pill users. Ectropion is a benign condition. Women on high-progestagen Pills may complain of vaginal dryness.

Candidiasis does not occur more commonly among users of modern low-oestrogen COCs than among control subjects. A complaint of vaginal discharge should be investigated to exclude lower genital tract infection and pelvic inflammatory disease, and these should be treated appropriately. Otherwise simple reassurance may help the woman accept this symptom.

Breast tenderness

Breasts may become tender and even slightly enlarged in the first cycle; however, these changes normally disappear in subsequent cycles.

Chloasma/melasma

Chloasma can occur with COCs, as in pregnancy, in light-skinned subjects and consists of irregularly shaped, brown-pigmented areas on the face, especially on the forehead and upper cheeks. This is believed to be directly related to the oestrogen component. It develops insidiously and only diminishes slowly on withdrawal of the hormonal preparation. Cosmetic masking may be required.

Immunity

Several studies have suggested that sex steroids can modify immune responses. The effects are of a similar nature but less marked than those seen in pregnancy. COCs have good effects on certain immune conditions and bad effects on others. An example of the former is thyroid disease and of the latter is tenosynovitis and systemic lupus erythematosus. Current knowledge allows the use of COCs in HIV infection, though the additional use of a condom is important (see page 140).

Extremes of reproductive life (see also page 210)

Puberty

Young nulliparous girls present a particular problem, and oral contraceptives should be used only after counselling in those with a history of irregular menstrual cycles. At the same time, it must be recognized that in some countries girls of 16 or younger are at risk of unwanted pregnancies. It may be necessary to prescribe oral contraceptives for them. In the absence of first-class pre-natal supervision, such pregnancies present a greater hazard to the health of both the mother and the baby than those in older women.

The climacteric

The administration of steroidal contraception near the time of the menopause should be regulated by the need for adequate contraception, attuned to declining fertility. Aspects to take into consideration include: the increased maternal and fetal risks of pregnancy, the observed rise in the incidence of thromboembolic disease in oral contraceptive users in this age group, particularly in those with risk factors (see page 53), and the need to deal with menopausal symptoms. Indeed, where there are added risk factors it has been recommended that oral contraceptives should not be used in women over 35. For other women over 35, the risk/benefit relationship should be carefully assessed. In many cases, low-dose COCs or progestagen-only Pills are to be preferred up to the age of 45. Over the age of 45 POPs continue to be a good choice.

Progestagen-only Pills (POPs)

Definition

POPs are oestrogen-free oral contraceptives containing a microdose of progestagen, either from the norethisterone or levonorgestrel group. The prototype Pill contained chlormadinone acetate and was introduced in 1969. Toxicity tests linked this progestagen to breast nodules in the beagle bitch and it was withdrawn in 1970. The POP is still under-used, probably because it requires maximum motivation by user and provider. The POP is taken regularly daily without breaks and regardless of bleeding patterns.

Mechanism of action

Progestagens in the dose used in the progestagen-only Pill exert their main action on cervical mucus, leading to the production of thick mucus with poor sperm penetrability. As an adjunct to this, biochemical changes are produced in the endometrium making it unfavourable for implantation. There is also a considerable effect in many women and in many cycles on ovulation. Because of the varying effects of POPs on ovarian function the cycle pattern can be disrupted and may range between regular cycles in some women and anovulatory amenorrhoea in others.

Efficacy

The efficacy is less than that of combined oral contraceptives and is age-related. Failure rates vary between 0.3 and 5.0 per 100 woman-years. Compliance in taking the progestagen-only Pill is essential. The time allowed for missing Pills is much more limited than with the combined Pill, as the main effect of the POP (namely on cervical mucus) is lost fairly quickly if a subsequent Pill is missed. The fact that POPs are taken on a daily basis, continuously without the seven-day break, makes it easier for the woman to adhere to a regular Pill-taking routine. On the other hand, the POP changes cervical mucus into a contraceptive barrier quickly, and 48 hours is probably adequate for the effect to be re-established.

The starting routine is similar to that of the combined oral contraceptive, namely on the first day of established menstruation. No additional contraceptive precautions need to be taken as the contraceptive effect is established within 48 hours. If a Pill is forgotten or taken more than three hours late, then extra contraceptive precautions should be used for 48 hours.

Antibiotics do not interfere with the effectiveness of the POP, apart from rifampicin, which like other enzyme-inducers is a contra-indication to the method.

Indications for the progestagen-only Pill

POPs combine good efficacy with lack of major side-effects and minimal alteration in metabolic variables, both for carbohydrate and lipid metabolism. There is no epidemiological evidence so far of increased risk of either circulatory disorders or neoplasia in POP users — nor of the absence of any effect.

Women for whom the POP would be a good choice include:

1. Those who have side-effects with, or contra-indications to, the combined OCs, in particular those believed to be oestrogen-related.

2. The older age group, mainly over age 45 who are non-smokers, but especially those over age 35 with risk factors (mainly cigarette smoking).

3. Diabetic and obese women.

4. Women with hypertension, either related to the combined oral contraceptives, or other varieties controlled by drugs.

5. Those with sickle-cell disease.

6. Migraine sufferers.

7. Most importantly during lactation.

The latter group is important, in that the combination of lactation and POPs is very effective. Moreover, the main drawback of POPs, namely irregular bleeding, is replaced by lactational amenorrhoea. The dose of progestagen is so small that the amount excreted in breast milk is negligible.

Contra-indications to the POP

1. Any severe condition likely to be worsened by steroidal contraception, such as past or current severe arterial disease or current high risk for cardiovascular disease.

2. Undiagnosed genital tract bleeding — can be confused with the irregular bleeding on POPs and therefore investigations must precede starting the POP.

3. Pregnancy — has to be excluded.

4. Recent trophoblastic disease until hCG is undetectable in blood as well as urine, since it may be the progestagen that increases the likelihood of chemotherapy being required.

5. Previous ectopic pregnancy. Some authorities consider this a relative contra-indication.

6. Functional ovarian cysts are commoner in POP users, and their presence is a relative contra-indication.

7. Any serious side-effect of the COC not certainly related solely to oestrogens (e.g. liver adenoma).

8. The woman's unrelieved anxiety about the POP method.

Side-effects and follow-up

The main side-effect of POPs is irregular bleeding. Users have to be counselled about it and asked to keep a menstrual record. The pattern often gradually returns to an acceptable routine. More than 50% of women will have a cycle length between 25 and 35 days, which they tolerate. Amenorrhoea may occur, especially in older women, and is usually caused by anovulation. After excluding pregnancy, the woman can be reassured. Persistent and/or heavy bleeding may require a change of progestagen or change of method. Mastalgia is an occasional problem; though transient, it may recur. A change to another progestagen may solve the problem.

Monitoring of blood pressure, breast examination and cervical cytology, when practicable, should be carried out in all women attending a family planning clinic.

The distribution and supervision of oral contraceptives

When oral contraceptives were first introduced, it was reasonable to restrict the use of these unknown and relatively powerful drugs to medical prescription. However, as experience from tens of millions of users was becoming available during the 1970s, it was becoming evident that this method of family planning is highly effective and relatively simple to use, and that the health benefits almost certainly outweigh the risks of use in nearly all cases. It has been found that the complications that do occur are difficult to predict by examination before use, but that access to follow-up facilities can be important, especially in enhancing continuation rates.

Continuation rates among oral contraceptive users have sometimes been disappointing, but the wide acceptability of the method enables it, by preventing unplanned pregnancy and induced abortion, and permitting the satisfactory spacing of children, to make a contribution towards reducing maternal mortality and increasing the quality of life for parents and their children.

The limitation of oral contraceptive distribution to doctors' prescribing makes the method geographically, economically and sometimes culturally inaccessible to many women. As a consequence, deaths and sickness of women and children, which might otherwise be avoided by the voluntary limitation of fertility, continue.

In many countries the regulations that are supposed to limit oral contraceptives to doctors' prescription are generally ignored. Those who can afford to purchase them from commercial outlets do so without medical supervision. However, national and international agencies abide by regulations, only distributing free or subsidized Pills through doctors. As a result there is discrimination against many of those more urgently in need of protection against unplanned pregnancy.

It was recognized that death due to thromboembolic disease is a rare but demonstrable complication of the use of oral contraceptives, and that certain endocrine and metabolic changes take place in some users. Nevertheless routine examination contributes little to reducing these risks because it is rarely possible to identify susceptible women. Some unknowns do remain concerning potential beneficial or harmful long-term side-effects, but these are most likely to be solved by case-control studies, which can be carried out independently of the method of distribution.

The IPPF believes that whoever normally meets the health needs of the community, whether doctor, nurse, traditional midwife, pharmacist or storekeeper, can be an appropriate person to distribute oral contraceptives. Many of the member associations of the IPPF, as well as other family planning providers, have set up responsible, simple methods of non-medical distribution of oral contraceptives (see page 311). In addition, their programmes continue to:

1. Pioneer innovative schemes for distribution of oral contraceptives (together with all other contraceptives).

2. Educate governments and the medical profession on the health benefits to women and children of non-medical methods of distributing oral contraceptives.

3. Plan programmes of information and education describing the use of oral contraceptives, relative contra-indications and possible side-effects.

4. Re-orientate clinic facilities so that the public has access to trained personnel in cases where the woman is uncertain about the use of oral contraceptives, has a complicating medical condition, or requires reassurance.

Community based distribution (see also page 311)

It is the experience of several countries, such as Brazil, Colombia, the People's Republic of China, Sri Lanka and Thailand, that oral contraceptive use can be enhanced when advice and supplies are provided by members of the community itself. Distributors, from villages or poor urban areas, are carefully selected, well trained, and appropriately supervised. They are linked into a chain of responsibility which allows access to medical skills if problems arise.

Early in the 1970s this type of distribution of oral contraceptives gave encouraging results in Thailand where auxiliary midwives were taught to take the woman's medical history and to use a simple examination check-list to decide when oral contraceptives might be given.

In 1974 a much more widespread community based distribution in Thailand was started under the direction of Mechai Viravaidya. This project, the Community Based Family Planning Services (CBFPS), had 140,000 cumulative oral contraceptive acceptors by September 1978, at which time there were 54,000 active users.

Nowadays, several other countries use examination check-lists for their community based distribution of oral contraceptives. They include Mexico, Sri Lanka, the Lebanon, Ghana and Barbados. A typical check-list is the one approved by the Sri Lankan Health Ministry. The following is an amended version.

History:
    Ask if the woman has had a history of any of the following:
    Yellow skin or yellow eyes
    Lump in the breast
    Discharge from the nipple
    Excessive menstrual periods
    Increased frequency of menstrual periods
    Bleeding after sexual intercourse
    Swelling or severe pains in the legs
    Severe chest pains
    Unusual shortness of breath after exertion
    Severe headaches

Examination:
 Yellow skin and yellow eye colour
 Lump in the breast
 Nipple discharge
 Varicose veins/leg oedema
 High blood pressure (Yes = above 150 systolic or 100 diastolic)
 Fast pulse (Yes = above 100)
 Sugar in urine
 Protein in urine
 (Some other lists include 'obesity' among items in the examination)

Instructions:
 If all the above are negative, the woman may receive oral contraceptives. If any of the above are positive, the woman must be seen by a
doctor before oral contraceptives may be prescribed.

Not only are procedures of this type practicable, but they may in
certain circumstances be more acceptable to potential users than
doctor and routine family planning clinic supervision. They allow the
possibility of taking oral contraceptives to the homes of potential
users. Encouraging experience has been found not only in developing
countries, but also in the USA, where family planning specialists with
only six months' training have been able to become responsible for
90% of the work involved in the distribution and supervision of oral
contraceptives in certain hospitals.

IMAP Statement on Steroidal Oral Contraception*

Introduction

Many millions of women have used oral contraceptives (OCs) since they
became available in the early 1960s. At present about 60 million women
are using this highly effective form of contraception. The first OCs to be
introduced contained high doses of oestrogen and progestagen. There has
been a gradual, but significant, reduction in both components since then
with even greater reduction in total dosage per cycle. Such reductions have
led to decreases in adverse effects.

---

*This statement is valid for those oral contraceptives currently distributed by IPPF.
The Panel reserves the right to amend this statement in the light of further
developments in the field of OCs when sufficient scientific information becomes
available.

Beneficial effects

During the time that OCs have been widely used, they have been studied more thoroughly than any other medication in common use. The great majority of women who have used OCs have done so safely, with protection from pregnancy and freedom from major side-effects. The benefits to health and well-being far outweigh the possible side-effects and infrequent complications which occur in a minority of users.

Ectopic pregnancies

The use of OCs protects against ectopic pregnancy, which is life-threatening, particularly where access to immediate surgical treatment is limited.

Pelvic inflammatory disease

A lower incidence of pelvic inflammatory disease is found in users of OCs when compared with non-users or users of other methods of contraception, with the exception of barrier methods.

Prevention of pregnancy

Prevention of pregnancy is the most obvious benefit and is the prime reason for the use of OCs. Used properly, they are virtually 100% effective. However, in actual use the failure rates are 2-4%. The prevention of unplanned pregnancies and the reduction of abortions and maternal mortality and morbidity associated with them has profoundly important health benefits.

Neoplasia

Use of OCs has a protective effect against cancer of the ovary and endometrium and also against benign breast tumours and benign ovarian cysts. Recent data show that OCs may also protect against the development of uterine fibroids.

Menstrual cycle

Blood loss is usually diminished with OCs, and this implies an added advantage in decreasing the chances of the development of anaemia, or of any increase in this condition. Where cycles have been irregular before, this is corrected. Mid-cycle pain, pre-menstrual tension and dysmenorrhoea are usually relieved. Acne, especially the pre-menstrual type, will usually improve.

Common minor side-effects

A number of symptoms associated with OCs resemble those found in early pregnancy. These include: nausea, vomiting, dizziness, breast tenderness, weight gain, headaches, fluid retention, inter-menstrual spotting, breakthrough bleeding and depression.

Adverse effects

Circulatory system disease

In developed countries an increased risk of disease of the circulatory system constitutes the most important adverse effect of combined OC use, although some of the information is conflicting. Studies are under way in developing countries where the incidence of these conditions is lower, and where the background risk factors may be different.

There is also evidence from developed countries that duration of use and ever-use are associated with later development of some cardiovascular diseases after discontinuation of use, but, again, the applicability to developing countries is not known.

The use of OCs is associated with changes in the serum lipid profile. Progestagens in general, and particularly those containing derivatives of 19-nortestosterone, are associated with an increase in low-density lipoprotein cholesterol and a decrease in high-density lipoprotein cholesterol, changes that can increase the risk of atherogenesis. Oestrogens, on the other hand, have the opposite effect, and as a consequence these effects are relatively balanced in low-dose combined pills.

Myocardial infarction: Data relating to myocardial infarction and use of OCs are not consistent, and most of the data are derived from women using the older higher dose formulations, which should not be in normal use. Nevertheless, there is no doubt that women in developed countries who use OCs and have one or more of the following risk factors, namely age over 40 years, smoking, hypertension, diabetes or hyperlipidaemia, show an excess death rate from this condition. It is probable that changes in plasma lipids related to high-dose OCs are involved. The relationship, if any, between currently used low-dose OCs, plasma lipids, and myocardial infarction requires further study.

Venous thromboembolism: Studies in developed countries show that OC users have a higher mortality than non-users from this cause. These deaths are mainly from pulmonary embolism. The oestrogen component of OCs is the main associated factor, having an adverse effect on specific clotting factors in the blood. Therefore OCs containing the lowest effective dose of oestrogen should be used. It is common medical practice to stop using OCs 2-6 weeks before major elective surgery and to restart OCs within four weeks of surgery. Alternative effective contraception should be advised during this time. In emergency procedures, the surgeon may consider the use of prophylactic anticoagulant measures. OCs can be restarted four weeks after surgery.

Subarachnoid haemorrhage: Although some data from developed countries suggest that this condition has been associated with OC use, these data are not conclusive. Some substantial studies show no such relationship.

Elevated blood pressure: Elevated blood pressure is sometimes observed in OC users. Several reports suggest that the progestagen component of OCs plays a part in determining the blood pressure effect. Certainly OCs containing the lowest effective dose of progestagen should be used. OC induced elevated blood pressure usually disappears on discontinuation of OCs. If persistent it almost always responds to treatment.

Liver disorders

It is recognized that the relative risk of developing a benign liver cell adenoma is increased in OC users. If it ruptures and haemorrhage occurs it can be life-threatening. It remains an extremely rare complication in developed countries; no data are yet available from developing countries.

Cholestatic jaundice may occur in some OC users, especially in those who have had cholestatic jaundice of pregnancy.

Possible carcinogenicity

The possible causal association between OCs and various cancers has been a major concern. Although much research has been done to clarify the possible links, results so far have been conflicting. Many of the cancers are caused by several factors acting singly or synergistically. They also have rather long latent periods. All of these factors make analysis of research findings and attribution of cause to any individual agent difficult. There are ongoing studies which it is hoped will help provide definitive answers in the future but this is likely to take many years. In the meantime the possible increased risks which have been noticed in a few studies are still small enough not to outweigh benefits nor to call for changes in current medical practice.

Breast

The relation between OCs and breast cancer has been studied extensively in developed and, more recently, in developing countries. Despite continued controversy about the risks in some sub-groups of women there is no conclusive evidence that OCs cause breast cancer.

Cervix

Recently completed studies in both developed and developing countries on the relation between OCs and cervical neoplasia are not conclusive, but some work suggests that prolonged OC use may be related to this condition. Indeed, it may never be possible to separate OCs as putative carcinogens from confounding factors such as age at first intercourse and number of sex partners for both the man and woman. Nevertheless, if an increased risk of cancer of the cervix exists it is small. Since invasive cancer of the cervix is largely a preventable disease, periodic cervical cytology should be offered to sexually active women when adequate treatment and follow-up facilities are available.

Melanoma

A slightly increased incidence of malignant melanoma in association with OCs has been reported. Recent definitive studies provide no support for this suggestion.

Liver

Recent data from a developed country suggest that long-term OC use may be associated with this extremely uncommmon cancer. Since the incidence of this disease is so low any increase, even if proven, would not be of public health importance. These findings should be confirmed by further studies, particularly in those developing countries where liver cancer is more common and has a different aetiology, being largely associated with hepatitis B virus. Unless such studies establish a significantly increased risk, there will be no reason to recommend a change in the use of OCs.

Other effects

Carbohydrate metabolism

Changes in plasma insulin and glucose tolerance in OC users have been consistently reported for many years. This may be a progestagen effect. There is no evidence of increased incidence of clinical diabetes; diabetic women may use OCs under close medical supervison.

Pituitary adenomas

Large studies have failed to reveal a causal relationship between use of OCs and pituitary adenomas. Nevertheless, if galactorrhoea is noted in a woman taking OCs, alternative methods of contraception should be used. If the galactorrhoea persists and particularly if there is subsequent disruption of the menstrual cycle, the woman should be referred for comprehensive investigation.

Gallbladder disease

The risk of gallbladder disease has been reported to be increased in some studies, but recent work suggests that OCs may simply accelerate the clinical presentation of previously sub-clinical diseases of the gallbladder.

Vitamins

Some changes in blood biochemical indicators of vitamin status take place during OC use. These changes are of no clinical significance and data suggest that there is no need for routine vitamin supplementation in OC users, even in populations where malnutrition is prevalent.

Return of menstruation and fertility

Incidence of post-OC amenorrhoea is low. By the end of six months after discontinuation less than 1% of users have amenorrhoea, and this group responds readily to treatment. There is no evidence of decreased fertility in former OC users, although there may be some delay in the return of fertility. By 24 months normal fertility levels are achieved.

Pregnancy outcome

A number of studies have demonstrated no excess rate of spontaneous abortion or fetal abnormalities in former users of OCs, including those who conceive soon after stopping OCs. In the rare situations where women have inadvertently taken OCs while pregnant or where the pregnancy occurred during OC use, an increased risk of fetal abnormalities has also not been proven.

Contraindications

Absolute contraindications include:

- malignancy of the breast
- malignancy of the genital tract
- venous thromboembolism
- cerebrovascular accident
- undiagnosed abnormal vaginal bleeding
- focal migraine
- familial hyperlipidaemia

Relative contraindications

There are other situations where medical assessment of risks and benefits should be made before a woman is put on OCs. The potential risks should be adequately explained and possible alternative contraceptive methods should be discussed. If OCs are chosen, it is particularly important that the woman be kept under medical supervision. These situations include: age over 40 years, smoking, mild hypertension or a history of hypertensive disease of pregnancy (toxaemia), epilepsy, diabetes mellitus, history of bouts of depression, recent history of oligomenorrhoea or amenorrhoea in nulliparous women, and gallbladder and liver disease.

Special situations

Lactation

Breast milk is the best source of nutrition for infants and also protects them against some diseases. Therefore it is important not to interfere with breastfeeding by inappropriate use of certain forms of contraception. Both high and low dose combined OCs containing oestrogen adversely affect the quantity and quality of breast milk, and reduce the duration of lactation.

If contraception is needed during lactation, progestagen-only OCs can be used. The combined OCs should be withheld until six months after delivery or till the infant is weaned, whichever is the earlier. Where they are the only available form of contraception, combined OCs may have to be started earlier, as a pregnancy during early lactation would be more detrimental to the health of the mother and her infant than a decrease in the milk supply. No deleterious effects have been reported so far from the transfer to the infant of small amounts of steroids in the milk.

Drug interaction

Rifampicin greatly reduces the efficacy of OCs, so women should use alternative contraception when taking this drug. There are a few reports of pregnancies in OC users being treated with other antibiotics (ampicillin, amoxycillin, tetracyclines and griseofulvin), with anticonvulsants (dilantin, phenytoin and phenobarbitone) and with laxatives. Except for rifampicin these findings may not be of sufficient importance to affect OC use but the possibility of interference with the effectiveness of OCs should be kept in mind.

Parasitic diseases

Because oral contraceptives are widely used in some developing countries their interaction with parasitic diseases common in those countries may be particularly significant. Research in such inter-relationships between the disease and/or drugs used in its treatment is sparse and needs to be encouraged. In uncomplicated schistosomiasis OC use does not alter the results of liver function tests. The same applies to the common Asian parasitic disease caused by the liver fluke (*Opisthorchis viverrini*).

Sickle cell disease

Sickle cell trait is not a contraindication to the use of OCs, and, although there are theoretical reasons to believe that women with sickle cell disease may be at increased risk of thrombosis and haemolytic disease, there is no

evidence to support this contention. Studies are in progress to confirm or
refute this.

Adolescence

In prescribing OCs for adolescents, caution is recommended until
menstruation is established (see IPPF policy on meeting the needs of
young people 2.2.2/01).

Post-coital contraception

The use of steroids for post-coital contraception has a limited place, only
in emergency situations (see IPPF statement on post-coital contraception
2.1.1.0/02).

Hormonal pregnancy tests

The use of oral steroids for pregnancy testing is not recommended (see
IPPF policy 2.1.9/01).

Types and selection of oral contraceptives

Oral contraceptives currently used are of two main types.

1. Combined oestrogen and progestagen.
    (*a*) Monophasic OCs.
    (*b*) Multiphasic OCs (biphasic and triphasic), a modification of the
        combined OC where varying combinations of oestrogen and
        progestagen are used throughout the cycle, with a lower total
        monthly steroidal dose.

2. The progestagen-only OCs.

Recommendations

Based on acceptable pharmacological principles, the lowest effective dose
of a compound should always be used.

It is recommended that not more than four combined formulations be
available in family planning programmes within the following ranges:

1. Between 30 and 50 μg of oestrogen, with the recommendation that the
    lower dose be given first, and either

2. 150 μg of levonorgestrel or desogestrel, or a progestagen from the

norethisterone group not exceeding 1 mg of norethisterone or its equivalent.

The progestagen-only OC, generally referred to as the mini-Pill, may have a place as an oral contraceptive in certain situations where the oestrogen component of the combined OC is contraindicated or not desirable. Examples include use during lactation and the years before the menopause.

Problems with the mini-Pill include reduced effectiveness, a relatively high incidence of ectopic pregnancy in contraceptive failure; and a higher incidence of menstrual disruption.

Duration of use

In women who are otherwise well, OC use may be continued for many years. There is no justification for periodic withdrawal of the use of OCs.

For women over the age of 40 the Pill should be prescribed with caution (see Relative Contraindications, page 73).

(This statement was approved by the IPPF Central Council in November 1986 following extensive review of the literature by the IPPF International Medical Advisory Panel.)

Chapter 5

Long-acting Hormonal Contraception

Introduction

The two main reasons for the development of long-acting hormonal contraceptives are convenience and freedom from the problem of 'missing' Pills. The long duration of action following a single administration is associated with other attributes such as increased long-term contraceptive efficacy in general use compared with oral contraceptives. Long-acting methods also often have a substantial safety margin in terms of timing of the next dose. Most of these methods can be administered in a relatively simple manner and, in most societies, are associated with high acceptability and high continuation rates.

The actual duration of action varies greatly with the particular method, from monthly administration with certain injectables, up to five or even seven years' duration with some subcutaneous implants. Long-acting methods have a considerable number of attributes, but some also have disadvantages. One of the most obvious of these is the fact that injectables, unlike implants, cannot be withdrawn from the body after administration. Their effects wear off naturally in two or three months. Other disadvantages and advantages of these methods are discussed below.

Family planning programme administration is a very important aspect of this fairly new methodology. All the methods involve relatively modern technology, and potential users need very careful instruction before starting the method. Increasingly, there has been a widespread realization of the major need for thorough training of counsellors who will be advising women who are intending to use long-acting methods. There is good evidence that detailed pre-treatment counselling substantially improves the acceptability and continuation rates. Recent field trials of injectable contraceptives have demonstrated that failure to provide very thorough counselling leads to large numbers of early discontinuations. There is also a need for ongoing reinforcement and counselling at subsequent visits. Most of these methods require well-trained staff to supervise them and in most places they are probably more suited to clinic-based distribution systems rather than community based systems. Nevertheless, mobile teams are able to provide them successfully in certain areas.

Different forms of long-acting hormonal contraception

Many different techniques have been studied, a few are already marketed, and a modest number of others are currently under clinical development.

First generation systems

The two most commonly used intramuscular injectable preparations are a three-monthly injection of depot medroxyprogesterone acetate (150 mg in a microcrystalline suspension; DMPA, Depo-Provera), and a two-monthly injection of norethisterone oenanthate (200 mg in oil; NET-OEN, Noristerat, Norigest).

Monthly injectable formulations, available in China and sold in some Latin American countries, usually contain a long-acting progestagen and a shorter-acting oestrogen. They are highly effective contraceptives which achieve more satisfactory menstrual bleeding patterns than the longer-acting methods. However, they have the disadvantage of requiring more frequent administration. Now monthly preparations are being used in advanced clinical trials in several countries.

Second generation systems

Subcutaneous implants with constant, slow release of a variety of different progestagens have been shown to provide excellent contraception. These have usually consisted of silastic capsules packed with crystalline steroid, but several attempts have also been made to perfect biodegradable polymers which will allow constant steroid release as they erode. Only the five to seven year levonorgestrel-releasing system developed by the Population Council (Norplant) has yet reached the stage of general marketing. This system suffers from the disadvantage that six silastic capsules, inserted through a small trocar, are required to provide adequate contraceptive blood levels. An implant system with two covered rods is currently under clinical trial in some countries. With these systems the capsules or rods can be removed at any time to end the contraceptive effect.

Silastic vaginal rings releasing constant, small amounts of progestagens are also nearing general availability. These systems also provide continuous low-dosage progestagen-only contraception, and have the advantage that they can be inserted and removed by the woman herself, if she so desires. The Progestasert is a progesterone-releasing intrauterine device, active for one year, and other IUDs containing progestagens (e.g. levonorgestrel) are under clinical trial. They provide another useful contraceptive option. A variety of other approaches to long-term hormonal action are being studied; these include such approaches as the micro encapsulation of contraceptive steroids (microspheres) in biodegradable polymers in a form which can be injected through a medium-sized needle.

Development and introduction of injectables

The possibility of prolonging the duration of the hormonal effect was first recognized with the synthesis of esters of different progestagens in the late 1950s, and with the discovery that formulation of medroxyprogesterone acetate as a microcrystalline suspension permitted slow release after injection into the body. DMPA was first studied as a contraceptive during the years 1963 to 1966, and came steadily into more widespread use thereafter. Since the early 1970s the development of new long-acting hormonal methods has been to some extent overshadowed by the stormy saga of the DMPA marketing application in the USA.

DMPA approval was initially deferred when high-dose toxicology studies in beagle bitches revealed an increase in breast tumours in this susceptible species. Other unresolved issues such as delay in return of fertility and a possible increase in cervical dysplasia in women, were sufficient to ensure that early approval would not be forthcoming. Eventually, the USA Food and Drug Administration (FDA) refused contraceptive marketing approval in 1978, but only after a positive recommendation in favour of marketing on two occasions from its own expert scientific advisory committee in obstetrics and gynaecology. A Public Board of Inquiry into Depo-Provera was eventually granted by the FDA and, in 1986, a final decision was left pending. The application by the manufacturer, Upjohn, was withdrawn, but a new one may be forthcoming.

A similar situation developed in the UK where political pressures led the Minister of Health to turn down a recommendation from the Committee for the Safety of Medicines for expanding the indications for the contraceptive use of Depo-Provera. Approval was eventually granted after a public hearing. It should be noted that almost every scientific body which has reviewed the use of Depo-Provera has recommended its wider use for contraceptive purposes. This includes the International Medical Advisory Panel of IPPF, which completed a thorough review in 1982 (see page 86). Nevertheless, there are still concerns in the international community about issues of informed consent for use of these long-acting methods, and their 'potential for abuse' in poorly educated and under-privileged groups.

In spite of these emotional and to a certain extent political concerns, DMPA is marketed for long-term contraception in about 100 countries, and there are very few countries where it is not registered for other indications such as treatment of endometrial cancer and endometriosis. DMPA is a thoroughly researched drug by any standards, with published data in more than 1,000 articles.

It is calculated that sufficient DMPA is marketed each year to provide contraception for more than two million women. NET-OEN is used by around a quarter of a million women per year. This use is rapidly increasing, and NET-OEN is marketed in a total of more than 40 countries.

Attempts to deliver contraceptive steroids by other routes and delivery systems have been intensified since the late 1960s when it was first demonstrated that relatively constant blood levels could be achieved from subcutaneous implants containing the concentrated steroid. Most attention has been focused on the uses of progestagens alone.

Pharmacology and mode of action

DMPA consists of a microcrystalline aqueous suspension which is best administered by deep intramuscular injection of 150 mg into the buttock or deltoid muscle. The injection site should not be massaged. The particles are 2-3 μm in diameter, have a very low aqueous solubility and erode very slowly at the surface over a period of several months. The effects of a dose of 150 mg are expected to last at least three months, and usually last for much longer. This provides an initially high plasma level around 5-10 nmol/l, which then gradually declines until the crystal has been totally eroded. Variability of absorption and metabolism contributes to the unpredictable delay in disappearance of the depot material and hence the unpredictable duration of action.

NET-OEN is a long-chain ester of norethisterone which is formulated in castor-oil/benzyl benzoate solution and given intramuscularly. The ester is distributed to adipose tissue throughout the body and slowly released back into the blood stream. Hydrolysis and release of the active steroid probably occurs mainly in the liver. High initial plasma levels are followed by a rapid exponential fall of variable duration. It is now recommended that NET-OEN 200 mg be given at eight-weekly intervals instead of 12-weekly regimes. At eight-weekly dosage intervals, contraceptive efficacy is maintained at a higher level, and there is no difference in the occurrence of amenorrhoea and minor side-effects with the more frequent dosage.

Most injectables act by inhibition of ovulation at a hypothalamic level with low-normal plasma levels of endogenous LH, FSH, and oestradiol. Subsidiary effects on luteal function, tubal function, endometrium and cervical mucus all contribute to the high efficacy of this contraceptive approach. Most of the newer delivery systems (subdermal implants and vaginal rings) concentrate on providing constant and so-called 'zero-order release' of progestagens. The amount of progestagen released per day can be tailored to produce blood levels which either inhibit ovulation or produce a low-dose 'minipill' type effect.

Clinical aspects

Efficacy

DMPA, monthly injectables and Norplant are among the most effective of all reversible contraceptives and have a higher use effectiveness than anything except sterilization. They are usually associated with fewer than 0.5 pregnancies per 100 woman-years, while NET-OEN has a failure rate around 1-1.5 per 100 woman-years. Efficacy of low-dose vaginal rings is slightly less.

In most societies acceptability of long-acting methods is high, in spite of the menstrual side-effects. In most published studies 50-90% of women will still be continuing their use after one year, which is equivalent to or better than most other contraceptive methods.

Adverse effects

Menstrual disturbance is an almost invariable accompaniment of progestagen-only contraception, and the worst disturbances occur with DMPA and NET-OEN. These disturbances are the most common medical causes of discontinuation. A spectrum of disturbances is seen, from amenorrhoea and oligomenorrhoea through occasional prolonged or frequent bleeding to rare heavy bleeding, the major problem being the unpredictability of the bleeding pattern. Monthly injectables and newer low-dose delivery systems cause less disturbance, but amenorrhoea and irregular bleeding are not uncommon.

Amenorrhoea is related to progressive endometrial atrophy, but the mechanism of the bleeding irregularities is not well understood. Management of the disturbances is unsatisfactory. It is known that cyclical oral oestrogen administration can induce regular withdrawal bleeding in those progestagen users with amenorrhoea, but this greatly complicates the method. Oestrogens (e.g. ethinyl oestradiol 50 μg daily or one combined Pill daily for 14 days or more) can also be used to stop an episode of prolonged, frequent or heavy bleeding. However, it is uncertain whether a single course of oestrogen treatment will improve the overall menstrual pattern.

It must be emphasized that pre-treatment counselling and community education combined with continued reassurance at follow-up visits, will ensure a high tolerance of these problems by most groups of women. This is by far and away the most critical part of the management of the menstrual disturbances with long-acting hormonal methods, and emphasizes the importance of employing well-trained and sympathetic staff in the supervision of women using these methods. Oestrogen usage is not generally recommended, and in most clinical trials has only occasionally been required. Curettage is rarely indicated to stop an episode of bleeding, but may be indicated for diagnostic purposes, especially in older women.

Delay in return of ovulation and fertility is the only other known side-effect of any consequence with the injectables. It appears that there is no delay in the return of fertility following removal of implants or vaginal rings. Large-scale studies indicate that the cumulative conception rate curve is displaced slightly to the right by DMPA, so that the median delay to conception is only five to seven months following the presumed end of contraceptive protection. This compares favourably with a 4.5 month delay for IUDs. Approximately 75% of couples will have achieved a pregnancy by 12-15 months and 92% by two years. There is no evidence of an adverse effect of prolonged use, or of permanent sterility in any group of users.

Other side-effects have not been a problem in any of the major trials, either in frequency or severity. Many different side-effects, such as weight gain, headaches, bloating, dizziness, fatigue, nervousness and other mood changes have been mentioned with varying frequencies in up to 15% of users. However, it is unusual for these to lead to discontinuation, and many are probably not directly related to hormonal treatment.

Minor biochemical changes can be detected in some users of injectable progestagens, but these are of a similar or lesser order than those seen with oral contraceptives and do not appear to be of major clinical significance.

Medical benefits

Progestagens may have substantial beneficial effects on the incidence and severity of pelvic inflammatory disease, crises in sickle cell anaemia, endometriosis, vaginal candidiasis and ovarian and endometrial neoplasia.

Progestagens on their own do not adversely affect clotting mechanisms and have been recommended as satisfactory contraceptives for women with a history of venous thromboembolism. Blood pressure does not appear to be affected by progestagens on their own, but in any given population some individuals may develop high blood pressure for other reasons and, therefore, this should be monitored.

Who should be using long-acting methods?

Contraceptive requirements vary with individual inclination, cultural pressures and stage of reproductive life. A number of differing long-acting methods have been developed to provide a new range of contraceptive options. Use of each will depend on local availability, as well as the availability of alternative methods. If a wide range of methods is available it is generally recommended that DMPA and, to a lesser extent, NET-OEN should not be used in nulliparous women or in women who are spacing their families, because of the rather unpredictable delay before fertility returns completely. In women who are breast feeding it is generally recommended that low-dose delivery systems are preferable, since a small amount of progestagen is transferred into the mother's milk. Apart from these cautions, the use of any particular method will depend upon individual preference.

Controversial issues

Debate about several issues is still continuing. In most cases this centres around possible theoretical, but very low levels of risk for long-term users.

Neoplasia

Extensive data are now available from combined oral contraceptive studies to indicate a major degree of protection against the development of endometrial and ovarian cancer with use of these agents. There is good reason to believe that a similar degree of protection will be found with progestagen-only methods. Available human epidemiological evidence does not suggest that DMPA increases the risk of breast cancer. The situation with regard to cervical neoplasia is less clear and the situation here may be similar to that found with combined oral contraceptives, where a small increase in risk has been demonstrated. This observed increase in risk can be explained by sexual risk factors. There is no evidence of an increased risk of any other type of tumour.

Teratogenesis

Since pregnancy rates with all these methods are so low, the risk of exposure of a fetus must be very small. The greatest risk is probably associated with inadvertent administration of the drug in the mid to late first trimester. Several investigators have published evidence which suggests that some synthetic progestagens may be very low-grade teratogens, but the majority of evidence indicates that they are safe. Nevertheless, 19-nortestosterone derivatives have occasionally been associated with some masculinization of the female fetus, and a small risk may be associated with inadvertent NET-OEN administration late in the first trimester.

Lactation and effects on offspring

One of the advantages of progestagen-only contraceptives is that they do not decrease, and may even increase milk yield. There is no good evidence to indicate any deleterious change in the composition of breast milk or any adverse effect on neonatal development. However, small quantities of progestagens and some of their metabolites can be transferred in measurable quantities into milk and into the infant's circulation. Exposure, however, is low, and lactating mothers can be reassured. However, most experts recommend that the first injection should ideally be deferred until approximately six to eight weeks following delivery to allow greater maturation of all neonatal systems. It has also been shown that injection of DMPA soon after delivery may lead to heavy bleeding.

Special considerations about Norplant

Since the Norplant subdermal contraceptive implant system consists of six small silicone rubber (silastic) capsules, their use needs a small incision under sterile conditions to place them under the skin and to remove them later. Each capsule is 3.4 cm long and 2.4 mm in diameter, and contains 36 mg of levonorgestrel. Other simpler systems with different hormones are under clinical trial at present.

Training for the persons who insert and remove the capsules is of the utmost importance. They must also be fully trained in counselling the women who are to receive the implants. This counselling should advise the women on how Norplant works (similarly to all progestagen-only contraceptives, but with the advantage of a non-fluctuating, constant low level of progestagen in the blood stream over the five-year life of the implant). Other important points to mention are: that the action of Norplant is completely reversible and fertility is restored as soon as the implant is removed; that the implant can be removed at any time the woman wants during the five years it is active; any possible side-effects, particularly the changes in the bleeding pattern; how it is inserted and removed; and comparisons of this method with other forms of contraception, including injectables (see page 23).

The Population Council, which developed Norplant, has established several training centres throughout the world, where personnel are sent by various FPAs and other bodies for training in insertion, removal and counselling techniques. The IPPF has approved Norplant as one of the contraceptives it supplies on request to its member associations in countries where the system is officially approved for clinical use (12 countries at present) or for use in clinical trials, and where FPA clinic workers have undergone proper training as mentioned above.

Conclusions

Long-acting contraceptives are highly effective in preventing pregnancy, have wide acceptability in most societies and have a number of other advantages. They each have a number of relative disadvantages and still face a number of incompletely resolved concerns. However, extensive information indicates that these concerns are no greater than those faced by oral and intrauterine contraceptives or surgical sterilization. IPPF believes that systems such as injectables and sub-dermal implants should be an integral part of the range of contraceptive choices in all societies.

IMAP Statement on Injectable Contraception*

Introduction

Injectable contraceptives have proved a welcome addition to family planning choices, and their currrent use prevents a measurable number of deaths from unplanned pregnancy and in particular from illegal abortion. Depot medroxyprogesterone acetate (DMPA) and norethisterone oenanthate (NET-EN) are the most widely used and studied of several injectable contraceptives available.

Injectable hormonal contraception with these two long-acting steroidal preparations provides an effective means of fertility regulation, and has become an important method of family planning. DMPA and NET-EN have several advantages which make them particularly suitable for some women and acceptable in family planning programmes. A single injection can provide highly effective contraception for two or more months, delivery is simple, independent of coitus, and ensures periodic contact with medical or other trained health personnel.

DMPA to date is registered as a therapeutic agent in nearly all countries and as a contraceptive agent in over 80 developed and developing countries. NET-EN is registered as a contraceptive in 40 countries. In some countries locally produced and untested formulations are also available and extensively used.

---

*This statement replaces earlier statements adopted in 1975, 1978, 1979 and 1980, and is valid for the injectables currently distributed by IPPF. The IPPF reserves the right to amend this statement in the light of further developments in the field of injectable contraception when sufficient scientific information becomes available.

Administration of injectable contraceptives

Administered by intramuscular injection in an aqueous microcrystalline suspension, DMPA exerts its contraceptive effect primarily by suppression of ovulation. However, its effects on the endometrium, the uterine tubes and the production of cervical mucus may also play a role in reducing fertility. DMPA as a contraceptive agent is generally given at a dosage of 150 mg every 90 days (three months). NET-EN, when administered as an intramuscular injection of an oily preparation at a dose of 200 mg, inhibits ovulation. It should be administered at eight-weekly intervals for the first six months of use, then at intervals of eight or twelve weeks. A slightly lower pregnancy rate has been observed with eight-weekly intervals, but this is accompanied by a slightly higher rate of discontinuation because of bleeding abnormalities.

Animal studies

Long-term animal studies with DMPA have been completed mainly on beagle bitches and rhesus monkeys, and similar studies with NET-EN are nearing completion. These studies have shown such side-effects as pyometra, mammary gland nodules, adenocarcinoma and acromegaly in beagles, and endometrial carcinoma in rhesus monkeys.

None of the findings in beagles is considered applicable to human populations because the beagle responds differently than humans to steroidal hormones. For example, the beagle endometrium is stimulated by DMPA, in some cases leading to pyometra and death, while in the human the endometrium becomes atrophic. Growth hormone levels are increased in the beagle, leading to acromegaly, while in the human there are no growth hormone changes. Of particular importance, there are different progesterone reception responses at the cellular level between the beagle and the human.

Therefore, the IPPF agrees with the conclusions of the WHO Toxicology Review Panel and the UK Committee on the Safety of Medicines that the beagle is an unsuitable model on which to observe potential adverse effects associated with the long-term effects of progestagens in women.

None of the deaths among rhesus monkeys was attributable to effects of the drug. Although endometrial carcinoma was found in two of the replacement monkeys given 50 times the human dose of DMPA and in one of the monkeys receiving a similar dose of NET-EN, it was also observed in some monkeys in control groups in two other studies. The number of animals is too small for statistically significant studies, and it is impossible to conclude whether DMPA or NET-EN caused these cancers or instead failed to prevent them.

Human data

Endometrium

Despite over 18 years of use and an estimated 13 million women who have ever used DMPA or NET-EN, no case has been recorded of endometrial malignancy in women so exposed — there is no evidence at this stage of a causal association, either anecdotal or scientific. It should be recalled that the situation was quite different with oral contraceptives. The first suggestions linking them to an increased risk of a cluster of cardiovascular side-effects were isolated case reports, which in turn led to the appropriately controlled studies confirming the association.

Endometrial cancer is the second most frequent malignancy of the female genital tract in many countries. When it arises spontaneously it does so usually in post-menopausal women, and is frequently found in a uterus where the unaffected endometrium is atrophic. Relatively short exposure to high levels of unopposed endogenous or exogenous oestrogens is associated with an increased incidence of carcinoma, after producing phases of widespread endometrial hyperplasia including adenomatous hyperplasia. It should also be noted that, in general, progestagens appear to be protective against this disease, and specifically that DMPA is used widely in the treatment of endometrial malignancy.

Finally, it should be reiterated that despite extensive and long-term experience, there is to date no human evidence to suggest the need to explore the morphology of the DMPA-exposed human endometrium. Present information does not indicate that DMPA causes endometrial malignancy. It is too early to know if it will always prevent it.

Cervix

Both the WHO and the Biometrics and Epidemiological Methodology Advisory Committee of the US Food and Drug Administration (USFDA) reviewed the available epidemiological and clinical data on malignant and pre-malignant disease of the uterine cervix in women on DMPA and found no evidence of an increased risk of such malignancy in DMPA users.

Fetus/Newborn/Lactation

There is sufficient evidence from investigations carried out in several countries that DMPA and NET-EN may increase both milk production and the duration of lactation. Only one study mentioned a decrease in lactation reported by fewer than 15% of DMPA users.

Although an increase in the quantity of milk may occur in women treated with injectable contraceptives, the question of possible consequences of the transfer of the steroid to the breast-fed infant has yet to be resolved.

It has been calculated that only small amounts (between 0.2 and 0.08 μg/kg/day) of medroxyprogesterone acetate (MPA) and/or its metabolites are ingested by the infant, and that only a small fraction of that is in fact absorbed because of an active intestinal metabolism and excretion. Recent studies have shown that the level of NET-EN in breast-milk is of the order of 3,000 pg/ml one week after injection, while by eight weeks it is usually undetectable. This is 0.05% of the maternal dose of NET-EN over the two-month interval of use. However, the amounts absorbed by the infant are infinitely smaller. Although these quantities are considered too small to affect the infant systems adversely, to date no proper, thorough follow-up studies of children breast-fed by mothers using injectable contraceptives have been carried out. However, several continuing studies indicate a lack of deleterious effects: data from infant growth equivalent in DMPA users and non-users, and data from Mexico suggest no adverse effects over a 13-year period. It should also be noted that the quantity of steroid received by the infant is considerably lower than the steroid to which children bottle-fed with cows' milk are exposed. In addition, it is worth noting that other toxic extraneous products such as organo-chlorine compounds are found in detectable quantities in breast milk.

When discussing possible risks to the infant, the inadvertent exposure to DMPA or NET-EN because of injections in women who are already pregnant must be considered. To prevent this, efforts are made to establish that the woman is not likely to be pregnant. The best time for starting a woman on injectable contraceptives is probably during the first seven days of a menstrual cycle. However, her request for injectable contraception at another time during the cycle should not be made a condition for rejecting her at that time if the possibility of a pregnancy can be ruled out. The risk of exposure of fetuses because of failure of an injectable contraceptive has to be considered minimal in view of the very high effectiveness of the drugs and the fact that escape ovulation will only occur when hormone levels are relatively very low.

Metabolic effects

Despite intensive biochemical research, the only clinical metabolic effect attributed to DMPA is weight gain. No other metabolic effect has associated clinical problems. Blood pressure, glucose tolerance, steroid metabolism and immune changes have been studied, and minor alterations have been observed which appeared to be of no clinical significance.

89

Changes in calcium uptake by bone and decreases in urinary calcium excretion have been documented, but no associated clinical problems, such as osteoporosis, have been identified. It should be emphasized that DMPA does not produce the type of changes in blood clotting factors and serum cholesterol which are associated with combined oral contraceptive use. Fewer data have been published on the metabolic effects of NET-EN but it appears not to affect most biochemical functions.

Menstrual irregularities/Return of fertility

NET-EN and DMPA are associated with disruptions of the menstrual cycle and irregular bleeding, but the occurrence of heavy vaginal bleeding requiring therapeutic intervention is extremely rare (found in about 0.5% of users). Oestrogen therapy or uterine curettage is rarely necessary and is seldom used. Fewer than one-third of women receiving DMPA report having normal menstrual cycles during the first year of use. Normal menses are slightly more common among women using NET-EN, with approximately half the users reporting at least one normal cycle during the first year. About half the women on DMPA will become amenorrhoeic at the end of one year. Menstrual cycles return to normal in most women within six months after the last injection.

Available data show that fertility is not impaired permanently. Cumulative pregnancy rates of 92-97% at the end of 24 months after discontinuation have been reported in a number of studies. Studies in the USA and Thailand showed a comparable pregnancy rate in oral contraceptive and intrauterine device users at 18 months. Fewer data are available on the return of fertility following use of NET-EN. The available data, however, suggest no impairment of fertility.

Conclusion

The International Medical Advisory Panel endorses the recommendations of the WHO, that it continues to be a responsible act to make DMPA and NET-EN available as contraceptives. The Panel concludes that careful long-term monitoring, including case-control, cohort and clinical studies, of injectables, as well as all other contraceptive methods, be continued.

(Statement by the IPPF International Medical Advisory Panel, October 1982; approved by the IPPF Central Council, November 1982.)

IMAP Statement on Norplant Subdermal Contraceptive Implant System*

The Norplant subdermal contraceptive implant system is a long-acting, reversible, low-dose, progestagen-only method. The drug levonorgestrel is delivered by means of six silastic capsules placed subdermally. The Norplant system was developed by the International Committee for Contraception Research (ICCR) of the Population Council (it is commercially manufactured at present by Huhtamaki Oy/Leiras Pharmaceuticals of Finland under licence from the Council). Clinical studies began in 1975 in seven countries and the device is currently being tested in pre-introductory trials in 19 countries, both developed and developing. More than 200,000 woman-months of experience have been collected to date and analysed.

The Norplant system has been registered for commercial use in Finland, the country of manufacture, and in Sweden (February 1985). Applications for registration are pending in numerous other countries. In October 1984, the World Health Organization (WHO) concluded after a specially-convened technical review that the Norplant system is "an effective and reversible long-term method of fertility regulation. It is considered suitable for use in family planning programmes along with other currently available contraceptive preparations and devices, since it provides an important option for women desiring long-term contraception".

Mode of action

As with other progestagen-only contraceptives, Norplant is thought to have three modes of action:

1. Levonorgestrel acts on the hypothalamus and pituitary and suppresses the LH surge responsible for ovulation. Progesterone levels consistent with ovulation occur in only about half the cycles. Oestrogen levels fluctuate and in the absence of elevated progesterone levels could indicate follicular activity without ovulation.

2. The effect of levonorgestrel on cervical mucus also contributes to its contraceptive efficacy. The mucus becomes viscous and scanty, making it less permeable to sperm.

---

*This statement is valid for the method of subdermal contraceptive implants described. The Panel reserves the right to amend this statement in the light of further developments in the field, when sufficient scientific information becomes available.

3. Finally, in most cases the endometrium shows signs of suppression.

Blood levels

Each capsule contains 36 mg of levonorgestrel and has a diameter of 2.4 mm and a length of 3.4 cm. The capsules release levonorgestrel at the rate of approximately 80 µg per 24 hours during the first few weeks of use, declining over the next 18 months to a constant rate of approximately 30 µg of levonorgestrel per 24 hours. The blood level is approximately equivalent to that attained daily by the use of progestagen-only mini-Pills, but in the latter case the blood levels fluctuate, with daily spikes. The steady release rate of Norplant, with a constant low level in the blood stream, probably accounts for much lower pregnancy failure rates than with the mini-Pill.

Clinical issues

Norplant is suitable for most women of reproductive age but is particularly recommended for use by women who wish to obtain long-term protection from pregnancy but who may desire another child in the future or do not wish to undergo sterilization. It is specially suited for women who should not take oestrogen and women who cannot use IUDs or oral or injectable contraceptives.

Contra-indications

Since Norplant is a new method of contraception, there has been insufficient time for large-scale, long-term studies, thus contra-indications and possible warnings regarding Norplant use must be based on extrapolation from information on other hormonal methods. Until further information is available it is inadvisable to use Norplant as a method of contraception for women undergoing anti-coagulant therapy, or with undiagnosed abnormal uterine bleeding, known or suspected pregnancy, haemorrhagic diathesis, or active hepatocellular disease.

Side-effects

A large number of clinical trials have been undertaken on Norplant. No serious side-effects have been shown to occur by these studies. Epidemiological studies on long-term safety are under way. The most frequently reported side-effect is irregularity of menstrual bleeding. About 60% of Norplant users report irregular bleeding patterns during the first year of use. Inter-menstrual spotting or amenorrhoea may also occur. There does not appear to be an increase in the total blood loss, and heavy bleeding is rarely encountered. The bleeding irregularities usually decrease with duration of use. Careful counselling of new acceptors has resulted in a high degree of satisfaction among the women and has diminished the number of removals because of bleeding problems.

When symptoms suggestive of pregnancy occur in the presence of amenorrhoea, steps should be taken to exclude pregnancy. If the woman is pregnant, the implant should be removed. Should a pregnancy be suspected, the possibility of an ectopic pregnancy must be borne in mind.

Infection at the site of the implant has been known to occur and can be minimized by the use of strict aseptic techniques and by keeping the implant site dry for three days.

Counselling

Counselling should include general information about Norplant (how it works, the length of protection provided, the fact that it is completely reversible, and the possible side-effects likely to occur), technical aspects of insertion and removal, the advantages and disadvantages of the method in relation to other contraceptive methods available, immediate post-insertion care, and possible problems that might arise with the method.

Insertion and removal of Norplant

Insertion should ideally be carried out during the first seven days after the onset of menstruation in order to minimize the risk of inserting Norplant in the presence of an undiagnosed pregnancy. Insertion can also be carried out immediately post-abortion, and immediately post-partum in non-breast-feeding women. With the current data available, it is not possible to make a recommendation on the use of Norplant in lactating women.

Sterile techniques should be maintained throughout the insertion and removal procedures. At the present time it is recommended that both procedures be performed in a clinic setting.

The preferred sites of insertion are the upper arm or forearm with only local anaesthesia. Capsules must be inserted subdermally, as deeper insertion makes removal more difficult. The incision is small and does not require sutures.

Capsules should be removed after five years of use, since effectiveness of the method declines after this time. No harmful effects are caused if the capsules are not removed at this time other than the risk of unplanned pregnancy. If a woman wants to continue using Norplant, a new set of implants should be inserted.

The capsules should also be removed if the woman becomes pregnant or for medical or personal reasons. A system must be established to ensure

that the woman can have Norplant removed at her request, and at no
additional cost.

Service issues

Although Norplant presents obvious advantages to family planning
programmes, its introduction poses a number of managerial challenges.
First, it is a clinic-based method and requires formal training in insertion
and removal. Second, it is a progestagen-only method, associated with
alteration of the menstrual cycle, requiring specific counselling for
potential acceptors. Accordingly, the training of medical personnel in the
use of the method, and of staff responsible for counselling potential
acceptors, is the most important factor in the successful introduction of
the Norplant method.

With reference to training, it is essential that all personnel involved with
the use of the method — from provider to potential user — be adequately
informed about the safety, efficacy, risks and benefits, and medical
procedures involved in its use, so that informed decisions on its selection
from the range of available methods can be made.

Doctors, nurses, midwives, and other health workers can perform
insertion and removal procedures provided they are formally trained.
These procedures are relatively easy to learn, but formal training will
minimize difficulties that may be encountered in removal if insertions are
not carried out correctly. Training programmes should place emphasis on
practical, hands-on experience in insertion and removal techniques.
Depending on the caseload and the number of personnel receiving training
during a session, trainers generally see that each trainee performs from 5
to 10 insertions and 3 or more removals.

Training in counselling is as important as technical training. The
introduction of Norplant into family planning programmes should be
preceded by pre-introductory trials, the setting-up of training centres and
the provision of back-up and referral facilities.

When introducing Norplant into family planning programmes,
administrators should ensure proper examination of availability of staff
ready to be trained, establishment of adequate mechanisms for training in
insertion and removal techniques, suitable clinic facilities and adequate
back-up systems. In the early period, efforts should be made to ascertain
acceptability patterns, and problems and difficulties in counselling and
follow-up.

A carefully designed public information programme is also important,
especially since Norplant represents a novel delivery system for
contraception. A variety of informational materials are needed for health
personnel, counsellors, potential users, and the general public. A clear and

concise explanation of the characteristics of the Norplant method is an essential element in wide-scale acceptance.

Effectiveness

Experience with more than 18,000 insertions with Norplant has shown a very low pregnancy rate. The annual pregnancy rates range from 0.2 to 1.3 per 100 women per year, during the five-year period. The cumulative pregnancy rate at five years is 2.6, a very low use-effectiveness rate for a reversible method. The method does not appear to increase the incidence of ectopic pregnancies. However, attention must be paid to the possibility of an ectopic pregnancy if clinical symptoms are suggestive. The Norplant system is considerably less effective after the five-year period. Effectiveness of the method compares favourably with oral contraceptives and IUDs.

Acceptability and continuation rates

Evidence shows a high initial acceptability. Counselling is a key factor in determining continued acceptability. The continuation rates at the end of the first year range from 60% to over 90%, and by the fifth year are around 50%; rates better than those commonly quoted for IUDs. Bleeding irregularities in some users are the main cause for discontinuation.

Safety

The two components of the Norplant system have been used extensively in humans. The use of silicone-rubber material for implants in humans began in 1950, and it is widely used in various surgical applications. Silastic (polydimethylsiloxane) has been used for more than 20 years for the long-term delivery of lipophilic drugs. Levonorgestrel is used extensively as a progestagen for contraception in combined progestagen-oestrogen oral contraceptives and the progestagen-only Pill, and is also the main progestagen being used in the steroid-releasing vaginal rings. Some women have used levonorgestrel continuously for up to nine or 10 years. The WHO Toxicology Group concluded that toxicological and teratological data on both levonorgestrel and silastic indicate that Norplant is safe for use in humans.

Reproductive system

There were no significant pathological changes in endometrial biopsies examined during nine years of Norplant use. There were no significant effects on the cervix, vagina or vulva. Transient ovarian enlargement was noted.

Metabolic effects

Several studies have been undertaken to determine the metabolic and biochemical effects of Norplant. Liver function has been evaluated at several centres, and has not been shown to be significantly affected. Measurements of urea nitrogen, uric acid, sodium, potassium, and calcium show no changes. Mean blood glucose levels have been shown to be elevated, but to be within the normal range.

While the data are limited, Norplant appears to have no deleterious effect on carbohydrate metabolism. Thyroid and adrenal functions were not significantly changed. Changes in some of the blood coagulation functions have been noted, but were significantly less than those observed in combined oral contraceptives. Further studies are still needed to clarify the effects of levonorgestrel released from Norplant on lipids and lipoproteins.

Return of fertility

The return of fertility is not delayed following the removal of Norplant. Of the women from whom Norplant was removd in order to conceive, 40% became pregnant by three months, 76% by one year, and 90% by 24 months.

Rare and long-term effects

The method is just beginning to be widely introduced. Epidemiological studies of long-term safety are under way. Surveillance of women with Norplant implants is important to gather information from as large a number of women as possible over a long period of time.

Future developments

The Population Council is developing a two-rod implant system, known as Norplant 2. This device is currently being tested in phase III clinical trials. Another implant being developed is a single biodegradable capsule containing levonorgestrel and effective for 18 months. This system is called Capronor, and is being jointly developed by US NIH and WHO.

(*Statement by the IPPF International Medical Advisory Panel, September 1985; approved by the IPPF Central Executive Committee April 1986.*)

Chapter 6

Post-coital Contraception

Introduction

Sexual intercourse without the intention of conceiving a child has taken place throughout history. Many post-coital techniques to prevent pregnancy after unprotected intercourse can be found in writings from the past.

For instance, in Persia in the eighth century post-coital sneezing and jumping backward the magical seven steps were supposed to dislodge the semen, while in the 18th century in France a post-coital douche was available in every better hotel.

But nowadays the uselessness of such methods is well understood. After intravaginal ejaculation sperm are mixed within 90 seconds with the cervical mucus. When the mucus is in a favourable state, sperm can reach the uterine tubes within five to 15 minutes after ejaculation. Therefore, unless proper contraceptives are used, the sperm cannot be prevented from reaching the uterine tubes after vaginal intercourse.

Indications for use of post-coital contraception

This method is meant to be used only to try to avoid pregnancy following a single unexpected and/or unprotected act of sexual intercourse. This includes cases of rape, and cases where no contraceptive has been used, or those where a condom has burst during use. Hormonal contraceptives used for this purpose are meant as a one-time procedure and not as a routine approach to contraception. However, when a woman asks for post-coital contraception, it is a good opportunity to discuss future long-term contraception.

In a country where post-coital contraception is available it is important that women needing this form of emergency treatment know where they can easily obtain it. This is because of the short time period (72 hours for the hormonal treatment and five days for the IUD insertion) during which post-coital contraception is likely to be effective. Likewise, doctors to whom these women may turn should either be able to give the treatment themselves or to refer the women as a matter of urgency to a clinic where they will be helped.

Post-coital methods

It was in 1964 that Haspels, in Holland, started to treat rape victims with high-dose ethinyl oestradiol (EO) in an attempt to prevent pregnancy, while in the same year Morris and Van Wagenen studied the effect of diethylstilboestrol (DES) in monkeys as a post-coital technique for preventing pregnancies. However, DES is associated with genital malformations and possible carcinogenesis in the offspring when accidentally used in pregnancy. If a single hormone is chosen, EO is preferred as the 'morning-after Pill'. Its correct use will reduce the probability of pregnancy after a single act of sexual intercourse to as low as 0.5-1%. Without such treatment, 5-20% would be expected to end in pregnancy. However, in most countries today, a low-dose combined oestrogen-progestagen combination is given in two doses with a 12-hour interval (see below).

Further research for alternative methods with less side-effects showed that a copper-bearing IUD inserted up to five days after the day of ovulation in the event of unprotected intercourse can prevent pregnancy. When used in selected cases, such a regimen compares well with high-dose oestrogen treatment. However, there are disadvantages. These include a risk of infection in such unprepared women, the possibility of interfering with an already existing very early pregnancy, or psychological distress after unprotected intercourse or rape which may not allow the insertion of an IUD. Also, the accepted disadvantages of fitting an IUD in a nullipara (a common candidate for post-coital contraception) must be remembered (see page 113). In Holland, a series of IUD fittings with 100% effectiveness against pregnancy has been published by Van Santen.

Though the insertion of a post-coital IUD is best carried out within five or at the most seven days of ovulation, there are reports of later insertion. This is not recommended, since there is a risk of septic abortion if an early pregnancy exists.

An anti-gonadotrophin, danazol, has been used as a post-coital contraceptive, but the failure rate of 3.7% is not acceptable.

Hormonal treatment with progestagens alone in doses ranging from 400 up to 1,000 µg post-coitally, and used several times per menstrual cycle as well, results in high pregnancy rates. Moreover, menstrual irregularities make such treatment unacceptable.

In Canada, in 1974, research was started with a low-dose oestrogen/ progestagen combination as a post-coital contraceptive. In a high school, after the introduction of such post-coital emergency treatment, a decrease in unplanned pregnancies was noted. A multicentre study was undertaken in 1982 by Yuzpe, with four tablets of 500 µg of norgestrel and 50 µg of ethinyl oestradiol, taken as two tablets at a time with a 12-hour interval between doses. There was a failure rate of about 1% in 700 women, a reduction of 84% in the expected number of pregnancies. The tablets should be started not more than 72 hours after intercourse. This clinical result has been confirmed for both hormonal treatments in a randomized comparative trial of the combined Pill versus high-dose oestrogens in Holland. Nowadays each of the four tablets used usually contains 250 µg levonorgestrel and 50 µg ethinyl oestradiol.

In the UK, Germany, France, USA and Canada, this Yuzpe regimen became known as the low-dose combination morning-after Pill, and has been used in these countries and many others since. Side-effects are low, but the success rates found differ considerably in various studies. Van Santen and Haspels found 39% nausea and 15% vomiting. The rates for side-effects are acceptably low and no prophylactic anti-emetic treatment is needed. The duration of complaints in this method was rather short; in 74% they lasted for only one day.

Recently some doubt has been expressed about the efficacy of this treatment. Yuzpe found a failure rate of 1.7% when multiple exposure had taken place. Other authors also found higher failure rates when this method is used post-coitally several times during one menstrual cycle.

It is often found that self-treatment with this regimen: "just take four tablets of the strip of contraceptive Pills of your friend" is common. Since frequently contraceptive tablets with oestrogen below 50 µg are taken, or this treatment is repeated several times a month, it is understandable that reports of frequent failures appear. In these cases it is attributable to user failure.

Synthetic progesterone molecules, modified at a single site on the steroid nucleus, act as anti-progesterones (see page 257). They bind strongly to progesterone receptors. Anti-progesterones induce menstrual bleeding in spite of a possible conception, just as if the progesterone had been withdrawn. In a pilot study in Holland and in

France this treatment has been tried within the luteal phase of the menstrual cycle to prevent implantation. This regimen can be used as a 'morning-after Pill' irrespective of the number of previous acts of intercourse and the time lapse passed before treatment is given. In a first report a failure rate of 3% is mentioned. Since at present no satisfactory 'morning-after' treatment exists beyond day 21 of the menstrual cycle, this failure rate is acceptable. For continuous use, as a once-a-month treatment, however, anti-progesterones cannot compare with the highly reliable regular forms of contraception.

Follow-up

It is important that the woman returns a month after the procedure to make sure that no pregnancy has occurred. If there is a pregnancy the woman should be counselled. She should be reassured, if high-dose oestrogen or combined oral contraceptives have been used as a post-coital method, that there is no evidence to link this with possible teratogenesis. Depending on the cause of the pregnancy, and if national laws permit it, an abortion can be discussed. Continuing with the pregnancy, keeping the baby or later having it adopted, are all options to be put to the woman (see page 252).

If there is no pregnancy, continuing contraception should be discussed again.

IMAP Statement on Post-coital Contraception*

There is still no ideal contraceptive to fit every circumstance. For the woman exposed to a single unexpected and/or unprotected act of sexual intercourse, post-coital contraception can be used to avoid an unwanted pregnancy. Since the mid-1960s, post-coital contraception using orally administered hormones has been shown to be highly effective in preventing pregnancy. *However, this should be considered as a one-time procedure, and not a routine approach to contraception.* There is no method of post-coital contraception where data on efficacy and safety allow a recommendation that such regimes are suitable for recurrent use in clinical practice. Repeated use should be restricted to well controlled clinical trials until

---

*This statement is valid for the methods of post-coital contraception described. The Panel reserves the right to amend this statement in the light of further developments in the field of post-coital contraception when sufficient scientific information becomes available.

further data are available. Evidence also suggests that a copper-containing IUD can act effectively as a post-coital contraceptive.

Recommended oral methods

Formulation

Combined oral contraceptives containing ethinyl oestradiol 50 µg and levonorgestrel 0.25 mg. (Other similar formulations may also have high efficacy.)

Dosage schedule

Two tablets at once followed by two tablets after 12 hours.

Indications for use

This method is indicated in women exposed to unexpected and/or unprotected sexual intercourse, such as cases of rape. It is effective *only* if instituted *within 72 hours* of the exposure. Data suggest this regime is as effective as diethylstilboestrol, but with fewer side-effects. During the first consultation, the woman's requirements for elective contraception should be discussed.

Contraindications

The standard contraindications to the use of hormonal contraception should be observed.

Possible side-effects

1. Nausea and vomiting
2. Irregular uterine bleeding
3. Breast tenderness
4. Headache.

Follow-up

The woman should be advised to return after one month to reinforce the need for elective contraception or, in the event of a failure, to diagnose pregnancy and initiate counselling.

In the event of a continuing pregnancy, the woman may be reassured that there is no evidence to associate this regime of oral contraceptive steroid administration with teratogenesis.

The use of copper-containing IUDs

Evidence indicates that effective post-coital contraception can be achieved by the insertion of a copper-containing IUD within five days of unexpected and/or unprotected sexual intercourse.

This method may be used where there is concern about the oral administration of oestrogen-containing preparations, or where there is a need for continuing contraception, but is subject to the contraindications which apply to IUD use. Special care should be taken when providing nulliparous women with IUDs post-coitally, bearing in mind the risks of pelvic inflammatory disease.

Effectiveness of post-coital contraception

Post-coital contraception is about 98% effective. However, the incidence of ectopic pregnancy appears to remain unchanged, although further data are needed. The use of post-coital contraception does not seem to impair future fertility.

(Adopted by the IPPF Central Council, November 1981, and amended by Central Council, November 1982 and November 1985.)

Chapter 7

Intrauterine Devices

Introduction

Since the publication of the fifth edition of this handbook in 1980 there has been further accumulation of data about intrauterine devices (IUDs) based on clinical experience, and also newer ideas and developments concerning this form of contraception. In this chapter an attempt will be made to bring up to date the current practice of IUD contraception.

It is estimated that at present about 60 million women are using IUDs throughout the world. The number of IUD users is steadily increasing, owing perhaps to the perceived disadvantages of alternative methods of contraception and the implementation of effective low-cost IUD family planning programmes. The IUD is an attractive method of contraception, since it requires very little in the way of user participation. Once the device is fitted sexual intercourse becomes unrelated to the method: it does not require pre-planning or daily Pill taking. Its further attraction is that the IUD can be left *in utero* for at least five years in the case of a copper-bearing IUD and indefinitely in the case of an inert plastic IUD. IUDs have some disadvantages. They require a trained person (not necessarily a doctor) to insert them and to provide follow-up care for women who use them. The failure rate with IUDs is around 3 per 100 woman-years. They also produce side-effects in some women (see page 113).

Research continues in the development and design of the IUD to improve its ability to prevent pregnancy and to deal effectively with the occasional problems of expulsion and bleeding. This research is concerned mainly with the testing of medicated devices (copper-bearing or hormone-containing) and those which are designed to 'fit' uterine configuration. However, epidemiological findings in many parts of the world suggest that factors associated with the person fitting the IUD may be of more importance in the continued use of the

103

IUD than its shape, composition or size. The relationship between whoever fits the device, the IUD user, and the IUD model itself is a complex one, and if effective IUD provision is to be attempted then this relationship must be understood. Care and sensitivity in fitting and follow-up are now seen to be of much more importance, and this, in part, explains the emphasis on adequate training for those responsible for providing an IUD service.

Views on the IUD have shifted during the last four decades from outright condemnation to relative acceptance. This acceptance is not complete, however, and arguments for and against the use of IUDs are still heard.

During 1986 several IUDs were removed from the market in the USA by their manufacturers for commercial and not for medical reasons such as concerns about safety or efficacy. They include the Lippes Loop, the Copper 7 and the Copper T 200. At that time, the only IUD still freely available in the USA was the Progestasert, a hormone-containing IUD. The IUDs withdrawn in 1986 are still approved by the US Food and Drug Administration (FDA) and recommended by WHO and other reputable international bodies. In June 1988, the T Cu 380 A IUD, previously approved by the US FDA, came on to the USA market.

Mechanism of action

This is still unclear and work continues to try and come to a firm conclusion about it. It is probable that the mechanism of action is complex. At the end of 1986 the WHO Scientific Group on the Mechanism of Action, Safety and Efficacy of IUDs looked into this aspect of the use of IUDs very thoroughly. Their main conclusions stated that all IUDs stimulate a foreign body reaction in the endometrium which is potentiated by the addition of copper, and progestagen-releasing IUDs produce endometrial suppression similar to that seen when the drug is administered by other routes, e.g. orally or by injection. They also said that it is unlikely that one single mechanism of action accounts for the anti-fertility effect of IUDs. They concluded that it is probable that alteration or inhibition of (*a*) sperm migration in the upper female genital tract, (*b*) fertilization and (*c*) ovum transport play a more important role in the human than the possibility of prevention of implantation.

Design

The design of an IUD should fulfil three basic requirements: first, the device must provide protection against pregnancy; second, it should be fitted easily and with minimal discomfort; and third, it should remain in place in the uterus until the woman wishes it removed. Unfortunately, devices that fulfil any one of these requirements are often unsatisfactory in relation to one or both of the other aspects. Small devices, for example, are easily placed in the uterus but are also expelled more easily, resulting in a complete loss of protection. Larger devices are more likely to stay in place but may cause an increase in unwanted uterine bleeding.

The composition, size and configuration of IUDs have developed rapidly in the last three decades (Fig. 2). Those IUDs made from catgut, polyethylene, plastic or stainless steel are often called first-generation devices, as they were the earliest of the modern devices to be developed. They are also sometimes called inert since they do not contain active metals or chemicals for slow release in the uterus as in the second-generation, bioactive or medicated devices. Some second-generation devices contain copper in the form of wire or bands, or copper wire over a silver core, and others contain hormones. Fashions come and go in IUD design, reflecting changing beliefs in the efficacy, for example, of devices possessing a broad surface area, or those that cannot be expelled, and of others that release copper ions, or progesterone or other hormones in small regular amounts. The medicated or bioactive devices, however, have a definite advantage, in that added copper or hormones allow smaller devices to be used. These avoid the problems related to the fitting of larger IUDs.

Disinfection of IUDs and inserters

Most IUDs, except when supplied in bulk, are now available, together with their introducers, already sterilized in prepacked containers. In other cases, the following advice applies:

For plastic or polyethylene devices

These cannot be sterilized by heat (dry or wet). They can be adequately disinfected, however, by immersion in various disinfectant fluids. These devices (and the plungers for use with the Lippes Loop)

Multiload

Copper 7

Copper T

Lippes Loop

TCu-380A

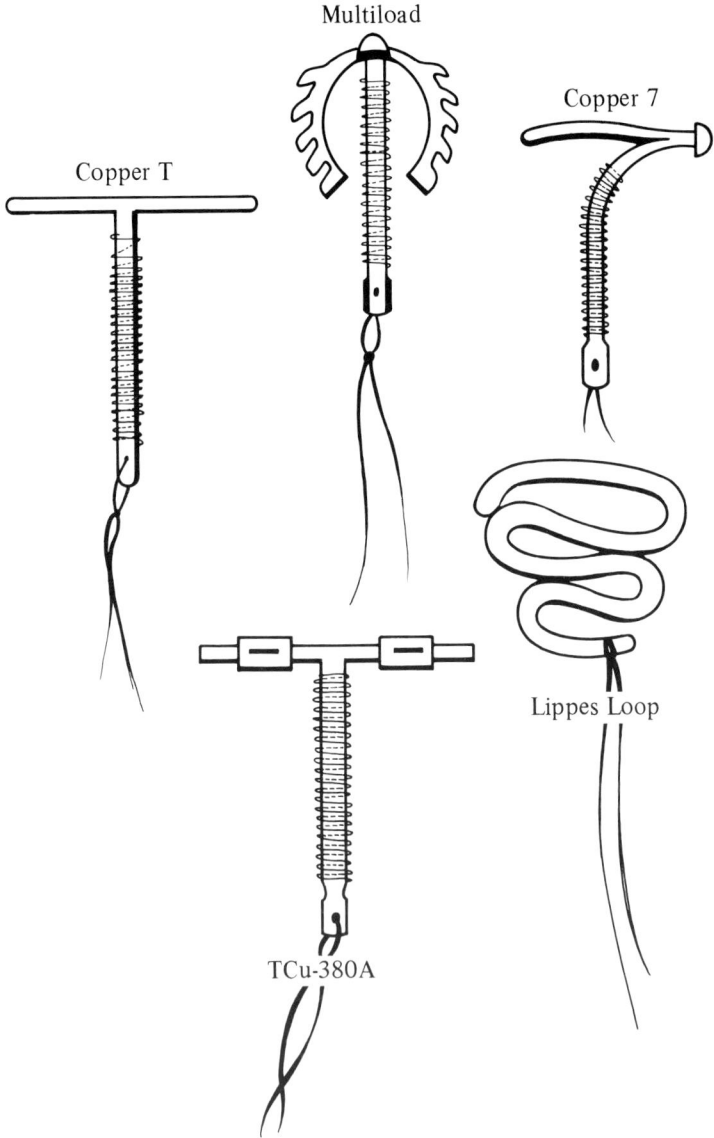

Fig. 2. *Various IUDs in common use.*

should be placed, for 20 minutes, in either of the following solutions before use:
1. Aqueous iodine 1:2,500 (a definite orange colour, not yellow or brown).
2. Isopropyl alcohol 75%.
Those not used at the end of the clinic session should be stored dry. The disinfecting liquid should be discarded, and a fresh solution used for the next session. Disinfection of the devices must be carried out with the greatest care.

For introducers and metal devices

The Lippes introducers can be boiled in the ordinary way, as can metal first-generation devices and their introducers.

For removal hooks

All removal hooks can be boiled or autoclaved.

Who should fit and remove IUDs?

Not only doctors, but also midwives, nurses and trained ancillary staff fit and remove IUDs in several countries from many parts of the world. The pregnancy, expulsion and removal rates following these insertions show little or no difference between the ability of the doctors and the others fitting IUDs. Adequate training is essential before the insertion of IUDs is undertaken — this applies to doctors and to other personnel alike. For an effective family planning service, the use of non-doctor personnel, trained in the insertion and removal of IUDs, has obvious advantages. In many communities such personnel are more readily available than doctors, and women who have problems after insertion can contact them more easily. When the work of IUD fitting is divided within the health team, doctors have more time to examine and treat the more difficult cases.

Technique before fitting of all devices

After a careful pelvic examination, the cervix is visualized with a speculum and swabbed with a sterile cottonwool ball dipped in an aqueous solution of iodine or other suitable disinfecting fluid.
A sterile sound should be inserted to confirm the direction and

depth of the uterine canal. A tenaculum or Allis-Chalmers forceps may be used to steady the cervix, especially if the cervical canal needs to be straightened or a cicatrized cervix needs dilation. The cervix needs dilating only in rare cases.

Since the linear devices tend to lose their 'memory' and straighten out if left in the introducer for too long before insertion, it is important not to load the introducer more than one or two minutes before insertion.

General advice on fitting devices

It is important to distinguish certain variations in technique with different devices. First, the introducer can be passed just beyond the internal cervical os and the device extruded gently (e.g. Lippes Loop, Cu 7) by means of a solid rod pushed up the hollow introducer tube. Second, the introducer can be passed as far as the fundus and then pulled back over the device and the solid rod which is held steady (Fig. 3). This allows the device to be left in the uterus rather than pushed into place (e.g. the Copper T and its derivatives). Third, insertion of the device may not require the use of a solid rod to act as a plunger, but uses a hollow tube alone, in which the IUD rests (e.g. Multiload, Progestasert).

Devices which are pushed out of the applicator (e.g. the Lippes Loop) are more likely to perforate, while withdrawal of the applicator leaving the device in place (e.g. Copper T group) is less likely to cause perforation and will ensure that the IUD is securely placed in the fundus of the uterus.

The person inserting an IUD must be properly instructed about which method to use with which device. Detailed instructions are included with individually packed devices. Scrupulous observance of the manufacturer's instructions for fitting will get the best results. IPPF International Office can supply instructions for bulk-packed IUDs. However, the IPPF is at present phasing out supplies of bulk-packed unsterilized IUDs to individual family planning associations.

Choice of IUD

All the IUDs available at present have advantages and disadvantages that must be weighed up when making a choice for the individual woman to be fitted. There are, however, certain general points that can be made:

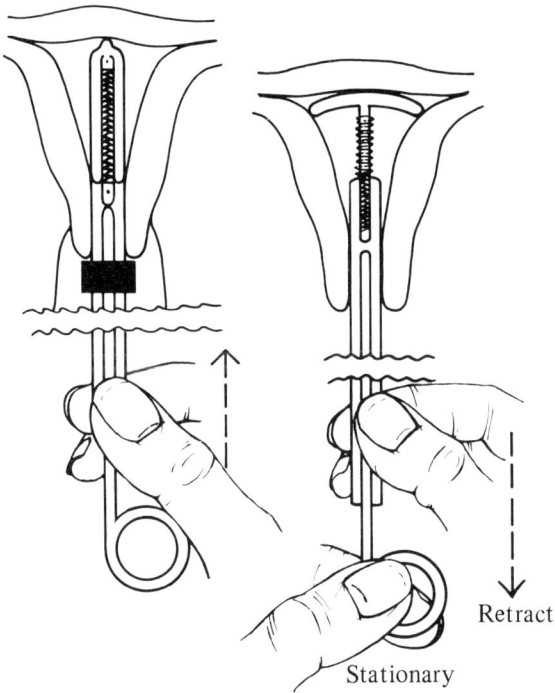

Fig. 3. *Insertion of copper T IUD and its derivatives.*

The newer copper-bearing IUDs have been shown to be safe and effective and to have a long duration of use. The trend nowadays is to recommend these devices rather than the inert ones. Also, the smaller copper-bearing IUDs usually cause less menstrual blood loss than the bulkier inert ones. Hormone-releasing IUDs have been shown to induce less bleeding.

Other factors to be considered include the IUD models available, the size and shape of the uterus, and the age and parity of the woman. Every effort should be made to tell her what IUD she has had fitted. This would help not only at follow-up, but also when removal is requested.

Note should be made not only of the device but also of the size and malleability of the IUD inserter. The size of the inserter varies according to the size and type of IUD being fitted.

Routine replacement after a set time interval is necessary in the case of the medicated devices (copper-bearing and hormone-containing

109

devices), and the choice of these devices will be affected by confidence in the woman's willingness or ability to return for follow-up visits.

In general, it is better to fit the IUD with which the person responsible for the fitting has skill and experience. Data collected from a large number of centres and personnel indicate that there is wider variation in successful IUD fitting and use between those doing the fitting than there is between different IUD models or sizes. Skill and regular practice are needed if the confidence of the woman is to be maintained.

Time of IUD fitting

During menstruation

An IUD can be fitted at any time during the menstrual cycle, but it may be preferable to do so during or just after menstruation. This makes it most unlikely that a pregnancy is present, and the cervix is easier to negotiate, being more patulous. The slight blood loss occurring as a result of the fitting procedure may be more acceptable to the woman at this time. However, any woman asked to wait to be fitted at her next menstrual period may be put at risk of becoming pregnant meanwhile. Indeed, some women come long distances to be fitted with an IUD, and if pregnancy can be ruled out they should not be turned away, but an IUD should be fitted at that visit, whatever the stage of the menstrual cycle. Consideration should also be given to the embarrassment some women may experience if they are requested to attend for an IUD fitting when they are menstruating.

After a pregnancy or abortion

After a full-term pregnancy, the IUD should ordinarily be fitted at the six weeks' post-partum examination. It is possible to fit an IUD immediately after delivery of the placenta, but the expulsion rate tends to be high.

In some situations, fitting post-partum (or post-abortion) may be the only opportunity to give any contraceptive protection to the woman. There is increased risk of perforation of the uterus if fitting is carried out later than the first week after delivery of the placenta and during lactation. After the first week, fitting should not be attempted until the six weeks' post-partum examination. Most doctors prefer not to fit an IUD at the end of a caesarean section, but to wait until the six weeks' follow-up examination. However, some do fit the IUD after caesarean section, especially if follow-up is unlikely.

Post-coital fitting

Where there has been no missed period, an IUD can be fitted in situations where a woman has been exposed to the risk of pregnancy as a result of unprotected sexual intercourse. A copper IUD can be fitted up to five days after sexual intercourse (see page 98). The IUD will provide continued protection against pregnancy as long as the device remains in place. In one study there were no pregnancies following fitting of a copper IUD post-coitally in 299 women after unprotected sexual intercourse around the time of ovulation. Risks and benefits of this form of post-coital contraception should be carefully weighed in nulliparas (see page 113).

Clinical management

Counselling and client selection

With careful selection of the woman using an IUD, its use effectiveness can be improved. It should be borne in mind that the most effective method of contraception may not be the most appropriate for a particular woman. It is therefore important that the woman should be carefully counselled in order to assess her feelings about using an IUD.

Some women will request an IUD because they may wish to have a change from other methods or may have heard good reports from friends who have used the IUD for many years without problems. In these cases it is worth while discussing their contraceptive needs, taking into account their parity, sexual history, age and marital status. They should be told about the other methods of contraception and be helped to make an informed choice.

In the case of some other women, the choice of an IUD may be dictated by circumstances. This group includes women who have developed complications while using hormonal contraception or other methods. They may have contra-indications particularly to hormonal methods. Again, they should be told about all methods, but may only be suitable candidates for IUDs, and may not be motivated to use methods such as barriers that require use associated with each act of sexual intercourse. All women being fitted with an IUD should be informed about the fitting procedure, the immediate side-effects that might occur should be explained and their likely duration mentioned. Possible delayed effects should be discussed. The most important of these is the slight chance of an ectopic pregnancy occurring, and the woman should be informed about the signs and symptoms to take note of (severe pelvic pain and sudden bleeding) and the importance of seeking medical advice if these occur. The possibility of the IUD being expelled should be mentioned, emphasizing that this is more likely at the time of menstruation or soon after.

The woman should be told which IUD has been fitted (see page 109), and, if it has to be removed later, how long it should remain in the uterus. She should know that it does not protect against sexually transmitted diseases, including HIV infection.

Medical history and examination

Before an IUD is inserted, a medical history should be taken to rule out such conditions as acute or chronic pelvic inflammation, menorrhagia severe enough to cause anaemia, intermenstrual bleeding or other discharges, or a recent septic abortion. These may constitute contra-indications until a diagnosis is made and the condition is treated and cured.

A pelvic examination should be carried out not only to assess whether the uterus is anteverted or retroverted, but also to exclude conditions which may contra-indicate the fitting of an IUD. It is important for a speculum examination to be carried out to identify significant vaginal discharge before a digital examination.

An attempt should be made to exclude the presence of *absolute* contra-indications such as:

1. Pregnancy.

2. Multiple fibroids, especially if these are impinging on the uterine cavity.

3. Congenital uterine abnormalities, affecting the shape of the uterine cavity.

4. Acute or sub-acute pelvic inflammatory disease (PID) or active vaginal inflammation.

5. Carcinoma of the cervix or body of the uterus.

6. Abnormal uterine bleeding, which should be investigated and corrected before IUD use.

There are also *relative* contra-indications which must be assessed individually in each case to decide if the benefits outweigh the risks. These conditions include: PID since the last pregnancy, a previous ectopic pregnancy, blood coagulation disorders, valvular heart disease with the danger of sub-acute bacterial endocarditis, heavy menstrual flow with anaemia, and severe dysmenorrhoea. Nulliparity is not an absolute contra-indication to the use of an IUD, but a nullipara with a history of pelvic infection or a previous ectopic pregnancy, or one with multiple sex partners, or whose partner has many sex partners, and who is thus liable to sexually transmitted infections, is not the best candidate for an IUD. Therefore nulliparas should be fully informed about other methods of contraception available to them.

Recent reports have suggested that the use of the IUD in diabetic women may be less effective in preventing pregnancies, but these reports are conflicting, and at the present time there is no reason why the device should not be fitted, if this is the acceptable method chosen by a diabetic patient.

After-care and side-effects occurring after fitting

Immediately after the device is fitted, the woman should be allowed to rest lying or sitting for a few minutes, to reduce any post-insertion symptoms. A six-weeks' follow-up check is advisable to discover if the woman is satisfied with the IUD, to assess pain and to ensure there is no infection. It is important to ensure that the device is *in situ* and not expelled, either partially or totally. Following this visit, checks at three months, six months and yearly thereafter, are advisable if they can be arranged. Where these may not be adhered to, at least yearly checks should be encouraged.

Bleeding

Following fitting of an IUD there is almost always a certain amount of bleeding. Women should be reassured that it is a normal reaction to the insertion.

Intermenstrual bleeding, usually in the form of spotting, or a serosanguinous discharge, may occur for a few weeks after fitting. This amount of bleeding is not a medical indication for removal of the device unless it continues for more than eight to 10 weeks, or the woman requests removal. Pre- and post-insertion counselling on the expected bleeding pattern will improve the woman's tolerance to any excess bleeding.

The first few menstrual periods after fitting may be heavier than previously and this change may last indefinitely, but does not usually become menorrhagic. However, if the bleeding is of any severity, causing anaemia, the device will have to be removed. Copper-bearing devices cause less bleeding than inert ones. Progesterone-releasing IUDs may decrease the amount of menstrual blood loss.

Various forms of treatment have been tried for the bleeding, but none has proved entirely satisfactory. These include: non-steroidal anti-inflammatory drugs, aminocaproic acid, mefenamic acid, ethamsylate, ergotrate, ascorbic acid, calcium, vitamins (especially vitamin K), hesperidin and ferrous sulphate, as well as progestagens in the second half of the cycle. The haemoglobin level should be ascertained at the annual check-up if possible.

Pain

Pain, usually in the form of uterine cramps, and occasionally as low backache, may occur soon after fitting, although the only complaint may be of some discomfort. Intermittent pain or discomfort is rarely present for more than the first few weeks and it is not as common as abnormal bleeding. Women should be warned that some discomfort or mild pain may be expected. Women vary greatly in their reaction to pain; psychological and cultural factors often affect this reaction.

Severe uterine cramps or syncope during the fitting of IUDs do occasionally occur, but these side-effects are rare and are usually found in nulliparas or in women who have not had a child for some years.

Analgesics may be given to some women who find IUD fitting painful, and can be suggested for recurrence of pain or discomfort later. Adequate counselling before fitting may lessen the impact of this symptom.

If pain persists or is associated with significant discharge or abnormal bleeding, further assessment is essential. It may mean there is infection and this will need treatment. Pain may be unrelated to the IUD and non-IUD causes of pain will certainly have to be excluded, for example endometriosis, ovarian cyst, cystitis, or bowel disorders.

Infection

Since IUDs were first used, there has been controversy about how much danger exists of associated pelvic inflammatory disease (PID). When the modern IUDs came into use in the early 1960s many doctors were concerned about possible ascending infection from the vagina along the transcervical threads. Others did not consider this a particular hazard. Also, reports of PID varied greatly from centre to centre, depending to a large extent on the definition of what constituted PID.

Modern bacteriological investigation shows that in almost all cases of IUDs with threads, some organisms similar to vaginal flora and other more virulent bacteria can be found in the uterine cavity after fitting. Mostly, these are overcome by the natural defences of the body, but can sometimes cause endometritis, cervicitis or occasionally more severe PID, such as salpingitis. This is particularly so in women at risk of contracting sexually transmitted diseases. A previously undiagnosed latent gonorrhoeal infection can be activated following the fitting of an IUD, causing a PID needing urgent treatment.

The difficulty of accurately diagnosing PID must be recognized, and care should be exercised in interpreting published data relating to the condition. About 2% of women can be expected to develop PID during the first year of use of an IUD. All such women should be screened for sexually transmitted diseases. Treatment with broad-spectrum antibiotics (including antibiotics active against both aerobic and anaerobic bacteria) is essential. After adequate treatment is instituted, the IUD should be removed.

Recent studies have shown that IUD users run a higher risk of PID than women using other forms of contraception. When IUD users are compared to those not using any form of contraception, the relative risk for IUD users is reduced. This can be explained by the protective effect against PID that has been found with hormonal and barrier contraceptives. Quantifying the relationship between IUD use and PID is difficult for two reasons: imprecise criteria for diagnosis of the disease, and lack of a standard reference group for comparison.

The risk of PID is higher not only immediately after insertion, but also for as long as the device remains in place. Among IUD users, young nulliparous women face a greater risk of PID than older women or multiparous women. Also, if PID occurs in nulliparous women, the chances of infertility resulting mean that the IUD is not the first choice of contraceptive in this group. PID associated with IUD use is unlikely in women in monogamous (mutually faithful) sexual relationships.

PID among IUD users has involved a number of different organisms. Measures have been taken to prevent or minimize the risk of IUD-related pelvic infection. Women with evidence of pelvic infection should not be fitted with an IUD until the infection has cleared. Young women under 30 who have multiple sexual partners and frequent sexual intercourse should be warned that IUD use will further increase the risk of PID.

It is good clinical practice to ensure that both the IUD and the insertion equipment are sterile or thoroughly disinfected at the time of fitting. This should prevent or reduce entry of bacteria into the uterus at this time. Some workers lubricate the tip of the inserter with an antiseptic or antibiotic cream as a routine to reduce the possibility of infection.

Infection is the most serious cause of morbidity among IUD users. Death from infection associated with IUD use has also been reported, mainly in women with septic incomplete abortion with the IUD *in situ*. Information from studies in the USA shows that deaths are associated with a range of IUD models. The mortality rate associated with IUD use has been estimated at between 1 and 10 per million users per year. The estimated rate among oral contraceptive users is between 22 and 45 per million users per year. The rate of hospitalization associated with IUD use is similar to that among oral contraceptive users, at between 0.3 and 1.0 per 100 women per year.

Actinomyces organisms in cervical smears in users of IUDs

There have been several reports of the finding of actinomyces-like organisms (ALO) in cervical smears in users of the IUD. Although some workers found a higher incidence in users of pure plastic IUDs compared with those using copper-bearing IUDs, this finding has not been substantiated by others. If these organisms are found in cervical smears and the women are completely asymptomatic with no evidence of significant discharge or pelvic tenderness, there is no need for antibiotic treatment or removal of the IUD. This is because this situation represents a superficial colonization of the cervix by these commensals. It is important, however, for these women to be followed up and if there is any clinical feature of infection, the IUD should be removed.

Pregnancy

When pregnancies occur during IUD use, two out of three are with the device in place; the remainder are associated with unnoticed expulsion or perforation. When an IUD fails and pregnancy occurs the pregnant woman needs the special attention of health care personnel.

When such pregnancies progress with the device *in situ*, the incidence of apparent spontaneous abortion is higher than in those where the device is expelled early in pregnancy. However, it is difficult to know how many of these abortions have been induced, since the pregnancies were obviously not planned or desired.

If a pregnancy occurs with a tailed device *in situ*, the risk of spontaneous abortion is greater if the device is left in place, than if it is removed. In the case of a tailless device, which requires removal by a hook inserted into the uterus, the risk of spontaneous abortion is less if the device is left *in situ* than if removal is attempted. If an abortion is requested it should be offered if national laws permit. Septic second trimester abortions are also a danger with an IUD *in situ*.

Other complications of pregnancy, including risks of premature delivery and stillbirth, may also be increased in pregnancies that occur with IUDs *in situ*. There is, however, no evidence that the pregnancy is more likely than usual to result in an infant with congenital anomalies.

Ectopic pregnancy

When a pregnancy occurs in an IUD user, it could be ectopic, which is a life-threatening condition.

The possibility of an ectopic pregnancy occurring means that health personnel should be alert to the chance of this serious condition. Careful diagnosis is especially important because some symptoms of ectopic pregnancy — abdominal pain or heavy bleeding — are often attributed initially to the IUD itself.

The higher ratio of ectopic to uterine pregnancies in IUD users than in non-users can perhaps be explained in two ways: (*a*) IUDs do not prevent ectopic pregnancy as well as they prevent uterine pregnancy, or (*b*) IUD-related inflammation or infection in the tubes interferes with the movement of the fertilized ovum, making ectopic pregnancy more likely. These theories are not mutually exclusive, and their relative role would affect the incidence of ectopic pregnancy in IUD

117

users. There is, however, no evidence that either inert or copper-bearing devices cause ectopic pregnancies.

Expulsion

A troublesome problem associated with the use of IUDs is their spontaneous expulsion from the uterus, especially in post-partum fitting. For all devices, the expulsion rate is highest during the first three months after fitting. Expulsion is less of a problem with the newer copper-bearing and hormone-releasing devices than with older copper and inert devices. Sometimes the woman is unaware that expulsion has taken place. Such unnoticed expulsions are often followed by a pregnancy.

Refitting with another IUD after expulsion is associated with a much higher risk of expulsion than a first fitting. About one-third of all such reinsertions also end in expulsion of the device. If possible, a device with a known lower expulsion rate should be used on refitting.

The skill and experience of the person carrying out the fitting is also an important factor in ensuring a low expulsion rate. Care should be taken to see that the device is entirely within the uterine cavity. Linear plastic or polyethylene devices should not be loaded into the introducer until immediately before fitting.

The lost IUD

The possibility of the device being expelled should be explained to the woman, together with the fact that it is more likely to occur at the time of menstruation or just after. Menstrual pads should be examined. Occasionally an expelled IUD can remain in the vaginal vault for some months. Many women can learn to insert a finger into the vagina to feel for the cervical tail; this manœuvre helps to determine if the device is still in position. The woman must be sure she feels the thread coming through the cervix and that the IUD is not lying in the vagina. Some women may find that feeling for the threads in the vagina is disagreeable and even upsetting to them.

If the cervical tail cannot be felt vaginally, the question will arise whether the threads have become detached or drawn up into the uterus, or whether the device has been expelled. In this case and with IUDs which do not have cervical tails, it cannot be certain if the IUD is in the uterus. Sometimes it can be felt in the uterus with a sterile sound. A straight X-ray will show up the IUD if it is made of or contains metal or if it contains barium sulphate. However, an X-ray should not be performed until it is certain the woman is not pregnant.

This will not necessarily confirm that the IUD is in the uterine cavity, unless at the time of the X-ray examination a metal sound is inserted, and postero-anterior and lateral films are taken. If perforation has occurred this procedure will confirm the intra-abdominal position of the IUD. On the other hand, the IUD may simply be lying in the vaginal vault if it has been expelled from the uterus. X-ray location of an IUD can be helped by double-contrast hysterosalpingography. Any X-ray examination is completely contra-indicated if there is a possibility of early pregnancy.

Ultrasonography is better than X-rays in confirming the presence of the IUD within the uterine cavity. It is also less invasive and if the woman is pregnant the fetus will suffer no exposure to radiation. If it is available it is therefore preferable to radiographic examination.

The fitting of a fresh device can be worth while, if the original one cannot be located. Radiography with a second IUD in place will help to outline the uterine cavity and show if the first IUD is intrauterine or extrauterine. This provides protection against pregnancy while the position of the first device is being investigated.

Perforation

Uterine perforation is a rare event. When it occurs it is usually at the time of fitting. Retrieval of the IUD should be attempted only by a gynaecologist. This may necessitate a laparoscopy or laparotomy for removal. Inert devices can be left in the peritoneal cavity unless there are symptoms or the woman requests removal. Medicated or closed devices must be removed. After perforation the woman is no longer protected against pregnancy.

Removal

At any time after fitting, the IUD may have to be removed because of the occurrence of a pregnancy, or severe bleeding or pain, or other medical reasons. A medicated IUD will need to be removed when its effective lifespan has expired. A woman may request removal because she is dissatisfied with the method, or because she plans pregnancy or for personal reasons, such as divorce or widowhood.

It is important to respect the woman's freedom to keep the IUD or to have it removed. At the same time it is also important that the provider counsels the woman adequately if she requests removal,

119

explaining the consequences and helping her to choose another appropriate form of contraception if necessary.

Moderate menorrhagia or abdominal pain need not, however, lead to the removal of the device. Reassurance and treatment often persuade the woman to keep the device *in situ* until the critical stage is past, which is usually within the first few months after fitting. Decision about removal for pain or bleeding must be related to the degree of insistence of the woman and an evaluation of her physical and psychological condition, particularly in the presence of anaemia.

Those IUDs possessing a tail are removed by gentle traction on the tail with any suitable instrument. Suction through a narrow cannula often helps to retrieve threads not visible at the cervix.

There are a number of different hooks or curettes which can be used to pick up the IUD inside the uterus if the tail is no longer present at or cannot be brought to the external os. A useful one is the disposable Mi-Mark Helix. It is disposable and cannot be used more than once, and is therefore expensive. This may be a drawback for its use on a large scale. The Novak or Sharman's curette and the Soonawala or Swartout hooks are among many other instruments developed to retrieve IUDs inside the uterus. Spencer Wells forceps may pick up the IUD if it is in the cervical canal without a tail. The cervical canal should only be dilated if removal proves difficult. An analgesic with an antispasmodic can be given to make removal less painful and to avoid occasional shock (syncope).

When an IUD, particularly a Lippes Loop, has to be removed with a hook (because the IUD has lost its threads) there may be difficulty in getting it out of the uterine cavity with ease if it is grasped by the hook near the fundus. The whole device may then bunch up without uncoiling so that it cannot be withdrawn through the cervical canal. Several suggestions have been made to overcome this problem. One is to make certain that the IUD is always grasped near the cervical end, so that it is pulled out uncoiled. Another is to twist the hook once it has caught the IUD at any level; this twist may help the IUD to uncoil.

The impacted IUD

Occasionally in an attempt to remove the IUD the thread breaks and the IUD cannot be retrieved in the clinic situation. It may be necessary to remove the IUD under general anaesthesia. This can still be difficult, as sometimes the IUD is embedded in the endometrium, especially if it has been *in utero* for many years. Curettage to remove superficial endometrium may be necessary before the device can be located. This procedure should be performed with extreme care, as the device may have partially perforated the uterus. It should only be undertaken by a gynaecologist.

Duration of effectiveness of IUDs

Copper IUDs remain effective for at least four years; some are effective for up to 10 years. Inert devices can remain *in situ* up to the menopause. The Progestasert hormone-containing IUD must be replaced annually, but longer-lasting hormonal devices are being developed.

Efficacy

Inert devices and the older copper-bearing IUDs (Cu 7 and Cu T 200) have failure rates above 2 per 100 woman-years. The lowest rates of pregnancy are among the newer copper-bearing devices (T Cu 220 C, T Cu 380 Ag, T Cu 380 A and Multiload 375). The Progestasert failure rate is about 2 per 100 woman-years.

Evaluation of intrauterine devices

Comprehensive reports have been published describing most of the commonly available devices. However, assessment of an IUD in a single country cannot always be extrapolated world-wide. Therefore care should be taken in the interpretation of event rates from only one country. Some investigations have shown that the performance of an IUD may be affected by the ethnic origin of a woman using the IUD or by her religious background. The sensitivity threshold to bleeding or pain in relation to the IUD may be closely bound to the cultural milieu to which the IUD user and the person undertaking the IUD fitting belong. In addition, some IUD centres are known to have a higher or lower rate of IUD removal than other centres. A review of the IUD research literature over the last two decades indicates that:

— Taking into consideration all three major undesired events that can occur with IUD use — pregnancy, expulsion and removal of the device following a complaint of bleeding and/or pain — the newer copper-bearing IUDs appear overall to be somewhat better than others that are currently available.

— The failure rate, in terms of the proportion of women accidentally becoming pregnant during the first year of use is usually between 1 and 3 per 100 woman-years.
— The single most common reason for IUD discontinuation is a complaint of excessive bleeding.
— The pregnancy and bleeding removal rates tend to fall slowly with time, while the expulsion rate falls dramatically with time, irrespective of the IUD design.
— Social and cultural factors appear to be important in influencing the demand for IUD removal and side-effects associated with bleeding.
— The skill and attitude of the doctor or other trained person fitting the IUD and his or her relationship with the woman appear to have a greater influence on side-effects than the type of IUD model being fitted.
— Continuation rates among women using the IUD tend to be higher than those among oral contraceptive users, over similar time periods.
— Women who become pregnant when using an IUD are more likely to have a greater ectopic pregnancy ratio than women who become pregnant when not using an IUD.
— Approximately one fitting per 1,000 results in a perforation of the uterine wall. Most evidence suggests that this perforation begins at the time of IUD fitting.
— Calcification of the IUD seems unrelated to the length of time that the device is left in the uterus. Individual characteristics of the woman seem more important.
— Pelvic inflammatory disease is increased among women with IUDs and the effect is more marked among nulliparous women.

At one time, the sole measure of effectiveness for any fertility regulation method was an estimation of the unplanned pregnancy rate. This interpretation no longer holds when contraceptive methods are used which may result in unwanted side-effects in addition to those associated with an unplanned pregnancy. Only negligible medical side-effects have been found to be associated with the older methods (e.g. allergy to rubber or reactions to certain spermicides), but the same cannot be said of oral contraceptives and IUDs. Safety, especially in terms of mortality, is a vital consideration. Apart from unplanned pregnancy and the possibility of septic abortion, the IUD may be expelled or require removal for a number of reasons. By including these events in the assessment of the IUD, the concept that social and psychological variables are present in IUD use is introduced. Skill in fitting the IUD is important, but so is the psychological effect of the interplay between the person fitting the device and the IUD acceptor — personal and cultural traits must NOT be ignored.

IMAP Statement on Intrauterine Devices (IUDs)*

Introduction

After more than two decades of widespread use, IUDs are now used by some 60 million women world-wide. They do not interfere with sexual activity and, for properly selected women, are a safe, effective and convenient reversible method of contraception.

The new copper- and hormone-releasing IUDs combine high continuation rates with low pregnancy rates. The recent removal by the manufacturers (in February 1986) of the Lippes Loop, the Copper 7 and the Copper T 200 from the US market was for commercial reasons and not for concerns about safety and efficacy. These IUDs are approved by the US Food and Drug Administration (FDA) and recommended by such agencies as the World Health Organization (WHO), the International Federation of Fertility Societies (IFFS), and the American College of Obstetricians and Gynecologists (ACOG). It seems likely that the already FDA-approved Copper T 380 A will be available in the USA during 1988.

Mechanism of action

The WHO scientific group on the mechanism of action, safety and efficacy of IUDs which met in December 1986 reviewed this topic extensively. Their main conclusions stated that all IUDs stimulate a foreign body reaction in the endometrium which is potentiated by the addition of copper, and progestagen-releasing IUDs produce endometrial suppression similar to that seen when the drug is administered by other routes, e.g. orally or by injection. They also said that it is unlikely that one single mechanism of action accounts for the anti-fertility effect of IUDs. They concluded that it is probable that alteration or inhibition of (*a*) sperm migration in the upper female genital tract, (*b*) fertilization and (*c*) ovum transport play a more important role in the human than the possibility of prevention of implantation.

---

*This statement is valid for those IUDs currently distributed by IPPF. IPPF reserves the right to amend this statement in the light of further developments in the field of IUDs when sufficient scientific information becomes available.

Contra-indications

IUDs, like other contraceptive methods, are not suitable for all women at all times. The following *absolute* contra-indications to IUD use are recognized:

1. Acute or chronic pelvic inflammatory disease
2. Known or suspected pregnancy
3. Abnormal uterine bleeding which needs to be investigated and treated before fitting an IUD
4. Confirmed or suspected malignancy of the genital tract
5. Congenital uterine abnormalities or fibroids distorting the cavity in a manner incompatible with proper IUD placement.

In addition, certain conditions must be weighed individually to determine whether the benefits outweigh the risks. These include a history of pelvic inflammatory disease since the last pregnancy, a previous ectopic pregnancy, blood coagulation disorders, valvular heart disease, heavy menstrual flow, particularly with anaemia, and severe dysmenorrhoea. Nulliparity is not an absolute contra-indication, but a history of pelvic infection, a previous ectopic pregnancy or multiple sex partners make the choice of an IUD inappropriate for such women. Women at risk of sexually transmitted diseases may not be suitable candidates for an IUD because of their higher risk of developing pelvic inflammatory disease.

Efficacy

Recent data show that inert devices and the older copper devices (the Copper 7 and Copper T 200) have failure rates above 2 per 100 women per year. The Nova T and Multiload 250 have failure rates of less than 1.5 per 100 and the newer copper devices (T Cu 220 C, T Cu 380 Ag, T Cu 380 A, and Multiload 375) have the lowest rates. Newer devices are superior to older devices. The failure rate of the available hormone device, Progestasert, is about 2 per 100.

Duration of use

The inert devices may be used up to the menopause, and need not be removed until then, except for specific indications. All copper devices have been shown to remain effective for at least four years, and some are effective for 10 or more years. The only currently available hormone-releasing device must be replaced every year, but longer-lasting hormone devices are under development.

Counselling

Good clinical management includes counselling the IUD user (giving all necessary information including information on alternative family planning methods) and informing her of the type of IUD to be inserted and the proper time for replacement if it is a medicated device. She should know that if she misses a period or is unable to locate the transcervical threads of the IUD she should return for follow-up care. She should also know signs of infection such as fever, pelvic pain or tenderness, unusual bleeding or unusually severe cramps, and she should be urged to seek help for these symptoms and signs. When a period is delayed, the health worker should keep in mind the possibility of an ectopic pregnancy.

IUD selection

Experience with the IUD throughout the world has demonstrated that within certain limits clinic and individual factors may have more impact on continuing IUD use than the design of the device itself. The skill of the health personnel, whether doctor, midwife, nurse or auxiliary in inserting the device, and the care and follow-up provided are of the utmost importance. Each of the currently available devices has advantages and disadvantages that must be weighed when making the selection for the individual woman. Certain generalities, however, can be stated:

1. The newer copper-bearing devices have been shown to be appropriate, safe and effective and have a prolonged duration of use. Therefore, the trend is to recommend the newer copper devices over the inert ones because they are appreciably safer and more effective.
2. The smaller, copper-bearing devices usually cause less menstrual blood loss than the bulkier inert devices. The hormone-releasing devices have been shown to induce less bleeding.

The IPPF reaffirms its 1975 policy that the Dalkon shield should not be used. All women still using the Dalkon shield should have the device removed because the Dalkon shield carries an extra risk to women during the second trimester of pregnancy when compared to other IUDs if a pregnancy occurs when an IUD is in place.

At the request of FPAs, IPPF will continue to supply inert and copper-bearing devices as approved by IMAP and as part of its contraceptive supplies service. Regular review of experience with these IUDs will continue in order to ensure that the latest scientific information is carefully processed and appropriate decisions are made.

Insertion

Importance of correct insertion

Correct insertion of an IUD is critical to its successful use, since it can affect all the major events that determine continuation of use—pregnancy, expulsion, bleeding, pain, uterine perforation and removal for other medical reasons. Expulsion rates decline as the skill and experience of the person performing the insertion increase. Evidence from many countries suggests that properly trained non-doctors can insert IUDs as well as doctors.

Timing of insertion

The IUD may be inserted at any time convenient to the user if it can reasonably be determined that she is not pregnant. There are certain advantages to insertion during the menstrual period: there is less likelihood of inserting the device into a pregnant uterus; because of a more patulous cervix, insertion is easier; and the bleeding associated with insertion is less likely to cause anxiety.

Post-abortion and post-partum insertions are appropriate, although special care should be taken with immediate and early post-partum insertion, immediate post-abortion insertion, and insertion during lactation, to ensure proper placement of the device and to avoid perforation. Immediate post-partum insertions result in more expulsions than those done at other times.

Insertion technique

The safest rule is to follow meticulously the manufacturer's instructions. IUDs should be inserted high in the uterus with care to avoid perforation. During IUD insertion the use of a sound to estimate the length of the uterus is good clinical practice, and a tenaculum may be useful to steady the cervix. The IUD and instruments inserted in the endocervical canal and/or uterus must be sterile. Of the two techniques for insertion, devices which are pushed out of the applicator are more likely to perforate, while withdrawal of the applicator leaving the device in place is less likely to cause perforation and will ensure better fundal placement of the device.

Disinfection of IUDs

The IPPF shall:
1. continue, where appropriate, to supply bulk package IUDs, with each packet containing clear instructions for methods of disinfection;
2. give guidelines on preferred methods of disinfection of IUDs;
3. supply the disinfecting solutions when requested to do so by FPAs;
4. ensure that FPAs adhere to the recommended techniques for disinfecting IUDs.

Not only the device but also the equipment used for insertion must be thoroughly disinfected.

Complications

(a) *Perforation*

Perforation is a rare event which almost always occurs at the time of insertion, when it may be accompanied by sudden pain and/or bleeding. There is a greater risk of perforation post-partum when the uterus is soft. Inert devices which have perforated need to be removed only if the woman has symptoms or requests removal; copper devices should always be removed. It must be remembered that following perforation the woman is no longer protected against pregnancy.

(b) *Bleeding and pain*

No standard effective medication is currently available for treatment of bleeding and pain in IUD users, although non-steroidal anti-inflammatory drugs and anti-fibrinolytic agents have been used with some success for bleeding, and prostaglandin antagonists for pain. Proper counselling, empathetic attention, together with reassurance, will improve the acceptability of these negative side-effects. Both bleeding and pain usually decrease after several cycles but, if not, the user is likely to want the IUD removed and will need advice on alternative methods of family planning.

A major concern of family planning providers in developing countries is the aggravation of existing anaemia in malnourished women who use IUDs for contraception. Treatment using oral iron has been shown in some cases to compensate for blood loss. The amount of increased bleeding associated with different devices varies, with the greatest amount from inert devices and less with copper-bearing IUDs. Hormone-releasing IUDs decrease the amount of bleeding below pre-insertion levels.

(c) Infection

In women at risk of sexually transmitted diseases (STDs) IUD use is associated with a measurably increased risk of pelvic infection. The usual symptoms of pelvic infection are vaginal discharge, pelvic pain or tenderness, abnormal bleeding, chills and fever, but the infection can be silent. All women with this diagnosis should be treated. If pelvic inflammatory disease occurs with an IUD in place, it should be removed once adequate antibiotic therapy that acts against aerobic and anaerobic pathogens has been instituted.

Pelvic inflammatory disease (PID) is a potentially severe health hazard in certain IUD users.

PID may pose a special problem for young nulliparous women as the infection is likely to impair their future fertility. When prescribing an IUD the woman's age, marital status, sexual habits, life style and previous history of pelvic infection must be taken into account, since women more at risk of sexually transmitted diseases are more likely to develop PID when using an IUD. Child-bearing considerations and the acceptability and appropriateness of other methods of contraception must also be considered. There is no evidence that IUDs affect subsequent fertility in properly selected women.

(d) Pregnancy

While many women have successfully completed pregnancy with an IUD *in situ*, the risks of spontaneous abortion and septic mid-trimester abortion are significantly greater if the device is not removed. When pregnancy is detected in a woman with an IUD in place, the device should be removed if the tail is accessible. If the tail is not visible termination of pregnancy should be offered where national laws permit. Particularly close supervision should be maintained if the woman elects to continue the pregnancy.

(e) Ectopic pregnancies

Since ectopic pregnancies can occur in women using IUDs, it is absolutely essential to rule out the possibility of an ectopic pregnancy, which is a life-threatening condition, in any woman exposed to the possibility of pregnancy, whether she is using an IUD or not, particularly if she has a history of pelvic infection. There is, however, no evidence that inert and copper IUDs cause ectopic pregnancies.

(f) *Expulsion*

Spontaneous expulsion may occur, particularly during menstruation and within the first three months of use. Expulsion is more likely if insertion is performed post-partum, and is less of a problem with the newer copper and hormone devices than with older copper and inert devices. Larger devices are more likely to be expelled than smaller ones.

Removal

Removal may be required for both medical and other indications. The medical indications are:

1. pregnancy
2. acute inflammatory disease
3. endometrial or cervical malignancy
4. perforation and partial expulsion of the IUD
5. abnormal or excessive bleeding if it is affecting the health of the woman.

Other indications are:

1. menopause — one year after last period
2. copper-bearing and hormonal IUDs when their effective lifespan has expired. The minimum period of effectiveness of copper-bearing IUDs is four years. No such time limit applies to non-medicated IUDs.

Follow-up care

Immediate post-insertion complications and long-term side-effects should be sympathetically managed. Wherever possible, it is useful to examine women three months after IUD insertion. Annual checks are useful to ensure the device is in place. Where regular follow-up care is not feasible, the user should be particularly advised regarding possible complications, and told of the nearest health facility to which she could go for help. When using medicated devices women should be told to return for removal and re-insertion at appropriate times.

(*This statement was drawn up by the IPPF International Medical Advisory Panel in April 1987 after extensive review of available data, and amended in November 1987. Adopted by the IPPF Central Council, November 1987.*)

Chapter 8

Barrier Contraception

Introduction

Before the widespread introduction of oral contraceptives (OCs) and intrauterine devices (IUDs), barrier methods were the most frequently employed means of fertility regulation. Many women switched to the newer techniques because of their high levels of effectiveness and because their use was not tied to sexual intercourse. However, as fears began to mount about the adverse side-effects of OCs and IUDs, often far out of proportion to the reality of the situation, many couples began to turn once again to the barrier methods. For instance, in the community based distribution programme in Guatemala, 10% of acceptors in 1976 chose condoms or spermicides, whereas two years later 27% of a larger number of acceptors chose these methods. In Colombia there was a notable increase in the use of barrier contraception in recent years. There has also been an increased reliance on barrier methods in the USA in the last few years. Similar increases in the use of barrier contraception are thought to be occurring in many other countries, although they have not all been documented. The methods discussed below are therefore once again becoming of greater importance in the field of family planning. About 40 million couples use barrier contraceptives (mainly condoms) throughout the world.

Barrier contraceptives act in one or more ways to prevent pregnancy. Spermicides kill and/or inactivate sperm on contact. Mechanical barriers (diaphragms, cervical caps and condoms) prevent the sperm from entering the endocervical canal. The vaginal contraceptive sponge which contains a spermicide, acts in both of the above ways, although it is mainly a vehicle for the spermicide. It also absorbs the sperm, bringing them into direct contact with the spermicide.

Caps include vaginal diaphragms, cervical caps, vault caps and vimule caps, made in various sizes and intended for repeated use with spermicides. Condoms are penile sheaths, intended for single use; reusable, washable sheaths are now practically obsolete. Spermicides include tubed creams and jellies, aerosols (foams), melting and foaming suppositories, foaming tablets and soluble films intended for use in the vagina. A 'female condom' is being developed.

Effectiveness

Good quality caps with spermicides, and condoms, are highly effective contraceptives, with theoretical pregnancy rates under 5 per 100 woman-years. Recent clinical trials have found pregnancy rates as low as 2 per 100 woman-years.

Spermicides used alone are fairly effective contraceptives, with theoretical pregnancy rates under 10 per 100 woman-years. Condoms used consistently with spermicides are therefore extremely effective contraceptives.

The use-effectiveness pregnancy rates of barrier contraceptives range widely, emphasizing the importance of consistent and correct use. For example, UK data show that, of recently married, comparably motivated couples, 5% of condom users, and 4% of oral contraceptive users, became pregnant in the first year of use.

Counselling

Before helping women or men to decide on a barrier method, they should be counselled on the use of contraception in general, as with any other method. The client should be told about other methods and their advantages and disadvantages. The status of the client should be taken into account (e.g. newly married, single, with children, near the menopause). All questions about barriers should be answered fully. Emphasis should be placed on the fact that they have to be used on each and every occasion of sexual intercourse and therefore the motivation to use them must be correspondingly high. The possible use of condoms needs special consideration, because they may be protective, if properly and consistently used, against most sexually transmitted diseases, including infection by the HIV virus (see page 140). Sometimes, in a high-risk situation, condoms may be advised in addition to another form of contraception, because of this protective effect.

Caps

Fitting a woman with a cap requires properly trained (though not necessarily medically qualified) health personnel. The medical prescription of caps is unnecessary.

The diaphragm

The *diaphragm* is the cap used most widely. It has a thin, nearly hemispherical, rubber dome, with a circular, rubber-covered, metal-spring reinforced rim in three different types — coil-spring, flat-spring and arcing (Fig. 4). The external diameter of the rim is the size of the

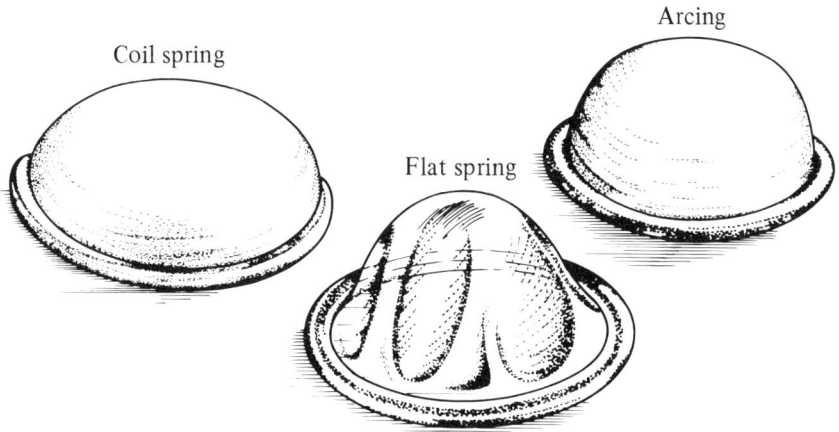

Fig. 4. *Diaphragms.*

diaphragm, ranging from 50 to 105 mm. The size of the softer, coil-spring diaphragm goes up in 5 mm steps, which the stiffer flat-spring diaphragm increases in 5 mm steps in the larger sizes (80-105 mm) and in 2.5 mm steps in the smaller sizes (55-75 mm); the 'half-sizes' are those between the 5 mm steps.

The diaphragm fits diagonally across the vagina, with opposite portions of the rim lodging in the posterior fornix, and behind the pubic symphysis, thereby covering the cervix (and much of the anterior vaginal wall), isolating it from penile contact during sexual intercourse. Whether the convex or concave side of the dome faces the cervix is a matter of individual choice: with the dome upwards, the concavity follows the vaginal contour; with the dome downwards, the diaphragm will be more difficult to remove. The diaphragm is held in place by the tension of the spring, and by the vaginal musculature. Since it is not sealed to the vaginal walls, its full effectivness depends on the previous application of a tubed spermicide (cream or jelly) to both sides of the diaphragm.

Clinic routine

After counselling (see page 131), the woman who has chosen the diaphragm should be asked to lie supine, while the person instructing her about correct insertion conducts a full, bimanual, pelvic examination, to find out the position and size of the uterus and the position of the cervix. The cervix should be visualized with a speculum, to observe any pathological condition, which should be treated if necessary. The instructor should then assess the strength of the muscles round the vaginal entrance, by placing two fingers in the vagina, and asking the woman to tighten on them: the tone should be such as to retain a diaphragm when the woman strains downwards. There must be a reasonably intact perineum. The diaphragm cannot be used where there is any condition (e.g. cystocele, prolapse) preventing retention of the rim. Use of the diaphragm is independent of the state of the cervix.

The correct size of diaphragm is estimated ('fitted') by inserting the index and middle fingers as far as they will go into the posterior fornix, and noting how far up the index finger the pubic symphysis comes. This length approximates the size of diaphragm required. (Special rings, of various diameters, are also available for this purpose.) A diaphragm of the corresponding diameter is selected and the rim compressed between thumb and fingers. The diaphragm is then inserted along the posterior vaginal wall as far as it will go into the posterior fornix, and the anterior rim is pushed up behind the pubic symphysis.

A correctly fitted diaphragm must cover the cervix, and not descend below the pubic symphysis when the woman strains downwards. A diaphragm that is too small or too large may allow the penis to pass between it and the anterior vaginal wall. If a woman is fitted with a diaphragm which is too small, she may insert it into the anterior fornix, leaving the cervix exposed to direct insemination. A diaphragm which is too large may be sensed by either or both partners, since the rim may buckle and not revert to its original circular shape. In addition, the rim may put undue pressure on the urethra, causing either acute or chronic urinary tract infection.

Teaching procedure

The woman should stand and place one foot on a chair, or squat. She should be taught to feel her cervix without the diaphragm in place. The diaphragm is inserted by the instructor, and then the woman is asked to feel for the anterior rim behind the pubic symphysis with her index or middle finger, hook the finger into the rim, and pull the diaphragm out straight downwards.

The woman is next asked to insert the diaphragm by herself. The diaphragm is held in one hand, while the fingers of the other hand separate the labia, and expose the vaginal extrance. The rim is compressed between the fingers and thumb, and the diaphragm is inserted along the posterior vaginal wall (backwards rather than upwards) as far as possible. The anterior rim is then pushed up behind the pubic symphysis with a fingertip.

The woman is taught to check the position of her diaphragm, as follows: the finger on the anterior rim should bend forwards to ensure that the rim is well up behind the pubic symphysis. The finger should then reach under the diaphragm to feel the cervix through the rubber dome (Fig. 5).

In some countries, special introducers are available, to make the insertion and removal of diaphragms easier, although they are rarely needed. Correctness of position must still be checked manually, either by the woman or her partner.

The woman should be advised on the use of tubed spermicide (cream or jelly) with the diaphragm, as follows: two 2.5 cm strips of spermicide are squeezed from the tube on to the convex side of the diaphragm, and smeared over the surface and round the rim. The diaphragm is turned over, and two further 2.5 cm strips of spermicide are applied in the same way to the concave surface. The diaphragm is then ready for insertion. The woman should also be advised on the cleaning and care of the diaphragm (see below).

At her first clinic visit, it is helpful to lend the woman a sub-standard ('fitting quality') diaphragm, and supply tubed spermicide, so that she can practise applying spermicide and inserting, removing and wearing the diaphragm, to ensure retention and comfort. At this stage, the diaphragm should not be relied on as a contraceptive.

At her second visit (a week or so later), the woman should return with the practice diaphragm in place, to check its position and size. The woman will tend to be more relaxed than at her first visit, and the

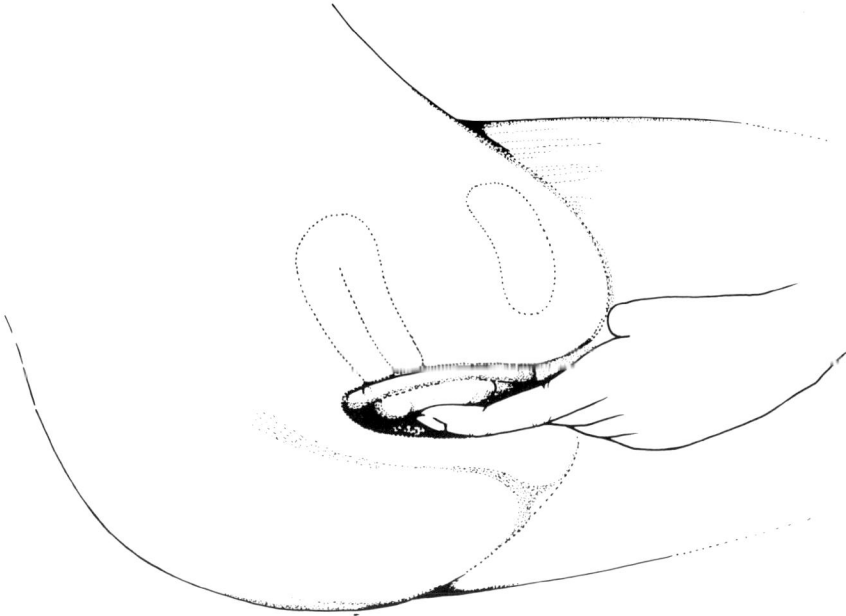

Fig. 5. *Feeling cervix through the diaphragm.*

correct size of her diaphragm may well be larger. She should then receive her own (first quality) diaphragm of the correct size, and tubed spermicide as required, for immediate use as a contraceptive. If a second visit is impracticable, then more time must be spent on teaching at the first visit, and the woman must receive her own diaphragm, and sufficient tubed spermicide, at that time.

Strict disinfection procedures should be carried out in the clinic, and all trial diaphragms, and those loaned to the women, must be thoroughly cleaned with soap and water and disinfected after use.

Diaphragm in use

The diaphragm may be inserted at any convenient time before sexual intercourse. If this is more than two hours, it is advisable that additional spermicide should be inserted in the vagina, as a cream, jelly or aerosol with an applicator, or as a non-oil-based suppository, without removing the diaphragm. The diaphragm may be removed at any convenient time after six hours have elapsed since the last act of sexual intercourse. It should then be washed with mild unscented soap and warm water, rinsed thoroughly and dried. The diaphragm may be dusted with corn starch before storage in its original container, but this dusting is not essential. Talc should never be used for this purpose. The diaphragm should be inspected occasionally for damage, and the rim kept circular. It should be kept in a cool place.

The woman should return to the clinic for a check-up every 6-12 months, as well as after delivery, any vaginal operation, or any substantial change in weight, and also during the menopause. In case of difficulty with the method she should return for advice. (If she has not previously had sexual intercourse or used a diaphragm, the woman should return six weeks after fitting.)

The arcing (bow bend) diaphragm has a rim which bends away from the fingers, when compressed across a diameter, helping the posterior rim to pass behind the cervix into the posterior fornix. The arcing diaphragm may also be useful for a woman with a cystocele or prolapse.

The cervical cap

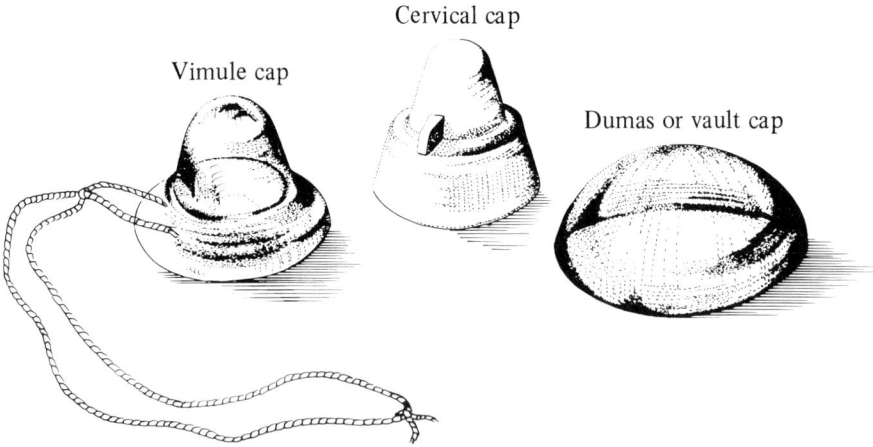

Fig. 6. *Various caps.*

The cervical cap (Fig. 6), made of rubber, plastic or metal, is a thimble-shaped bowl with an expanded rim, fitting snugly over the cervix, which must be healthy, parallel-sided, sufficiently long to protrude into the bowl, and accessible to the woman's fingers. The cervical cap is useful for women unable to retain a diaphragm. The internal diameter of the rim is the size of the cervical cap, ranging from 22 to

Barrier Contraception

31 mm in 3 mm steps. The correct size has the same diameter as the base of the vaginal portion of the cervix.

For insertion, the cervical cap is held rim upwards, compressed (if made of rubber) between thumb and index finger, and guided along the posterior vaginal wall, till the posterior rim is just behind the cervix. The rim is allowed to open, the thumb removed, and the cervical cap pushed upwards, on to the cervix, with the index and middle fingertips. Correctness of position is checked by feeling the cervix through the bowl of the (rubber) cervical cap.

Before it is inserted, a 5 cm strip of tubed spermicide should be applied to each side of the cervical cap, and smeared over the convex surface. Alternatively, the bowl of the cervical cap may be one-third filled with 5 cm of tubed spermicide, the cap inserted and the vaginal dose put around the cap as a cream, jelly or aerosol with an applicator, or as a non-oil-based suppository.

The cervical cap is removed by inserting a fingertip between the rim and the cervix, easing off the cap, and withdrawing it with the index and middle fingers. Alternatively, a thread may be attached to the rim, to make removal easier. Post-menstrual insertion, with retention till the next menstruation, is not recommended. The cervical cap may be removed at any convenient time after six hours have elapsed since the last act of sexual intercourse.

The vault (Dumas) cap

The vault cap (Fig. 6), made of rubber, is a nearly hemispherical bowl, with a thin dome, and a thick rim. It covers the cervix, and clings by suction to the vaginal vault. The cervix must be healthy, short enough to be accommodated in the shallow bowl, and accessible to the woman's fingers. The vault cap is useful for women unable to retain a diaphragm. The external diameter of the rim is the size of the vault cap, ranging from 50 to 75 mm in 5 mm steps. The correct size is the smallest which will fit evenly into the vaginal vault.

For insertion, the vault cap is held rim upwards, compressed between thumb and index finger, and guided along the posterior vaginal wall into the posterior fornix, till the posterior rim lies behind the cervix. Then the centre of the dome is pushed firmly upwards into the vaginal vault to develop suction, and so retain the cap in place. Correctness of position is checked by feeling the cervix through the dome of the vault cap. Straining downwards may dislodge the vault cap, the position of which may require subsequent adjustment.

137

Before it is inserted, a 5 cm strip of tubed spermicide should be applied to each side of the vault cap, and smeared over the surface, avoiding the rim (spermicide here would hinder suction). Alternatively, the bowl of the vault cap is one-third filled with 5 cm of tubed spermicide, the cap inserted, and the vaginal dose put in as a cream, jelly or aerosol with an applicator, or as a non-oil-based suppository. The vault cap is removed by inserting the thumb or middle finger under the rim to break the suction, then withdrawing the cap with the index and middle fingers. The vault cap should be left in place for at least six hours after the last act of sexual intercourse.

The vimule cap

The vimule cap (Fig. 6), made of rubber, is a combination of cervical and vault caps, with a thimble-shaped portion to accommodate the cervix, and a wide flanged rim, clinging by suction to the vaginal vault. The cervix must be accessible to the woman's fingers. The vimule cap is useful for women unable to retain a diaphragm or a cervical or vault cap, e.g. women with prolapse or a cystocele. The external diameter of the rim is the size of the vimule cap, ranging from 45 to 51 mm in 3 mm steps. The correct size is the smallest which will comfortably accommodate the cervix, and fit evenly into the vaginal vault.

For insertion, the vimule cap is held rim upwards, compressed between thumb and index finger and guided along the posterior vaginal wall on to the cervix. The centre of the dome is pushed upwards into the vaginal vault. Correctness of position is checked by feeling the cervix through the bowl of the vimule cap.

Before it is inserted, a 5 cm strip of tubed spermicide should be applied to each side of the vimule cap, and smeared over the surface (avoiding the rim). Alternatively, the bowl of the vimule cap is one-third filled with 5 cm of tubed spermicide, the cap inserted, and the vaginal dose put in as a cream, jelly or aerosol with an applicator, or as a non-oil-based suppository. The vimule cap is removed by inserting the thumb or finger under the rim to break the suction, then withdrawing the cap with the index and middle fingers. Alternatively, a thread may be attached to the rim to make removal easier. The vimule cap should be left in place for at least six hours after the last act of sexual intercourse.

If the vimule cap is left in place for several days it may produce a higher frequency of cervical and vaginal abrasions and lacerations than other cervical caps.

Condoms

Latex rubber condoms, also known as French letters, prophylactics, protectives, rubbers or sheaths, and by brand names, are intended to envelop the penis during sexual intercourse. Manufactured in various shapes and colours, condoms are essentially circular cylinders, 15-20 cm in length, 3-3.5 cm in diameter, and 0.003-0.007 cm in thickness; closed at one end (plain- or teat-ended), and open at the other end, with an integral rim (Fig. 7). Condoms are packaged rolled on to

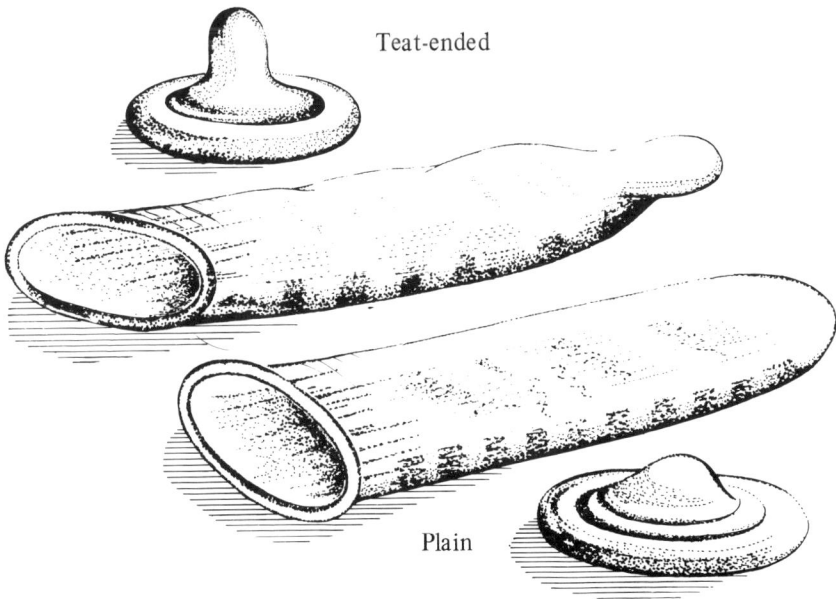

Fig. 7. *Condoms — rolled and unrolled, teat-ended and plain.*

the rim, sometimes lubricated, and usually sealed hermetically in metal and/or plastic foil, in packets containing between one and 12 (usually three) condoms. Use entails breaking open the foil, and unrolling the rolled-up condom over the entire length of the erect penis shortly before sexual intercourse, making sure to leave an airless pocket at the closed end to contain the semen.

Condoms are usually supplied in one size only. They are widely available commercially, through various retail outlets, including vending machines. Directions for use do not always accompany

139

condoms, though they are largely self-evident. The essential rules are that the condom should be rolled on to the erect penis, leaving space for the ejaculate to collect, and that, during penile withdrawal after ejaculation, the rim of the condom should be held against the man's body, to avoid any semen escaping on to the vulva and possibly into the vagina at this time. The penis should be dried before further genital contact. Condoms should be stored in a cool place, and should not be used more than once. They should not be used at all after the date of expiry, or more than five years after date of manufacture.

Condoms are one of the few contraceptives currently available which offer some protection against the spread of sexually transmitted diseases (STDs).

Laboratory studies have shown that many of the pathogens causing STDs do not penetrate through the wall of the condom. This includes a number of the viral infections for which there is no effective treatment at the present time. Among these, great attention is focused on the acquired immuno-deficiency syndrome (AIDS) (see page 277). It is, therefore, important that individuals at high risk for STDs be counselled to use condoms, in addition to another contraceptive method such as oral contraceptives.

Because condom use is part of the 'safer sex' campaign in various countries, there is great interest in them at present. Ways of getting more couples, especially young couples, to use them are constantly being put forward, and more open advertising of them (e.g. on television) is now taking place in many countries. It is important to emphasize that condoms of a high standard of manufacture should be used, with less chance of breakage or bursting in use, e.g. those with the British Standard kite mark in the UK. Also, times of expiry should be strictly adhered to, particularly in hot countries, since they may otherwise deteriorate and break.

Coloured condoms and condoms in various 'titillating' shapes are manufactured, intended to appeal mainly to adolescents. If they achieve this object and are used properly and consistently, this will be important both as a part of family planning campaigns and in the fight against HIV and other sexually transmitted infections.

Condoms are unlikely to fail merely from semen leaking through a small hole. The main cause of failure is condom breakage, discharging most of the ejaculate into the vagina. Unlike the incidence of holes, the bursting propensity of condoms is unpredictable. Care in removing each condom from its packet, lubrication (preferably with spermicide), care in placing the condom on the penis well before ejaculation, care in leaving space for the semen at ejaculation, and care in avoiding semen leakage past the rim thereafter, should maximize contraceptive effectiveness. It has been shown in laboratory studies that the addition of a spermicide to condoms decreases the number of viable sperm before artificial rupture.

Vegetable-oil-based suppositories reduce the tensile strength of condoms. However, it remains unclear whether they weaken condoms sufficiently to increase their bursting propensity, during the limited contact they have with disposable condoms. (The same consideration may apply to non-spermicidal, oil-based lubricants, e.g. petroleum jelly.) Non-oil-based suppositories, aerosols, and tubed spermicides do not affect the tensile strength of condoms. (Foaming tablets do not lubricate condoms.) Condoms packed already lubricated with a spermicide may be slightly more effective than other condoms.

Skin condoms, made from sheep intestines, available in very few countries now, are more expensive than rubber condoms, though they may be re-used a few times, if washed carefully and kept moist. They are placed on the erect penis like a sock, and do not need to be unrolled. They are not recommended for general use.

Short, glans condoms (called in some countries 'American tips'), covering only the glans penis, may either slip off, or fit too tightly, and should not be used as contraceptives. Urethral contraceptives, consisting of a small bag, with a stem for insertion into the man's urethra, may harm the user and are not recommended.

Spermicides

Spermicides (chemical contraceptives) are intended for insertion into the vaginal vault, as close to the cervix as possible, shortly before sexual intercourse. They are widely available commercially. Use with mechanical contraceptives entails greater effectiveness than spermicidal or mechanical contraceptives used alone. Spermicides offer some protection against certain sexually transmitted diseases. In the laboratory, spermicides containing nonoxynol-9 have been shown to destroy the HIV virus. Their use in women at risk of infection with this virus is being investigated. The following types of spermicides are available:

Tubed products (creams and jellies) are contained in soft metal or plastic tubes, from which they may be expressed on to caps, or into applicators, before vaginal insertion.

Aerosols (foams) are contained under pressure in strong bottles, from which they may be released into an applicator, by pressing a valve, for insertion deep in the vagina.

Suppositories ('soluble pessaries') incorporate an active spermicide in a base melting at body temperature, for manual insertion close to the cervix.

Foaming tablets incorporate an active spermicide with foaming ingredients, which effervesce in contact with vaginal moisture, and are placed deep in the vagina close to the cervix.

Plastic films are available which are impregnated with a spermicide. The film is water soluble and disintegrates in the vagina. It is placed deep in the vagina, covering the cervix if possible. Earlier it was suggested that either partner could use the film, the man placing it on the tip of the penis before insertion, but this has proved unsatisfactory.

Vaginal sponges

Vaginal sponges incorporate an active spermicide in a polyurethane mushroom-shaped vehicle (Fig. 8). The spermicide is released by

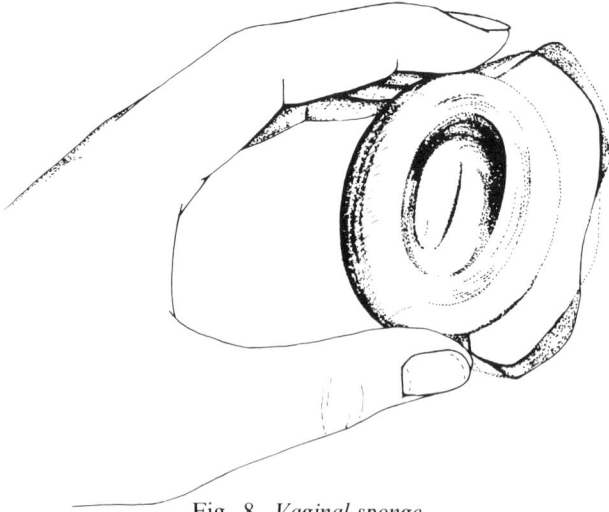

Fig. 8. *Vaginal sponge.*

wetting the sponge before manual insertion close to the cervix, and also by continued contact with the vaginal secretions.

The sponge may be inserted up to 24 hours before sexual intercourse. It allows intercourse immediately after insertion and may be used for multiple acts of intercourse within 24 hours following insertion. It should be removed six hours after the last act of intercourse.

The sponge is looked on as a carrier for spermicide and has the same range of effectiveness as spermicides. It is disposable and less messy than some spermicides. The spermicide it contains may offer at least partial protection against the transmission of some STDs.

The vaginal shield or 'female condom'

Still under investigation at the time this book is being prepared, this innovative barrier method has interesting possibilities for the future. It is a tube of strong elastic polyurethane plastic, closed at one end, about 15 cm (6 in.) long and 7 cm ($2\frac{1}{2}$ in.) in diameter. At the open end is a soft ring which holds the shield against the vulva. The other end contains a flexible ring which helps to keep the shield in the vagina during sexual intercourse. It is intended for use once only.

The vaginal shield is said to interfere less with sexual pleasure in both sexes than the condom. It has other advantages, such as being under the control of the female partner, and it can be inserted well before intercourse. It may be protective, like the condom, against sexually transmitted disease organisms, including viruses.

The shield is under research in several institutions, including the Margaret Pyke Centre in London. If it does not produce unexpected disadvantages, it should be a useful addition to the barrier methods now in use.

Home-made barriers

Where necessary, barrier contraceptives may be improvised. Vaginal pads, tampons or sponges may be used, soaked or smeared with domestically available (or preferably manufactured) spermicides, and inserted deep in the vagina, to cover the cervix before sexual intercourse, and may be washed in soapy water, rinsed, dried and used again.

Pads may be made from 15 cm square pieces of clean, soft, white cloth, folded with the frayed edges inside, and sewn together with a thread, leaving a free end to assist removal. Clean cotton or silk waste may be cut, and rolled into tampons about the size of a hen's egg, held together with a thread for removal. Small sponges either naturally occurring, or cut from foam rubber or plastic, may be enclosed in a net, and a thread attached. Commercially available menstrual tampons may also be used.

Spermicides may be fashioned from vinegar or lemon juice (1 part) mixed with boiled water (20 parts); mild soap (1 cm cube) dissolved in warm, boiled water (1 litre); or any edible oil or fat. Strong soap, soap powder, detergents, mustard oil and strong salt solutions will irritate or injure the vaginal walls and should not be used.

Post-coital douche

Although water is spermicidal, flooding the vagina (e.g. with a special syringe) immediately after unprotected sexual intercourse, to wash out the semen, is ineffective as a contraceptive, and is not recommended.

Direct insemination of the cervix deposits sperm in the endocervical canal within a few seconds of ejaculation. In addition, sperm can be found in the uterine cavity and uterine tubes 90 seconds after ejaculation.

It is for this reason that post-coital douches should not be used as a form of contraception.

Quality testing

The quality of barrier contraceptives should be checked in the factory. Diaphragms may be inflated with air and inspected visually to eliminate those with gross holes or other flaws. Disposable rubber condoms are usually 'electronically tested' (i.e. sorted), to eliminate those with holes or weak patches, before packaging. Such testing of each condom should be distinguished from sample testing, which essentially checks the efficiency of electronic sorting in eliminating defective condoms.

Sample testing of barrier contraceptives should also be distinguished from clinical testing, intended to evaluate contraceptive effectiveness. *In vitro* quality requirements may bear little relation to *in vivo* conditions of practical use. Condoms satisfying high standards have not been shown to be more effective contraceptives than condoms satisfying lower standards.

Spermicides passing or failing an *in vitro* test may show no corresponding difference in contraceptive effectiveness. While barrier contraceptives satisfying quality requirements may be intuitively preferable to other barriers, any difference in theoretical effectiveness may well be exceeded by differences in consumer acceptability (e.g. affected by imaginative packaging), which is decisive in determining use effectiveness.

Only a few countries have national standards for the quality of diaphragms and there are no such standards for cervical, vault or vimule caps. An international standard for diaphragms is at present being considered by the International Organization for Standardization (ISO).

On the other hand, there are many national standards for the quality of rubber condoms. These vary from country to country and the ISO is working towards an international condom standard.

No national standards exist for spermicidal effectiveness.

IMAP Statement on Barrier Methods of Contraception*

Introduction

Barrier methods of contraception are safe and fairly reliable for couples who are sufficiently motivated to use them consistently. Although they are not as effective as other available contraceptives, barrier methods can play an important role in family planning programmes. Their use often constitutes a first step in contraceptive practice, the user gradually moving towards more reliable methods. IPPF should promote wider use of barrier methods, emphasizing the need for adequate education to ensure their effective use.

The main advantages of barrier contraceptives are that their action is not systemic, they have no known serious short- or long-term side-effects, and they do not interfere with lactation. Spermicides and condoms have an additional advantage in that they can be distributed through non-clinical programmes. The major drawback of barrier contraceptives is that they tend to be used inconsistently and incorrectly, with a resultant high failure rate. The use of barrier methods has the practical drawback that they are all related to coitus and consequently require a high level of motivation. Some couples relying on methods of ovulation detection to identify the fertile period of the cycle may wish to use contraceptives only

---

*This statement is valid for barrier methods of contraception currently distributed by IPPF. The Panel reserves the right to amend this statement in the light of further developments in the field of barrier contraception, when sufficient scientific information becomes available.

during that time. For them, the consistent use of barrier contraceptives during the fertile period may have a place.

The effectiveness of all barrier contraceptives also depends on their quality, both at the point of manufacture and in the field. If they are stored under inappropriate conditions, their quality can seriously deteriorate. IPPF encourages the use of standards developed by the International Organization for Standardization (ISO) for diaphragms and condoms in the manufacture and quality testing of these products.

Diaphragms

The most widely used female barrier method is the diaphragm. There is a need for further research to resolve specific issues relevant to diaphragm use, such as whether its contraceptive effect is chiefly due to its role as a barrier to sperm, or as a carrier for spermicide. The relative importance of the fit has also been called into question. Until more evidence becomes available, diaphragms should be used together with spermicides in order to ensure maximum contraceptive protection. Spermicides can also act as a lubricant. Diaphragms should be fitted by trained personnel, as a pelvic examination is necessary. A second visit is recommended after the diaphragm has been fitted, in order to check the client's ability to use the diaphragm correctly. Following childbirth, diaphragm size should be checked.

Contraindications to the use of diaphragms include anatomical anomalies, such as uterine prolapse, which prevent adequate fitting.

If sexual intercourse takes place more than three hours after inserting the diaphragm, more spermicide should be inserted, without removing the diaphragm. It should be left in place for at least six hours after intercourse to allow time for any sperm remaining in the vagina to become inactive. It can be left in longer, but not for more than 24 hours without being removed and cleaned. The user needs to know how to check the condition of her diaphragm, and how to clean and store it. This may present problems in certain settings, where a source of clean water is not readily available.

Cervical caps

The cervical cap may be more suitable for some women than the diaphragm; however, it is not widely used, and there are no reliable data on its effectiveness.

Contraindications to its use include anatomical features that might make effective fitting difficult. It is recommended that cervical caps should not be left in place for longer than three days before being removed and cleaned, otherwise unpleasant odour or infection may result.

Spermicides

Spermicidal products (creams, jellies, foams in pressurized containers, foaming tablets or suppositories) when used on their own, are not as effective as other contraceptives, but they do provide additional protection when used in conjunction with the condom or diaphragm. Spermicides can also be useful as back-up contraceptive protection for couples relying on lactational amenorrhoea or using IUDs.

Spermicides are well suited for commercial and non-medical distribution, as they have no proven systemic side-effects or serious local reactions. Furthermore, evidence suggests that they have a protective effect against certain sexually transmitted diseases. Some recent reports have suggested an increase in birth abnormalities in the case of accidental pregnancies following the use of spermicides. However, the data are equivocal, and there is a need for more research into this question.

Spermicides containing phenylmercuric acetate should not be used because of the potential toxicity of mercuric compounds.

Condoms

Condoms can be a highly effective method of contraception if they are used correctly at every act of coitus and should be promoted more in family planning programmes. They are particularly suited to non-medical distribution systems and probably offer the best contraceptive option for adolescents. Condoms provide the man with the opportunity of being the active partner in sharing fertility regulation responsibilities. Condoms can also play an important role in the prevention of sexually transmitted diseases.

Sponges

A recent addition to the range of barrier contraceptives has been the sponge, impregnated with spermicide, which is now available in some countries. Its effectiveness is still under review, and no reliable data are yet available.

(Adopted by the IPPF Central Council, November 1983, and amended by the Central Council, November 1984.)

Chapter 9

Periodic Abstinence

Introduction

Family planning by periodic abstinence from sexual intercourse has a long and somewhat chequered history. Recently, its use has been strongly promoted by certain religious groups, especially members of the Catholic Church.

The reproductive cycle in a woman is controlled by the follicle stimulating hormone (FSH) and the luteinizing hormone (LH) from the pituitary gland. These hormones control the production of the ovarian hormones oestrogen and progesterone. Oestrogen is mainly active in the early part of the cycle. During this time follicles ripen in the ovary and the endometrium builds up under the influence of the oestrogen produced by the ripening follicles. A surge of LH then triggers ovulation. During the post-ovulatory phase of the cycle the dominant influence is progesterone produced by the corpus luteum (resulting from the ripened follicle). This causes the endometrium to build up further in preparation for implantation of a fertilized ovum. If an ovum is not fertilized and does not implant, the endometrium is shed, thus producing the menstrual bleeding.

Oestrogen and progesterone have a wide range of other effects, some of which can be readily observed. Oestrogen produces physico-chemical alterations in the cervical mucus which changes from a thick, opaque sticky plug to a thin, clear, lubricant substance as ovulation approaches. Progesterone is thermogenic, producing a rise in basal body temperature (BBT) after ovulation. It is the observation and recording of these phenomena which provide the physiological basis for the modern approach to periodic abstinence. They provide markers as to the stage of development of the cycle under scrutiny. In this they differ fundamentally from the older approach based on predicting the time of ovulation solely on the basis of the length of previous cycles (calendar or rhythm method).

None of this would be of practical value were it not for the limited life of both the ovum and the sperm. The ovum can only be fertilized during approximately 12 hours after release. The life of sperm is longer and more susceptible to variation, but averages about three days. Thus, if sexual intercourse is to lead to conception it must take place around the time of ovulation during the fertile phase of the cycle. Before and after that time are the infertile phases. Confining intercourse to the infertile phases, especially that after ovulation, greatly reduces the chance of conception.

Basal body temperature method

This was the first scientific method based on periodic abstinence to be developed. Essentially, a woman records her temperature immediately on waking each morning to get a basal reading. Following menstruation during the early part of the cycle the BBT remains at a lower level. At ovulation it rises by about 0.2°C-0.4°C and then maintains a higher level or plateau until the onset of the next menstruation. The shift of temperature from a lower to a higher level is the marker of ovulation. By waiting until three consecutive daily temperatures at the higher level have been recorded, the woman can then start intercourse with very little risk of conception. This is because of the short life of the ovum. The post-ovulatory infertile phase continues until the next menstruation.

The BBT gives no indication of the approach of ovulation, and since sperm may survive on average for three days, intercourse cannot take place in the first part of the cycle between menstruation and ovulation despite the fact that part of that time the woman will be infertile.

Practical instruction

For best results the following instructions should be carefully observed:

1. The BBT must be recorded immediately on waking before undertaking any activity.

2. A special 'ovulation' or 'fertility' thermometer, though not essential, is extremely helpful, since the markings are widely spaced at 0.1°C intervals, making it easy to read. If the mercury stops between two marks, the lower mark should be used for recording on the chart (see 4 below).

3. The temperature may be taken by various routes: orally, rectally

or vaginally, the thermometer being left in position for at least three minutes. The same route must be used throughout a menstrual cycle. Oral temperatures, although useful, give the least satisfactory record because they are more susceptible to minor irregularities.

4. The temperature should be recorded on a chart designed specially for the purpose of easy identification of the shift and of displaying the rise of temperature to the best advantage (Fig. 9).

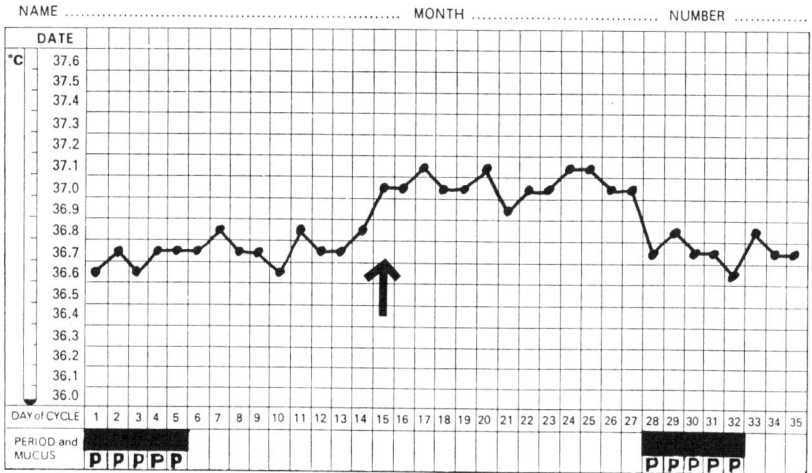

Fig. 9. *Temperature chart showing rise of temperature on Day 15 (arrow) indicating that ovulation probably occurred on Day 13 or 14.*

5. The post-ovulatory infertile phase starts after three consecutive daily temperatures, all of which are above the level of the immediately preceding six consecutive daily temperatures, have been recorded.

6. This can be recognized graphically by drawing a cross on the lines of the chart showing three daily temperatures in the top right square and six in the bottom left square (Fig. 10).

7. There must be abstinence from intercourse throughout the early part of the cycle, from the onset of menstruation to the day on which the third temperature at the higher level has been recorded. Intercourse can take place from that point to the onset of the next menstruation.

Advantages and disadvantages

The BBT method, when used alone, clearly requires a long period of abstinence in each cycle. On the other hand, it offers a high degree of reliability. An unexpected pregnancy rate of less than one to about six

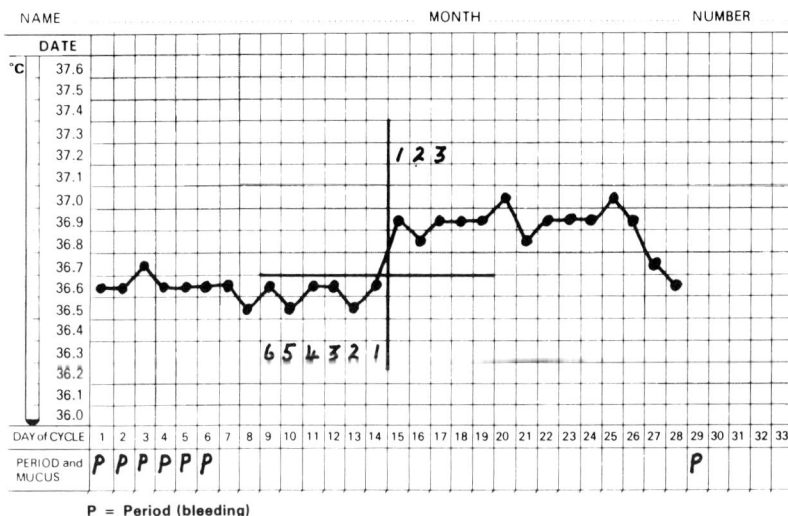

Fig. 10. *Basal body temperature chart with acute rise due to ovulation demonstrated by the three over six rule.*

per 100 woman-years of use can be achieved, according to the standard of instruction and motivation of the couple. Since the BBT method requires the identification of ovulation before sexual intercourse can resume, it is not a very useful or appropriate method for women with very irregular cycles. Also, thermometer breaking and replacing can be a problem for some women.

Cervical mucus method

Recognition of the value of monitoring changes in cervical mucus to identify the fertile phase of the menstrual cycle came later than the BBT method. Following the end of menstruation there may be a number of 'dry days'. During this time the cervical mucus consists of a thick plug at the cervix, with none flowing down the vagina. The woman experiences a positive sensation of dryness at the vaginal entrance. Under the influence of the rising level of oestrogen, the mucus changes first to a thick, sticky, opaque substance which reaches the vaginal entrance and can be detected there, either by the sensation it produces or by visual observation. The change continues until the mucus is thin, clear and slippery, giving rise to a sensation of 'wetness' and 'lubrication'. The last day of this type of mucus marks the estimated day of ovulation after which the mucus reverts to a thick,

151

dry state or disappears entirely. The last day on which the mucus is not necessarily most abundant, but most slippery and lubricative is known as 'peak' day which can only be detected retrospectively, i.e. on the day after, when it no longer possesses these characteristics.

Practical instructions

1. Observations should be made throughout the day at convenient times, for instance, when going to the toilet.

2. Observation can include both the sensation experienced and visual inspection of mucus which appears at the vulva.

3. Sensation will be of positive dryness, changing to absence of dryness, then to a feeling of wetness, followed again by an absence of dryness.

4. Inspection shows a change from a thick, sticky, opaque substance to a thin, clear, watery, slippery substance. In the latter state, the mucus can be stretched as an unbroken thread between the fingers or between folded leaves of toilet tissue.

5. The results of the observations throughout the day should be recorded each evening on a chart.

6. Intercourse can take place during the dry days following menstruation. It is recommended that intercourse only takes place on alternate dry days, to avoid the risk of residual semen masking the first appearance of mucus. Not every woman has dry days following menstruation; sometimes mucus appears immediately, in which case abstinence during this phase is necessary.

7. Once mucus appears there must be abstinence from intercourse, if the intention is to avoid pregnancy.

8. The day of peak mucus — that is the last day when mucus is slippery and lubricative — is marked by a cross on the chart.

9. Intercourse can be resumed on the fourth day after peak. Thus, if peak day is marked by a cross and the next three days numbered 1, 2, 3, intercourse begins on the first unmarked day (Fig. 11). It can continue as often as desired until the next menstrual period.

Advantages and disadvantages

For those women who experience 'dry days' after menstruation, the cervical mucus method has the advantage of allowing intercourse at this time, thus reducing the duration of abstinence. It also has the advantage of requiring nothing beyond a means of recording the

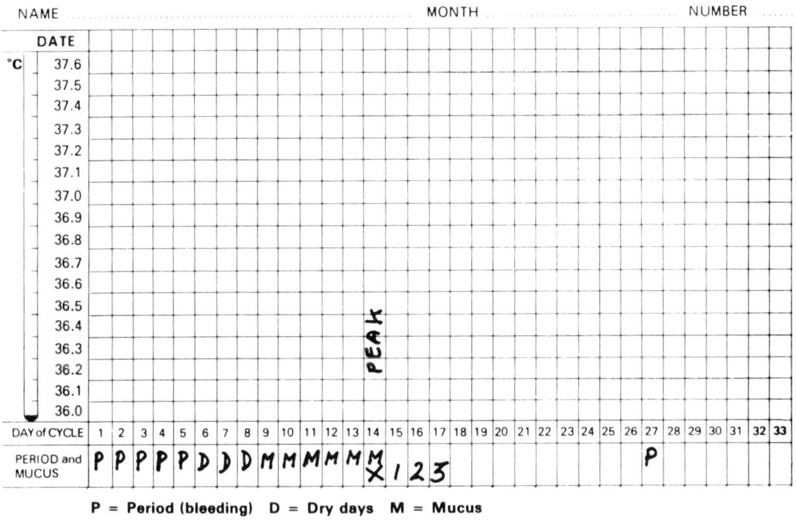

Fig. 11. *Chart showing convention for marking peak mucus.*

observations. However, the frequency of unexpected pregnancies is higher than with BBT, and has ranged from five up to 35 pregnancies per 100 woman-years of use.

Sympto-thermal method

Combining BBT and mucus observations has the obvious advantages of using two markers of ovulation, which should increase the accurate identification of the fertile period. The mucus method is used to determine the pre-ovulatory infertile phase, while the start of the post-ovulatory infertile phase is determined both by mucus and temperature shift. The rule for resuming intercourse with the mucus method is fourth day after peak and for the BBT method after three consecutive daily temperatures at the higher level have been recorded. The two, however, frequently coincide because the peak tends to precede and the temperature shift to follow ovulation. When there is discrepancy the later day should be followed, to make the sympto-thermal method as effective as possible. Some women using this approach also monitor one or more secondary signs or symptoms to help to determine the fertile phase of the cycle. These include intermenstrual pain ('Mittelschmerz'), intermenstrual bleeding, breast

153

tenderness, oedema and mood changes. These are uncommon and inconsistent, and are not often used on their own.

Advantages and disadvantages

In studies of the sympto-thermal method pregnancy rates have ranged from four to 26 per 100 woman-years. Effectiveness is therefore not much different from the cervical mucus method, but both methods require less abstinence than the BBT method. The longer abstinence of the BBT method helps to contribute to its greater effectiveness. The major disadvantage of the sympto-thermal method is that it requires more time and motivation on the woman's part in recording and interpreting several signs and symptoms of ovulation.

Cervical palpation

Self-palpation of the cervix has attracted increasing interest. This is best done standing, with the right foot on a chair while the middle finger of the right hand is inserted into the vagina. In the early part of the cycle after menstruation the cervix is low in the vagina and can easily be felt. It is firm with a consistency rather like the tip of the nose. The cervical os is closed. As ovulation approaches, the cervix becomes soft; its consistency is that of the lips rather than the tip of the nose. The os begins to open and is felt as a dimple, and as the cervix is higher in the vagina it is more difficult to reach. After ovulation the changes revert to give a low, firm cervix with a closed os. Sufficient studies have not yet been conducted to demonstrate the percentage of women who can learn this method. Also there is no clear indication of its effectiveness in preventing pregnancy.

General considerations

Motivation is the essence of successful family planning of any kind. Nowhere is this more true than in the practice of periodic abstinence. Motivation is best secured through a thorough understanding of the method.

Prescription of a set of rules to be followed blindly is unlikely to work. A couple must understand what they are doing and why. The background knowledge required for the practice of periodic abstinence promotes this understanding. The physiological principles

154

need not be couched in highly technical terms; a simplified version of the phases of the cycle can be grasped by anyone.

Couples appreciate learning about phenomena which they have already observed, the significance of which they have not understood. They enjoy knowing more about their bodies and their fertility. The need to acquire this knowledge means that couples are making a positive choice to learn and use the methods, which in turn strengthens their motivation. This knowledge is best conveyed by other successful users who have been specially trained for the task. Their personal experience combined with their training as teachers of the method make them credible. These methods, though inexpensive in terms of equipment, are costly in terms of personnel. However, most organizations teaching the methods use trained volunteers.

Many studies have shown that most women who want to learn these methods are able to do so, regardless of their educational level. It appears that when the methods are taught and followed correctly they can be very effective in preventing unplanned pregnancies. The methods can also be used to advantage in timing sexual intercourse so as to improve the chances of conception when a pregnancy is desired.

Side-effects

Periods of abstinence may, when used positively, enhance rather than detract from a relationship. In strongly motivated couples they may strengthen the bonds between them. However, in some instances there may be psychological strain on the relationship, especially if one partner is more highly motivated than the other. Couples may, in these circumstances, use barrier methods during the fertile phase of the cycle, so that sexual intercourse can continue. It is essential if the method is to be effective that the woman observes her signs of fertility and infertility with the same care as she would if abstaining during the fertile phase.

That a possibility of harmful side-effects in the mother and offspring exists, can neither be confirmed nor completely dismissed on available evidence. There is strong evidence from animal studies that if fertilization involving ageing gametes does occur, there is a raised possibility of congenital abnormalities in the offspring. If pregnancy occurs as a failure in the correct use of these methods there will be a more than usual chance that the sperm or ovum will have been in the female tract for an abnormally long time. This theoretical possibility is being watched closely, and at least one prospective or cohort study is underway to try to resolve the question.

The suggestion has also been made that if fertilization takes place late in the menstrual cycle, there may be a higher than usual probability of ectopic pregnancy and placenta praevia, with their associated risks for the mother and infant. This hypothesis, though supported by some observational data, has not been confirmed.

Conclusion

Knowledge of the most fertile, least fertile and infertile phases of the human menstrual cycle is important knowledge which women should understand whether they wish to conceive, to use periodic abstinence for fertility regulation, or whether they wish to use coitus interruptus and/or barrier methods only at the time when conception is most likely.

IMAP Statement on Periodic Abstinence for Family Planning*

Results of recent, properly conducted trials show conclusively that periodic abstinence (sometimes inaccurately referred to as 'natural family planning') is much less effective than other available family planning methods. This method depends on identifying the fertile phase of the menstrual cycle which occurs around the time of ovulation. In order to avoid pregnancy, abstinence from sexual intercourse during the fertile phase has to be observed. Owing to the difficulty of accurately predicting the fertile phase, abstinence sometimes has to be observed for a large part of the menstrual cycle. Present techniques, which include the calendar method, basal body temperature method, cervical mucus method or a combination of these, such as the sympto-thermal method, may be used for identifying the time of ovulation and deducing from it the fertile phase.

Although theoretical calculations may suggest that these techniques can be relatively effective, in practice the failure rates are high. In recent major studies, almost 20% of women using the sympto-thermal method became pregnant within a year, as did about 25% of those using the cervical mucus method, compared with less than 5% of those using oral

---

*This statement is valid for the currently available methods for identifying the fertile phase of the menstrual cycle. IPPF reserves the right to amend the statement in the light of further developments in this field.

contraceptives or intrauterine devices. While the sympto-thermal method appears to be more effective than the cervical mucus method, the two methods show wide and overlapping ranges of pregnancy and discontinuation rates among different groups of women. Failure and discontinuation rates at this level are unusually high as compared with other methods. IPPF therefore does not advise that periodic abstinence be considered as an equal alternative to other more effective family planning methods.

Nevertheless, periodic abstinence can be the only choice for individuals and couples who cannot or do not want to use other methods of fertility regulation for a variety of reasons. Family planning associations should therefore familiarize themselves with the techniques and be prepared to teach them if a demand can be demonstrated. Couples electing to use periodic abstinence should be clearly informed that the method is not considered an effective method of family planning, although the method may be very effective in highly motivated couples.

It should be recognized that periodic abstinence as a method is better than no method at all. There are also various benefits to be obtained from an understanding of the reproductive cycle. It provides an opportunity for women to learn about their physiology. The identification of the fertile phase is the basis for one contraceptive practice whereby couples choose to use barrier methods only during those days estimated to be the fertile phase of the woman's cycle. It may also be a starting point for the use of more effective contraception. Finally, methods for the detection of ovulation have been used and continue to be valuable in the diagnosis and, more importantly, in the treatment of infertility.

(Statement by the IPPF International Medical Advisory Panel, October 1982; approved by the IPPF Central Council, November 1982, and amended in November 1983.)

Chapter 10

Coitus Interruptus

History and acceptability

Coitus interruptus or male withdrawal is the oldest method of reversible contraception. It remains the commonest method in countries such as Italy, and was partially responsible for the decline in fertility, measurable from the 17th and 18th centuries onwards, in European countries such as France. In most of contemporary Eastern Europe its use is very popular and is associated with large reductions in the birth rate. In Britain it is the third most common method, exceeded only by oral contraceptives and condoms.

World Fertility Survey data show that coitus interruptus is used by one in four contraceptive users in the Philippines and almost half the contraceptors in countries such as Kenya and Turkey.

Its use appears to be known in most human cultures, although in some Oriental societies it is not as widely used as in Christian or Muslim societies.

Coitus interruptus was used in Muslim society at the time of the Prophet. A companion of the Prophet related the following: "We used to practise coitus interruptus during the time of the Prophet. The Prophet came to know about it but did not forbid us. The Prophet, however, insisted that the wife should give her consent to the practice".

The Biblical story of Onan became the basis of St Augustine's condemnation of contraception, beginning the train of thought that eventually led to *Humanae Vitae*. However, it is not clear if Onan's 'sin' (to 'spill his seed on the ground' when he had to have sexual intercourse with his dead brother's wife) was to practise coitus interruptus or to disobey his father.

Euphemisms

In surveys of contraceptive practice and use, or in counselling the individual couple, the use of withdrawal is easy to overlook. In response to the question, "Do you use a method of contraception?" the answer may be "No", while in answer to the question, "Are you being careful?" the answer may be "Yes". Euphemisms to describe the method are common. Four thousand years ago it was described by a Jewish writer as 'threshing inside and winnowing outside'. Common euphemisms used nowadays include 'pulling out', 'using self control', 'being considerate'. Travelling euphemisms are common, incorporating the idea of getting off a vehicle or aeroplane one stop before the end of the journey, e.g. 'flying to Bangladesh, but getting off at Bombay'.

Effectiveness and side-effects

Coitus interruptus has not been scientifically studied to the extent that so widespread and significant a practice deserves. The few studies on failure rates that are available suggest a moderate effectiveness, which in certain circumstances can become high. In one USA study the failure rate was 10 pregnancies per 100 woman-years of use (three pregnancies per 100 in high-income groups) compared with an average of 12 per 100 for all other methods. In the 1949 Royal Commission on Population in Britain no difference was found in the average family size of those using mechanical methods of contraception and those using withdrawal. In 1970, 38% of British users of coitus interruptus claimed they were completely satisfied with the method and 41% fairly satisfied. Approximately twice as many couples who had tried coitus interruptus persisted in its use compared with those who had tried a vaginal diaphragm.

Effectiveness depends on the man's ability to withdraw his penis before ejaculation. However, it is sometimes claimed that the pre-ejaculatory fluid contains fertilizing sperm. No scientific studies are known to have been carried out to prove or disprove this contention. Probably satisfied users of the method never seek professional advice, while those who are dissatisfied with the technique or have had failure attend a family planning clinic, quite reasonably seeking an alternative contraceptive method.

Psychologically the method has been credited as the cause of numerous possible neurotic symptoms, but again there is no objective evidence linking the use of coitus interruptus with any adverse emotional effects. Indeed, the widespread use of the method suggests that it is unassociated with serious side-effects while, conversely, its commonness makes it likely that people complaining of any neurotic symptoms may have adopted the method simply by coincidence.

Who should use it?

Coitus interruptus is simple, moderately effective, and appears widely acceptable to large numbers of people. Many well-adjusted and well-motivated couples enjoy a fulfilled sex life using this method with understanding.

Men who are well able to control their build-up to ejaculation so that they can withdraw in time are obviously the most suitable users of the method. If they can help to bring their partners to orgasm before or after withdrawal the couple can enjoy a good sex life. Adolescent males are unlikely to be the best users of coitus interruptus, since they may not have sufficient control over ejaculation. Men who have a tendency to premature ejaculation are also not good candidates.

Conclusion

Coitus interruptus has the advantage of not requiring any professional supervision, it cannot be left at home when the couple goes on holiday, it cannot be picked up and eaten by the children, it cannot be taxed or its importation forbidden by the government, and it does not cause menorrhagia or weight gain. Certainly, more couples use this method than vaginal barriers or hormone injections, although these later methods have accumulated a research literature that is literally one thousand times larger.

Those who counsel individuals on family planning are unlikely to find themselves advocating the method, but their professional wisdom and usefulness will be increased if they have a general understanding of the method and the characteristics of those who use it.

Chapter 11

Male and Female Sterilization

The role of sterilization in fertility regulation

Sterilization, male or female, sometimes called 'surgical contraception', is often the best choice when the desired family size has been achieved. It is the most effective contraceptive method available. It is a one-time procedure which is relatively simple in either sex. It does not require constant use of a method, a check-up at regular intervals, or the cost of contraceptive supplies. The risk of complications or death is minimal if the procedure is performed according to strict medical standards.

Apart from its value in purely family planning terms, sterilization is appropriate to offer, from an obstetric point of view, to the following high-risk groups: women of parity three and above, women older than 35 years of age, women with a history of obstetric complications or several caesarean sections, and women with health problems that may be contra-indications to pregnancy or to the use of other family planning methods. In all these cases, circumstances may sometimes suggest that the male partner should have a vasectomy in preference to the female partner being sterilized, e.g. if the woman is too ill to undergo the operation.

Sterilization operations usually demand a somewhat greater investment in skill, training, and equipment than temporary methods of contraception. However, they usually give many years of complete protection against pregnancy and are therefore generally more cost-effective than reversible methods of fertility regulation.

Legal and ethical aspects

Sterilization is now legal in nearly all countries, either through special provisions or, more frequently, because no law prohibits it. In some parts of the world there are cultural or religious differences within the medical profession in attitudes towards both male and female sterilization. On the one hand, doctors have a right not to engage in procedures that offend their conscience. On the other hand, the medical community as a whole has an obligation to make sure that services are available to all men and women who may choose to use them. The primary ethical responsibility of the operator and the counsellor is to ensure that the individual gives mature, informed, voluntary, unpressured consent to the operation, and is legally and socially competent to give that consent (see page 340).

Male or female sterilization?

When couples are considering sterilization, many factors are involved in the decision as to which partner should be sterilized. Often it is simply a matter of mutually agreed preference. However, if there are health reasons why one partner rather than the other should be sterilized, these should override most other factors.

Both male and female sterilization can be performed quickly, safely, with local anaesthesia, on an outpatient basis, and in free-standing facilities. As a general principle, family planning workers should look at the needs of the couple and try to help them to decide which partner is most suitable for the sterilization operation (Table I). Vasectomy is the much easier technique and one with fewer potential difficulties. However, if there are medical indications for the woman to cease child bearing, it is generally sensible to recommend that she is the more logical candidate for sterilization, unless her medical condition is such that the operation would be risky from the surgical or anaesthetic point of view.

Counselling

Counselling is essential to ensure that consent is truly voluntary and informed and that the individual or the couple fully appreciate both the permanent nature and the small risk of failure of sterilization. It is a checkpoint between the client's request for the procedure and follow-through to surgery. Counselling sessions before the sterilization procedure are occasions for assessing what the individual or couple know about family planning, providing information on all forms of contraception and, when necessary, helping the individual or couple to reach a firm and comfortable decision. The psychological readiness and emotional fitness of individuals for sterilization can be assessed by listening to them carefully, with particular attention to

TABLE I. Comparison of vasectomy and female sterilization

Vasectomy	Female Sterilization
Effectiveness	
Very effective, but slightly higher rate of spontaneous recanalization and pregnancy.	Very effective; slightly lower failure rate.
Effective 6 to 10 weeks after surgery.	Effective immediately.
Early complications	
Procedure involves almost no risk of internal injury or other life-threatening complications. Small risk of haematomas.	Procedure involves slight risk of serious internal injuries and other life-threatening complications.
Very slight possibility of serious infection, including tetanus under conditions of poor hygiene.	Slight possibility of serious infection.
No anaesthesia-related deaths.	Few anaesthesia-related deaths.
Acceptability	
Minute scar.	Scar can be small but still visible.
Less expensive.	More acceptable in many cultures.
Personnel	
Can be performed by one trained person with or without an assistant.	Team needed, including one doctor, possibly one trained anaesthetist, and at least two assistants with more training than needed for vasectomy assistant.
Safely performed by nurses and trained paramedical personnel.	More difficult for paramedicals to learn and perform.
	Usually only doctors with training in gynaecology can perform laparoscopy and laparotomy. Minilaparotomy is simpler.
Equipment	
Requires no specialized equipment. Equipment readily available.	Laparoscopy requires expensive, complex equipment, which needs to be carefully maintained. Mini-laparotomy requires only simple, standard surgical instruments.
Possible long-term side-effects or late complications	
None demonstrated. Increase in sperm antibodies, not associated with medical problems.	Slight risk of ectopic pregnancy.

Adapted from *Population Reports*, Series D, Number 4, November–December 1983.

signs of doubt, conflict, misunderstanding, or unrealistic expectations about the procedure.

Because surgical contraception is intended to end permanently an individual's ability to have children, it is always preferable to counsel both the client and the partner, as a couple and individually. However, spousal consent should not be a prerequisite for receiving services unless it is a legal requirement.

The counsellor should encourage clients' questions, and should answer them clearly and directly in terms they can easily understand. In some circumstances it may be advisable for the counsellor to be of the same sex as the client and even of the same ethnic group. The counsellor must, of course, speak a language the client can understand, or use an interpreter. It is important that counselling be objective and that the counsellor avoid expressing any bias for or against sterilization or any other family planning method.

Clients may ask about the possibility of a reversal operation. They should be told that it is important for them to look on sterilization as permanent, but that in some instances reversal can be carried out, although the certainty of a pregnancy following such a procedure cannot be guaranteed (see page 186).

Counselling may be done at any time. However, an individual should have time to reflect on his or her decision concerning sterilization before the procedure, and the decision should not be made when his or her judgment may be impaired.

It is not in the best interests of the client to impose a strict time interval between his or her request for sterilization and the operation, as long as the client has the opportunity to review the decision to end fertility and to change his or her mind before the operation.

When a woman is pregnant and interested in sterilization the operation can be discussed with her during the pregnancy, well before the date of delivery. Some women, of course, are only seen immediately before or even during labour, and may have to be counselled at this stage. However, wherever possible, the sterilization decision should be avoided immediately before, during or after delivery or abortion. Tubal occlusion is sometimes carried out at the time of an induced abortion, but its acceptance should never be made a prerequisite for the performance of an abortion.

It is important, should sterilization be scheduled as an interval procedure (weeks or months after a pregnancy or abortion) that a woman be advised to use contraception until the time she is to be sterilized. It is possible for conception to have occurred earlier in the cycle in which a sterilization operation is carried out. The doctor would not know that the woman had recently conceived, and this would account for some post-operative pregnancies. It is thus useful, if circumstances allow, to carry out an interval sterilization during or just after menstruation. This is especially so if the woman is not using any contraception.

Sterilization should not be recommended when a marriage is unstable, because sterilization seldom proves to be a stabilizing influence, and reversal may be requested after divorce and remarriage. Inquiry should also be made about the health of the children and the age of the youngest, as the first year of life is still the most dangerous.

During information and counselling sessions, counsellors can assess what the individual already knows about sterilization and family planning so that information gaps can be filled. A significant proportion of couples do not know how sterilization is performed, how it prevents pregnancy, or what happens to the sperm or ova after the vasa or tubes have been obstructed. Some believe sterilization is easily reversed. Many confuse vasectomy with castration.

Clients should be told that sterilization does not affect normal sexual functioning, physical health, or mental health. They should understand the possibility and consequences of failures (i.e. pregnancy). Vasectomy clients must be advised of the importance of using reversible contraception until azoospermia occurs (see page 172).

Prospective clients should know of the benefits and risks of available temporary and permanent methods of contraception. Special attention should be given to failure rates, types of possible complications, specific side-effects, and the suitability of each method for the characteristics and contraceptive needs of the client.

If the individual is prepared and eligible for the sterilization procedure, discussion should include specific information as to what to expect during surgery and what the possible operative, anaesthetic, and post-operative complications and side-effects may be.

Elective sterilization

Sterilization should be made available based on what is best for the individual and not strictly on the criteria of age, parity, or marital status. While these factors may be weighed in judging whether to provide a sterilization, an arbitrary formula based on specific age, parity, or marital criteria is not an adequate basis for providing or denying a sterilization. As long as the individual is not being pressured to have it done, and as long as the person involved is legally competent and has enough information to make this important decision voluntarily, it should be the individual's own decision to undergo sterilization. However, the doctor must remain aware of his or her right to decline a request for an elective procedure. Where the doctor is not convinced that a sterilization is advisable, he or she should be prepared to obtain the opinion of a colleague.

Informed consent

Informed consent is the voluntary decision by an individual for a surgical procedure to be performed after he or she has been fully informed about the procedure and its consequences. The client is considered to be informed when he or she has been given information on and understands the following important points:

1. The exact type of operation, including risks and benefits.

2. Alternative methods of family planning which are available to the individual.

3. If successful, the operation will prevent the client from having any more children.

4. Sterilization should be considered permanent.

5. There are occasional failures subsequent to the operation.

6. Any individual may refuse consent to sterilization without loss of medical or financial benefits.

In many countries a client's signature on an informed consent form is legal authorization for the procedure to be performed. However, a signature on a form is not in itself a guarantee of a free and informed decision. This can only be assured after careful counselling.

The consent form must be readily understandable in the individual's own language. For clients who can read and write, the informed consent form should be read and signed by the client and the attending doctor or his or her delegated assistant. For illiterate clients, a witness chosen by the client should also sign or mark the form.

Consent should not be obtained when physical or emotional factors may compromise a client's ability to make a carefully considered decision about contraception – specifically, when a client is sedated, when a woman is in labour, and when a woman is experiencing stress before, during, or after a pregnancy-related event or procedure. If a woman is to be sterilized immediately post-partum or at caesarean section, the consent should be obtained, where possible, long before the birth. Steps must be taken to make sure that no person in any way coerces the woman into being sterilized.

Male sterilization (vasectomy)

Vasectomy is a simple, minor surgical procedure. The vas deferens can usually be readily identified by palpation before incising the skin, the scrotum heals rapidly, and the operation has the advantage that its success can be checked, though only after at least 12 ejaculations.

Pre-operative assessment and preparation

Local skin infections or genital tract infections must be treated before a vasectomy is performed. Local conditions that can make a vasectomy difficult or increase risks include: a varicocele, a large hydrocele, local scar tissue, an inguinal hernia, filariasis, cryptorchidism, previous scrotal surgery, and an intrascrotal mass. Some systemic disorders require special precautions and possible hospitalization for the vasectomy. These include severe anaemia, bleeding disorders, diabetes, and heart disease.

Pre-operative information and instructions are important to ensure the safety of the procedure and to inform and reassure the client. The following points should be covered: steps of the operation, instructions for wound care, what pain and discomfort the client might experience, common complications and what to do/where to go if they arise, how to use any medicine prescribed after surgery, when the client can return to work and when he can resume sexual relations. There is no strict rule when sexual intercourse can be resumed after the operation. The client's own feeling of well-being will be an adequate regulator. Clients should be advised of the need to use some form of efficient contraception for at least 20 ejaculations.

To prepare for the operation, the client should wash the operative site with soap and water and bring with him a clean, tight-fitting undergarment to act as a scrotal support. Shaving or clipping of hair at the operative site is optional. However, if hair obstructs the operation, it should be removed. Clipping is preferred to shaving. If the client shaves or clips the pubic and scrotal hairs, he should be told to do so carefully, without abrading the skin.

Some doctors wash the operative area with an antiseptic, such as chlorhexidine. At a minimum, the site should be thoroughly washed with soap and water. In all sterilization procedures, an antiseptic agent should be applied to the skin immediately before the operation. Care should be taken to avoid materials that will irritate the skin or cause discomfort. Water-based iodine preparations such as povidone-iodine or, alternatively, chlorhexidine, are excellent antiseptic agents for the genitalia. Alcohol-containing preparations should not be applied to the sensitive genitalia.

The doctor must scrub up as for any surgical procedure and wear surgical gloves. Even if the no-touch technique is used in which only properly sterilized instruments touch the vas, sterile gloves must be worn. Gowns, caps, and masks need not be worn for vasectomy procedures when other aseptic practices are strictly followed.

Technique

The information given here is not intended as a practical guide to carrying out the operation, but rather as an outline of important steps. A full description of the technique can be found in the IPPF handbook *Vasectomy*.

The most important step is to locate, isolate, and firmly anchor the vas before injecting the local anaesthetic and making the incision. The vas should be identified in the upper portion of the scrotum where it is easily palpated. To separate the vas from the rest of the spermatic cord, the operator gently pulls the testis downward to draw the cord out. Manipulation of the vas should be gentle to avoid discomfort.

Anaesthesia

Vasectomy is preferably performed using local anaesthesia. General anaesthesia exposes the client to unnecessary risk and is indicated only in a complicated procedure associated with scrotal abnormality or other surgery.

Adequate anaesthesia of the skin can be obtained by raising a small wheal with subcutaneous lignocaine. The needle is then introduced deeper, and 2-5 ml is injected as close as possible to the vas, which is held away from the other structures of the cord. Adrenaline must not be used with the local anaesthetic because such infiltration may cause prolonged ischaemia and post-operative ache of the testis.

Delivery and cutting of the vas

The operator may make one or two incisions. The two-incision technique is recommended for all those not experienced in vasectomy. When using the single-incision technique, the operator must carefully identify each vas to avoid operating twice on the same structure.

With the vas firmly held, a vertical incision 0.5-1 cm is made in the skin and the deeper dartos layer. The tissues are separated with mosquito forceps and the vas is grasped with tissue forceps (Fig. 12).

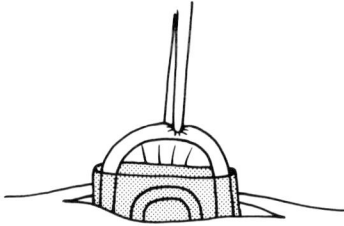

Fig. 12. *Vas with its mesentery being pulled out of its sheath.*

The vas sheath is incised in an avascular area until the pearly-white vas is seen. To make sure that the sheath is fully divided, the incision is carried slightly into the vas itself. The exposed vas is held with a second forceps (Fig. 13) or with a specially designed vasectomy hook.

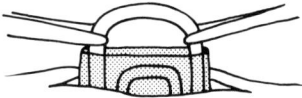

Fig. 13. *Segment of vas to be excised clamped at both ends.*

If the man experiences discomfort at any point, the operator should inject additional local anaesthetic into the vas sheath or surrounding tissue.

Once the vas is isolated, it is divided. The cut ends are fulgurated with a needle electrode or ligated to occlude the vas. It is not necessary to remove a segment of the vas, although most operators do to increase the separation of the cut ends. Before concluding the operation, the ends of the vas are pulled out (when ligatures are used) to look for bleeders which will have oozed blood with the relaxed tension. When a single-incision technique is used, it is useful to leave the ligatures long on the first vas until the second has been isolated. Some operators create a fascial barrier between the cut ends by pulling the sheath over one end of the vas and suturing it. This is to prevent or minimize re-canalization.

Modifications of the technique

A recent modification of the standard technique performed by a few operators is to leave open the proximal (testicular) end of the vas (open-ended vasectomy). This appears to reduce symptoms of epididymal congestion. Some doctors report increased failure rates, but the technique may improve the reversal success rate.

A modified technique developed in the People's Republic of China may reduce the incidence of haematomas by not using a scalpel. Two different instruments are used — an extracutaneous ringed forceps for fixing the vas, and a sharp-pointed curved haemostat as a dissecting forceps. After the vas is grasped with three fingers and infiltrated with a local anaesthetic, it is encircled and stabilized with the ringed forceps without penetrating the skin. The sharp haemostat punctures the scrotal skin down to the vas, and by spreading the blades of the haemostat, all layers from the skin to the vas are separated, exposing the vas. It is delivered through the puncture opening, and the ringed forceps released and reapplied to the vas.

Closing the incision

After the operation, the operator should carefully check for bleeders and return the vas to the scrotum. Small skin incisions are not sutured by some surgeons who feel that avoiding sutures helps prevent haematoma formation. If the skin is sutured, an absorbable catgut suture should be used.

The wound should be covered with a sterile dressing, held in place by adhesive tape or a scrotal support. The man should not bathe or wash the scrotum for 24 hours; he can then remove the dressing. He should be told that any skin sutures will fall out by themselves. Routine use of prophylactic antibiotics is not recommended.

It is common to get a dragging sensation in the testes after the operation, and a tight scrotal support will ease this feeling. This support should be worn for up to a week, or less if the man himself feels it is no longer needed. He should be told to avoid heavy lifting for two days.

Complications and side-effects

Immediate complications

Allergic reactions to the antiseptic or the local anaesthetic are rare, especially if the anaesthetic is lignocaine. Toxic reactions to lignocaine may be manifested as convulsions. In such cases, sedation and controlled ventilation are required.

In rare instances traction or manipulation of the vas, spermatic cord, testes or bowel may produce stimulation of the vagus nerve with hypotension and bradycardia.

Complications in the first week

Short-term post-operative side-effects are minor and usually subside within one or two weeks. The most common complaints are swelling of the scrotal tissue, bruising, and pain. While these symptoms generally disappear without treatment, ice packs, a scrotal support, and simple analgesics provide relief.

The common short-term complications of vasectomy that require active treatment are post-operative *bleeding* and *infection*. Looseness of the scrotal skin and a persistent bleeding vessel can combine to form a slowly enlarging haematoma that can attain the size of a grapefruit. Haemostasis must be absolute at the end of the procedure. The risk of post-operative bleeding can be reduced further by ensuring that the man rests for some time after the operation and refrains from heavy manual work for two days.

Small haematomas usually resorb completely with bedrest. The treatment of large haematomas depends on the situation and the judgment of the operator. Drainage may be appropriate if the scrotum is tense and painful or the haematoma is infected.

Infection is usually less common than haematoma formation. Most are superficial skin infections, usually around the site of the incision or the skin suture. Treatment depends on the severity of the infection. Superficial infections at the wound site often heal without treatment. If pus has formed, it should be allowed to drain freely, if necessary by removal of a skin suture.

If antibiotics are required, cultures should be taken, if facilities exist, and a broad-spectrum antibiotic should be used. In rare instances an abscess may need to be opened and drained.

Tetanus infection following vasectomy has occurred. Strict aseptic technique combined with proper disinfection and sterilization of equipment are the most appropriate methods for preventing tetanus.

Granulomas may form at the site of the occluded vas. The majority of granulomas noticed by patients are symptomless and respond to conservative treatment with simple analgesics or anti-inflammatory drugs. Infrequently, a persistent and painful granuloma may necessitate surgical intervention.

Long-term complications

Large-scale studies in men have consistently shown no adverse effects of vasectomy. Specifically, they show no increased incidence of heart disease, hypertension, or other signs of atherosclerosis. A large proportion of men develop antisperm antibodies in the first year after vasectomy. The significance of these antibodies is unknown. However, long-term studies of a number of conditions that could be caused by antibodies have so far failed to identify any adverse consequences.

Medico-legal and social problems may arise if a man fathers a child after vasectomy. A seminal analysis can be done in all such cases. The doctor should be sensitive to the possibility that the woman may have had another sexual partner. If the seminal fluid is sperm-free, the doctor should make his or her personal decision whether to divulge the information and to whom. If sperm are present, the vasa will require to be re-explored.

Checking the operation

Varying advice has been given concerning the number of ejaculations that should occur or the length of time that should elapse before investigating the semen. At least 12 ejaculations should take place before testing for the first sperm-free specimen.

Two sperm-free specimens should be obtained after vasectomy before saying that the operation was a success. It is not necessary to perform a full seminal analysis. All that is required is to collect the semen, place several loopfuls on a slide under a coverslip and, with the low-power lens of a microscope, determine if there are any sperm present. It is not necessary to count sperm or to comment on their motility or normality. The man should use effective contraception until two sperm-free specimens have been obtained.

172

In situations where it is not possible to rely on the man to return for investigations, or facilities for doing a semen examination are not available, 20 condoms should be provided, to be used with the first 20 acts of sexual intercourse after vasectomy.

Female sterilization

Female sterilization is accomplished by occluding the uterine tubes. The operation is simple, and it is rarely necessary to employ a large incision. To reach the tubes, most doctors use an abdominal approach. There are many ways of occluding the tubes. Those methods which are most effective may be more difficult to reverse if this is requested later. A brief description of the various approaches and methods of occlusion can be found in the IPPF booklet, *Female Sterilization.*

Because clients may change their minds, surgeons should consider using procedures that have an acceptable efficacy rate, but that cause the least damage to the tubes, particularly in young and in low-parity women. However, it is important that the woman and her partner accept the operation as permanent when it is done.

Pre-operative assessment and preparation

As with any surgery, proper medical screening of clients is critical. A physical examination, medical history, and appropriate laboratory work are required.

Active pelvic infection and pregnancy are absolute temporary contra-indications to female sterilization. Conditions that may increase the risks or difficulty of female sterilization include: heart disease, irregular pulse, respiratory problems, hypertension, diabetes, bleeding disorders, severe nutritional disorders, severe anaemia, mass in the pelvic area, pelvic or abdominal adhesions, and obesity. When any of these conditions is present the operation should only be performed in properly equipped medical facilities.

Additional conditions that may increase the risks for post-partum women include: puerperal fever, ante-partum or post-partum haemorrhage, prolonged or difficult labour, and infection or an increased risk of infection after delivery.

Pre-operative information and instructions are important to ensure the safety of the procedure and to inform and reassure the client. The outline of what should be discussed has been set out under 'Male sterilization' (see page 167). Apart from the fact that the male operation is not immediately effective, the information and instructions apply broadly to the woman as well.

To prepare for the operation, the client should wash the operative site with soap and water and wear clean, loose clothing when coming for the operation. The client should be told to fast for eight hours before the operation.

Shaving or clipping of hair at the operative site is optional, but hair should be removed if it obstructs the operating area. Clipping is preferred to shaving. The site should be thoroughly washed with soap and water. An antiseptic agent should be applied to the skin before surgery. Water-based iodine preparations such as povidone-iodine or, alternatively, chlorhexidine are excellent antiseptic agents for both abdomen and the genitals. Alcohol-containing preparations should not be applied to the sensitive genitalia; however, a solution of iodine and alcohol is an excellent antiseptic for the abdominal skin.

The operator must scrub up as for any surgical procedure and wear surgical gloves. Surgical mask, cap, and gown are also required.

Anaesthesia

General and spinal anaesthesia may cause serious problems more easily than properly administered local anaesthesia. Whenever general anaesthesia is used, there could be the possibility of anoxia, cardiac arrhythmia, bronchial aspiration and other complications. Local anaesthesia makes the monitoring of the woman safer. There is a more rapid recovery after local anaesthesia because there is little drowsiness or respiratory depression, and no sore throat or laryngitis from intubation. No matter what type of anaesthesia is used, monitoring and recording of vital signs must take place before, during and after the operation until the client is discharged.

Because the client is fully conscious during properly administered local anaesthesia, pre-operative preparation is extremely important to ensure the co-operation of the client and to minimize her fears. The conscious client is an excellent monitor of analgesic effects and can provide early indications of a complication.

Local anaesthetic regimens consist of three types of drugs: systemic agents that sedate the woman and block pain, local anaesthetics that relieve pain at the incision site, and systemic drugs that prevent nausea or disturbances of heart function.

It is essential that the operator wait for analgesia and anaesthesia to take effect. Layer-by-layer infiltration should be done slowly. Ten to 15 ml of 1% lignocaine is generally adequate. If only 2% lignocaine is available, dilute to 1% to achieve better effectiveness and safety within the maximum dose limits. The operator starts from the skin so that by the time the lower levels are injected, the skin is already numb. With laparoscopy, infiltrate the abdominal wall layers down to the peritoneum in a diamond-shaped pattern until a local field block is established. A gentle massage of the incision site helps to spread the anaesthetic. Before making an incision the adequacy of the anaesthesia can be tested by pinching the skin with an Allis clamp and by talking to the client. To achieve local analgesia for the tubes, 5 ml of 1% lignocaine is applied to each tube. If the client still experiences discomfort, the operator should increase systemic analgesia or local anaesthesia. However, the maximum safe dose of lignocaine (without adrenaline) is 5 mg per kg body weight.

Approaches to the tubes

Minilaparotomy

In the minilaparotomy approach, the uterine (fallopian) tubes are occluded through an abdominal incision measuring 2 to 5 cm. Minilaparotomy is usually carried out under local anaesthesia with light sedation. It can be performed immediately after abortion or within the first 48 hours after uncomplicated childbirth or abortion. It may also be performed any time once the uterus has returned to its normal size in the pelvis. Minilaparotomy may be difficult when the woman is obese or when her tubes have been damaged by infection or surgery and are immobilized by pelvic adhesions.

Interval sterilization

With interval minilaparotomy the bladder should be emptied by voiding immediately before the operation or by catheterization, and the woman put into the lithotomy position. A pelvic examination must be done. If the uterus is not anteverted, this position should be achieved by bimanual manipulation or by inserting a uterine manipulator into the uterus through the vagina (Fig. 14).

Proper placement of the incision is essential to avoid difficulty or injury. In interval procedures, if the incision is too high the tubes will

175

be difficult to reach, and if it is too low, the bladder may be damaged. A transverse incision 2 to 5 cm in length is made over the uterine fundus, usually slightly above the pubic hairline (Fig. 14). The

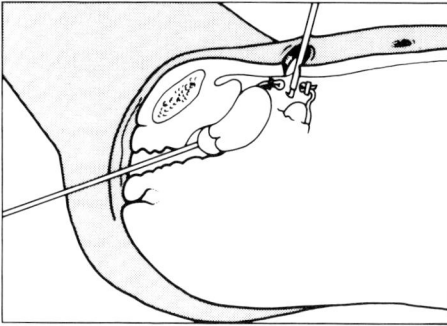

Fig. 14. *Interval minilaparotomy.*

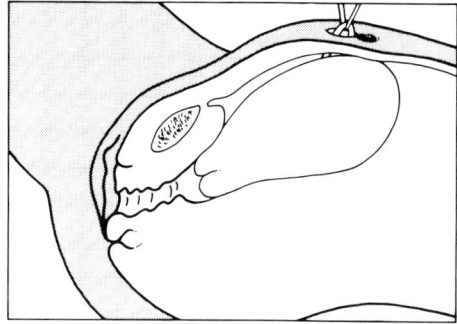

Fig. 15. *Post-partum minilaparotomy.*

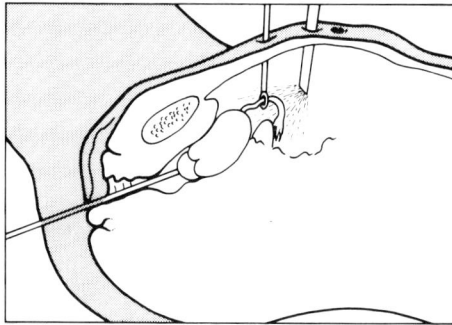

Fig. 16. *Laparoscopic sterilization.*

subcutaneous tissues are separated through blunt dissection to minimize bleeding. The fascia is then elevated and incised. The underlying rectus muscles are separated bluntly, and the peritoneum is very carefully lifted, inspected, and opened. The patient may then be placed in a Trendelenburg position (not exceeding 20°). Using the uterine elevator, the operator moves the uterus to bring each uterine tube under the abdominal incision. Part of each tube is lifted out of the abdomen with a clamp, hook, or the operator's finger, occluded and replaced in the abdomen. All manipulation should be very gentle and care should be taken to identify the tube properly by observing the tubal fimbria. The abdominal incision is closed with absorbable or non-absorbable sutures.

176

Post-partum sterilization

Compared with the uterus of a woman who has not recently been pregnant, the uterus immediately after delivery is high in the abdomen and the uterine tubes are easily accessible — especially within 48 hours of the birth. For immediate post-partum minilaparotomy, a 1.5 to 3 cm half-circle incision is made within the lower rim of the umbilicus (Fig. 15). The technique is similar to the interval procedure except that no uterine manipulator is used, and lithotomy and Trendelenburg positions are not required. Extra care should be exercised so that the bowels are not inadvertently incised when entering the peritoneal cavity or vessels torn when handling the tubes. Bladder injury is virtually eliminated. Because the abdominal wall is loose, the incision site can be moved to the side, above the area where the tube lies. Alternatively, the uterus can be moved by pushing it gently to bring the uterine tubes towards the incision.

When local anaesthesia with light sedation is used, the routine hospital stay for a normal vaginal delivery is not extended because of the sterilization. In some hospitals, discharge occurs less than 24 hours after delivery.

Laparotomy

Laparotomy by definition is an incision larger than 5 cm. General or regional anaesthesia is usually necessary. Instead of bringing the tubes to the incision, as with interval minilaparotomy, the instruments are introduced into the abdominal cavity to reach the tubes. Obese women may require a larger incision to expose the pelvic organs as may those who have had pelvic disease or previous pelvic surgery. Laparotomy incisions may prolong recovery time and are more visible than minilaparotomy incisions when healed. Laparotomy incisions are also associated with a greater risk of complications.

Laparoscopy

Laparoscopic sterilization involves inserting a laparoscope, essentially a telescope combined with a light, into the abdomen. The design of some laparoscopes permits operating instruments to be inserted through them to enter the abdomen. If such a laparoscope is used, one incision is sufficient. Otherwise a second puncture is made in the lower abdomen for ancillary instruments to manipulate organs or occlude the tubes. To begin the procedure, place the woman in a Trendelenburg position (not exceeding 15°) and insufflate the abdomen with carbon dioxide, nitrous oxide, or room air. The volume should be the minimum necessary to visualize the pelvic structures (usually 1-2 litres). A 1-1.5 cm sub-umbilical incision is made and a sharp trocar and cannula (sleeve) is pushed through the abdominal wall into the abdominal cavity. The trocar is removed and the laparoscope inserted through the cannula. To make the approach to the uterine tubes easier, uterine manipulation, as used in minilaparotomy, is commonly employed (Fig. 16).

Open laparoscopy, which combines the minilaparotomy and standard laparoscopy approaches, was developed to reduce the chances of bowel or blood vessel injury when the insufflator needle or the trocar is inserted into the abdomen. A small incision is made either through the lower part of the umbilicus or just below, and the abdominal cavity is opened under direct vision. Most surgeons use the standard (closed) technique, outlined above.

The laparoscopic route may be used with general or local anaesthesia. However, the equipment is expensive and delicate, and the surgeon should be skilled and specially trained in laparoscopy. Because the punctures in the abdominal cavity are 'blind' with the standard technique, women selected should ideally be free of abdominal scars and should not have a history of severe pelvic or peritoneal infection. Gross obesity makes the procedure much more difficult. Severe heart or lung disease are also contra-indications. There is a risk of intra-abdominal trauma, including visceral insufflation and perforation, arterial tears, and puncture of the vessels. Bowel and bladder burns were a concern with unipolar cautery, which has largely been replaced by bipolar cautery, silastic rings, and clips.

The vaginal approach

With colpotomy or culdoscopy, the tubes are reached through an incision made high in the vagina posterior to the cervix. Vaginal approaches are not as safe or effective as minilaparotomy or laparoscopy. They are generally more difficult to perform and require more training. Owing to the higher complication and failure rates associated with vaginal approaches, colpotomy and culdoscopy

178

should only be used in exceptional cases, such as in conjunction with vaginal surgery and at clinics or hospitals well equipped for major gynaecological surgery.

The transcervical approach

Hysteroscopic techniques require a great deal of skill, and the equipment is expensive and delicate. Because of this and high failure rates, they are not currently recommended.

Non-surgical sterilization is still experimental. It includes closing the uterine tubes by introducing a chemical (such as a phenol compound, quinacrine, or methylcyanoacrylate) or another substance (a plug) through the cervix.

Methods of occlusion

Once the surgeon has access to the uterine tubes, the tubes can be occluded in a number of ways.

Tubal ligation

The Pomeroy technique is the most widely used ligation technique. A loop of each uterine tube is ligated in two places with a plain catgut suture, and the top of the loop is resected. This permits the ends to separate when the suture is absorbed. The technique has low failure and complication rates. It is preferred over the Madlener technique (where the ligated loop is not excised), fimbriectomy (which is totally irreversible), and salpingectomy (a much bigger operation). The Pomeroy operation is simpler to perform than the Uchida technique (where the uterine end of the cut tube is buried in the mesosalpinx), and the Irving technique (where the proximal end of the cut tube is buried in the wall of the uterus and the distal end in the mesosalpinx). Both these more extensive operations are more effective than the Pomeroy, and, in addition, the Irving technique is useful when sterilization is performed at the same time as a caesarean section.

Occlusive bands or rings

Falope rings (Yoon bands) are applied with a special applicator, usually through a laparoscope or the Laprocator, but rings can also be applied during minilaparotomy. A loop of the isthmic portion of

179

the tube is grasped, and a small silastic band is placed over the loop, rendering it avascular. A ring destroys 1-3 cm of tube. Adhesions or tubal hypertrophy make the application of silastic rings difficult. The tube may be cut, resulting in bleeding that may require a ring on each transected end or further surgery to obtain haemostasis. Rings carry the risk of tearing the mesosalpinx and its vessels, with possible bleeding.

Occlusive clips

Occlusive clips destroy the smallest segment of tube, about 6-8 mm, and offer the greatest potential for reversal. They are effective in the hands of skilled surgeons who can place the clip fully over the isthmus of the tube, 1.5-2.5 cm from the uterus. Placement further from the uterus, on the ampullary portion of the tube, has resulted in failures. If the operator is uncertain whether the entire tube has been captured by the clip, a second one may be placed immediately adjacent to the first. Ectopic pregnancies have been rare when there is failure of a clip, and this may prove to be an important advantage. Clips are usually applied by laparoscope, but can also be used during minilaparotomy.

The Filshie (Nottingham) clip is made of titanium metal with a silicone rubber lining that continues to compress the tube after the open end is locked closed. Compression forces are sufficient to occlude the tube when it is thickened or enlarged, and even when the ovarian or round ligament may also have been captured by the clip.

The Hulka-Clemens (Rocket) clip is a spring-loaded clip consisting of two plastic jaws with interlocking teeth. The jaws are held together by a gold-plated stainless steel spring, which is pushed forward to lock the clip in place. Compression forces are less than for the Filshie clip and it is best suited for normal-sized tubes. It must be placed on a right angle to the tube to be effective. Some operators routinely use two Hulka-Clemens clips on each tube.

Other clips have been associated with high failure rates and are no longer used.

Tubal diathermy (thermocoagulation)

With tubal diathermy a unipolar or bipolar electric current is applied to the tube until it is burned. This method is traditionally used in conjunction with the laparoscope. About 3-4 cm of each tube is coagulated. Bipolar coagulation is considered safer than unipolar coagulation, but it has been associated with more failures than unipolar. Both methods have been associated with higher ectopic pregnancy rates following surgery. The possibility of reversal depends on the extent of tubal destruction, but is usually poor.

Hysterectomy

Hysterectomy, removal of the uterus, carries a much higher risk of morbidity and mortality than other forms of sterilization and should not be used unless the woman has a gynaecological disease that requires removal of the uterus.

Complications

Immediate complications

The immediate complications of sterilization are few and are usually related to the scale of the operation and the type of anaesthesia used. With both interval and immediate post-partum minilaparotomy, during the surgery bleeding from the mesosalpinx or injury to the bowel may occur. Bladder and uterine injuries are generally related to interval procedures.

Laparoscopy may cause certain complications that do not occur with minilaparotomy or laparotomy. Insufflation of the abdomen can lead to gas embolism, subcutaneous emphysema, or respiratory or cardiac arrest. Lacerations of blood vessels or abdominal organs can occur from the insufflation needle or the trocar.

Pelvic infection can occur after tubal occlusion, and predisposing factors include a history of previous sepsis or surgery, or a pelvic infection undiagnosed before surgery. A careful pelvic examination is essential before interval procedures.

Wound infections are usually, but not always, minor and can be frequent if the umbilicus is not thoroughly scrubbed to remove all debris. An effective topical antiseptic should be used before laparoscopy or minilaparotomy.

Some complications are unique to ring or band application or to diathermy (see above).

Some discomfort is common after surgery. Women undergoing laparoscopy may feel chest and shoulder pain for one to two days because of insufflation of the abdomen and trapped gas afterwards.

Lower abdominal pain is common and usually relieved by aspirin or other mild analgesics.

Among tubal occlusion techniques, rings (bands) appear to cause more post-operative pain than others. This may occur because nerve endings in the avascular loop do not die for several days. Applying lignocaine to the tubes during ring or band sterilization reduces pain temporarily.

There is a small but definite risk of anaesthetic problems during sterilization procedures. These include cardiac arrhythmias, inhalation of gastric contents, and hypersensitivity reactions to the anaesthetic used. In some countries anaesthetic complications are the main cause of the rare deaths associated with female sterilization.

Late complications

All occlusion methods have a failure rate, however slight, and these pregnancies carry a high risk of being ectopic. These require immediate attention and usually surgical intervention.

Causes of pregnancy include:
— The woman may have become pregnant in the same cycle in which the operation was carried out (pre-operative conception). This is not a sterilization failure since she was already pregnant.
— Failure to operate on the appropriate structure. This is an operator error and usually involves the round ligament. It can be avoided by following the tube to the fimbrial end for positive identification.
— Equipment failure.
— The ends of the uterine tube reconnect spontaneously (recanalization). This may occur with any technique used.
— The uterine end of the tube may develop a fistula with the peritoneal cavity. This may permit sperm to pass, and the resulting pregnancy is often ectopic.

The approach to the tubes can also affect failure rates. Minilaparotomy may be slightly more effective than laparoscopy. With laparoscopy, equipment problems and surgical errors, especially by surgeons just learning the technique, account partially for the slightly higher pregnancy rates.

Some gynaecologists believe that a sterilization procedure increases the risk of subsequent dysfunctional uterine bleeding. However, objective assessment of this condition, which includes prospective analysis of the quality and quantity of subsequent menses, has failed to demonstrate any change up to two years following the operation. Many reported changes in menstrual patterns after sterilization are actually caused by discontinuing oral contraceptives or IUDs.

Choice of procedure

Selection of the approach to the tubes, as well as the method of occlusion, is influenced by multiple factors. Minilaparotomy can be performed by non-specialized doctors or appropriately trained and supervised nurses or paramedical personnel. However, back-up facilities should be easily available. The instruments are inexpensive and easy to maintain.

From the point of view of convenience and acceptability to the woman, laparoscopy is popular in some countries, but the complexity of the equipment and the surgical skill required are drawbacks. Laparoscopy demands a supply of insufflating gas, electricity, and facilities for maintaining delicate equipment. Although complications are uncommon, when they do occur they are more likely to be serious, requiring experienced surgical intervention. To be used safely, the laparoscope must be used frequently, so that the skills of the operating-room team are kept at a high level. Trainees in laparoscopy should be doctors with a minimum of three years' experience in abdominal and pelvic surgery.

The timing of the sterilization procedure also influences the choice of approach. In the immediate post-partum period, minilaparotomy is the preferred approach, with occlusion of the tubes by the Pomeroy technique, or sometimes with clips or rings. With proper selection criteria, post-partum sterilization within 48 hours entails no more risk than interval sterilization and has several advantages. Technically, there is easy access to the uterus because of its size and abdominal position. There is less risk of bladder injury, usually the incision is smaller, and less local anaesthetic is needed. However, engorged tubes and the mesosalpinx will bleed more if injured during an immediate post-partum procedure. Equipment needs are less (no uterine elevator or special table with drop end). Combining post-partum and post-operative convalescence means there is no additional hospitalization when local anaesthesia with light sedation is used. This is more economical and also helps those women who find it difficult to return to the hospital some time after the baby's birth because of obligations

183

at home or at work. However, special care is necessary to ensure that the woman's decision for the sterilization was not made under the stress of the end of the pregnancy or during labour. Also, when post-partum sterilization is discussed, the possibility of death in its first year of the infant just born should be kept in mind. This is a particular hazard in developing countries.

Sterilization during caesarean section is also convenient, but it should never be used as the sole indication for a caesarean section, because of the increased risk of morbidity.

Reversal

Sterilization should be considered permanent, but unforeseen events such as the death of a child, divorce, remarriage, or the desire for more children, may lead a sterilization acceptor to seek a reversal procedure. The current demand for sterilization reversal appears to be low, but the number of reversal requests is likely to increase as the number of sterilization acceptors world-wide increases, and the mean age and parity of acceptors fall.

Effective handling of reversal requests is important. Failure to counsel requests for reversal adequately may have adverse effects on a programme far beyond the individual concerned. Whenever possible, adequate facilities for attempting reversals should be available to those who have chosen sterilization. Reversal services are better provided by a few highly specialized, well-equipped centres than a broad group of local institutions.

It is extremely important that while the possibility of reversal is recognized, and while an effort is made to create realistic services in this field, a guarantee of reversibility should never be given to any man or woman undergoing sterilization. Over-optimistic estimates of success of reversibility should not be used as an inducement towards acceptance of sterilization.

Counselling for reversal

With both male and female sterilization reversal requests, it is important to understand the reasons for the request and to explain all the factors involved carefully, including:

— Reversal involves complicated and difficult surgery, requiring great skill.

184

— Of those individuals who request reversal, some may be inappropriate because of age or fertility impairments, such as infertility of the spouse or insufficient length of tube or vas for reversal.

— Even for clients who are suitable candidates for reversal, functional success (pregnancy), as opposed to anatomical success, cannot be assured, even when the reversal procedure is performed by a highly skilled surgeon using the most advanced surgical techniques.

— Reversal procedures are costly.

The risks of the procedure must be fully explained. The risks of vasectomy reversal are much the same as for vasectomy. However, haematoma is more common after reversal and there is a greater chance of infection.

For female reversal surgery, the risks include those usually associated with major abdominal and pelvic surgery. The most important risks are the risks of general or spinal anaesthesia and of deep-vein thrombosis and pulmonary embolism. There is also an increased risk of ectopic pregnancy after reversal. In recent studies ectopic pregnancies occurred in 5% of women after electrocoagulation reversal compared with 2% or less for reversal of other methods.

Selection of clients for reversal

Screening is an integral part of providing reversal services. Evaluation of the health and potential fertility of the couple is important before recommending a client for restorative surgery. This should include a physical examination, medical history, laboratory screening, review of the sterilization operative report, and evaluation of the partner's fertility. Consideration should be given to the client's age, since fertility declines with age; for women, obstetric risks of further pregnancies need careful assessment. The length of time since the sterilization can also be important. Vasectomy reversal is usually more successful when done not more than 10 years after the vasectomy.

For female reversals, most surgeons will not operate if less than 4 cm of viable tube remains. If a female client decides to proceed with a reversal following counselling, a laparoscopy should be done to determine the condition of the tube when sterilization was by coagulation or when the operative report is unavailable or ambiguous. Some surgeons perform a hysterosalpingogram to ascertain the integrity of the uterus and the proximal part of the tube.

Results

Male

Although the anatomical success of reversal in the male (with the appearance of sperm in the semen) is greater than in the female, experienced surgeons have reported restoring fertility, as measured by a full-term pregnancy, in an average of only 50% of cases, and success rates for less experienced surgeons are probably lower. Magnification is an important factor in a successful reversal, and pregnancy rates as high as 82% have been reported after use of a microscope in the hands of a highly skilled surgeon.

The success of reversal depends not only upon the skill and technique of the surgeon, but also upon the original procedure done, the length and position of the segment of vas removed, the method of occlusion of the vas and the time elapsed since the vasectomy.

Female

Methods of tubal occlusion that cause the least damage to the tubes have the best chance of being reversed. Because clips damage the smallest length of tube, they are the most easily reversed, and intrauterine pregnancy rates average 90%. Results of reversals by ring have averaged 72%. Ligation techniques have pregnancy rates on reversal of between 35% and 73%, with the average being 56%. Results of reversals of electrocoagulation have ranged from 16% to 70% with the average being 52%. Success rates must be interpreted with caution, however, since many women seeking reversal, especially after electrocoagulation, are screened out as poor candidates for reversal surgery (up to 70% in some studies). Also, many surgeons who have low success rates do not publish their results.

Methods of reversing sterilization

Sterilization reversal is achieving greater success since the introduction of microsurgery. Microsurgery improves operative results by minimizing tissue trauma and assuring accurate dissection, realignment and suturing. Microsurgery employs a combination of the following techniques:

— use of magnification (loupe, operating microscope)
— electrocoagulation to minimize bleeding
— accurate realignment of tubal segments and placement of sutures
— use of fine, non-tissue-reactive suture material and fine needles
— special care to avoid leaving foreign matter
— constant irrigation of the operating site to keep tissues moist

For female reversal procedures, the use of loupes or operating microscopes give similar pregnancy rates. Loupes, however, are considerably less expensive than operating microscopes.

More important than the type of magnification used, the tissue handling, meticulous haemostasis, the use of special instruments and fine sutures to permit careful dissection, and accurate tissue approximation are the major factors in restoring anatomical continuity.

For clients who are poor candidates for reversal surgery, *in-vitro* fertilization, if available, may be presented as an alternative. However, the success rate is low, less than 20%, and the cost is 10 times that of reversal surgery.

IMAP Statement on Voluntary Sterilization*

Introduction

Voluntary surgical sterilization has become an extremely popular and well-established contraceptive procedure, providing the most effective protection against pregnancy for couples desiring no more children. It offers many advantages over other contraceptive methods in that it is a once-only procedure which eliminates the risk of unwanted pregnancy and the sequelae of induced abortion almost completely. It does not entail regular check-ups or the need for or expense of continued contraceptive supplies, and does not rely on the sustained motivation of the user for its effectiveness. Also, the risk of complications is small if the procedure is performed according to accepted medical standards.

*This statement is valid for the methods of male and female sterilization described. IPPF reserves the right to amend this statement in the light of further developments in the field of voluntary sterilization when sufficient scientific information becomes available.

Counselling

Counselling is an important component of any family planning programme. It is particularly important in the case of voluntary sterilization where the individual concerned is accepting a permanent form of contraception. The counsellor should be trained in counselling techniques and have full knowledge about sterilization and all other methods of contraception. Counselling should include (*a*) a discussion of all contraceptive methods available, including their risks and benefits; (*b*) emphasis on the expected permanent nature of the operation and the small risk of failure; (*c*) discussion of all aspects of the various procedures of sterilization and types of anaesthetic available.

Counselling should ensure voluntary, informed consent. Wherever possible, an adequate time interval should be allowed after counselling before the actual procedure is carried out. The person concerned should understand that he or she can change the decision at any time before the operation. Even though the partner's consent is not obligatory, it is advisable that both partners be counselled, irrespective of which one has the operation. A consent form should be signed by the person undergoing the procedure.

Female sterilization can be done as an interval procedure, post-partum, or at the time of an abortion. However, the decision to be sterilized should where possible be made a reasonable time beforehand and not at a time of emotional stress, including that of labour or abortion. No woman should be forced to have a sterilization in order to have an abortion.

Techniques of sterilization

When sterilization is being considered by the couple, many factors are involved in the decision as to which partner should be sterilized. Often it is simply a matter of agreed preference. Clinically, vasectomy is preferred because the technique is simpler and safer.

Anaesthesia

Usually both male and female sterilization can be carried out under a local anaesthetic with mild sedation. However, in some circumstances a general anaesthetic may be required. Whenever a general anaesthetic is given there are important rules to be followed. The patient should be in the hands of a health professional trained in anaesthesia. Fasting for at least six hours pre-operatively is essential. Intubation and positive-pressure ventilation are recommended. Anaesthesia remains the most important cause of morbidity and mortality associated with female sterilization operations. Equipment for emergency resuscitation must always be available.

Vasectomy

This is a simple operation which can be performed as an outpatient procedure. When carried out under a local anaesthetic and using a strict aseptic technique, it should have no risk of mortality. The operation is not immediately effective and another method of contraception is needed for a period of time, usually until approximately 15 ejaculations have taken place.

Female sterilization

Post-partum tubal occlusion remains a widely used method of female sterilization. During the past decade new approaches to female sterilization have been developed which allow programmes to offer interval sterilization procedures. Of these, two have become most common, namely laparoscopy and minilaparotomy.

Laparoscopy is a procedure which requires rather costly and sophisticated equipment and training. In most cases, specialist obstetrician-gynaecologists are needed and the procedure is best carried out in hospitals with specialized equipment and staff, where it can also be used for diagnostic purposes. Although complications are uncommon, when they do occur they may be of a serious nature, requiring experienced surgical intervention. With the use of the new technique of open laparoscopy the chance of puncture of abdominal viscera or blood vessels may be minimized.

Minilaparotomy is a relatively simple procedure which is perhaps more appropriate for most family planning programmes. The equipment required is inexpensive and the training is straightforward for any professional capable of doing abdominal surgery. Even health auxiliaries and medical students have been trained to perform this operation.

Both procedures can be carried out under either a local or general anaesthetic, and women can be discharged home the same day as surgery is performed, with relatively minor post-operative symptoms.

Vaginal approaches to the tubes can also be carried out—direct vision through an incision in the vaginal vault (colpotomy) or by insertion of an endoscopic instrument through the posterior vaginal fornix (culdoscopy). However, these approaches may be associated with a higher degree of major complications, including post-operative pelvic infection, than the abdominal route, and are much less frequently used.

Having reached the tubes, there are several ways of occluding or ligating them. These include the use of rings, clips, coagulation, ligation (e.g. the

Pomeroy operation), and the use of sclerosing agents. Studies are currently under way to assess the relative advantages and disadvantages, including failure rates, of each of these methods. For the present the Pomeroy technique seems to be most satisfactory when used with the minilaparotomy procedure, and rings or clips with the laparoscopy procedure. The method of occlusion can have a significant effect on the potential for reversal.

Complications

Vasectomy

Early complications of vasectomy include pain, scrotal haematoma and local infection. Late complications include orchitis, spermatic granuloma, and spontaneous reanastomosis of the vas. Antisperm antibodies can occur, but have not been shown to have deleterious effects in the human. They have been implicated in some cases of infertility after reanastomosis. In some monkey studies they have been associated with atheromatous changes in the blood vessels. Data from human studies so far do not give any evidence of increased risk of cardiovascular disease.

Where vasectomy has not been carried out under strict aseptic conditions, tetanus infection has occasionally occurred.

Female sterilization

Immediate complications include wound infection and haematoma formation, pelvic infection and intraperitoneal haemorrhage. Occasionally trauma to the intra-abdominal viscera and blood vessels can occur. With electrocoagulation, burns to the bowel have occurred. Puncture of large blood vessels and other potentially fatal complications have been reported as major hazards of laparoscopy.

Among the late complications the most important is failure of sterilization with a consequent pregnancy, which may be ectopic. There may be psychological or emotional sequelae associated with regret at having had the operation.

Reversal

As mentioned in the counselling section, sterilization procedures, both male and female, should be regarded as permanent. Nevertheless, up to 1% of those sterilized request a reversal operation at some time for a variety of reasons, mainly remarriage or loss of existing children. There are various techniques for reversal which require specialized training. It is possible to reunite the vas or tube satisfactorily in many cases, but pregnancy rates are lower.

(*Statement by the IPPF International Medical Advisory Panel, October 1982; approved by the IPPF Central Council, November 1982.*)

Chapter 12

Breast Feeding, Fertility and Contraception

Introduction

Lactation is part of the reproductive cycle and, before the use of modern forms of contraception, was the major factor in ensuring adequate intervals between births. This effect was recognized by traditional societies for thousands of years. Until the end of the last century, breast feeding, often for prolonged periods of time, was extremely widespread in almost all countries. In the present century, modern technology has given us the 'formula feed', and this revolutionized the practices of infant feeding. Artificial feeds were first introduced into the more developed countries and it soon became clear that breast feeding had more functions than infant nutrition alone. Breast feeding confers protection against infections in the baby, may prevent some forms of allergic illness, can reinforce the natural feelings of affection which a mother has towards her baby, and lead to a strong mother/infant bonding.

One important function of breast feeding is the inhibition of fertility, and this aspect is the main topic of this chapter. Although breast feeding has had a moderate resurgence in developed countries, mainly among more highly educated mothers, the reverse trend has been seen in many developing countries. This is particularly unfortunate in countries with high infant mortality rates and low rates of contraceptive usage, because the abandonment of breast feeding increases the health risk for the infants and may add a further upward twist to the population growth spiral.

There are three reasons why the relationship between breast feeding and fertility is of interest to those who are involved in family planning. These are:

1. Breast feeding still plays a major role in fertility control in most countries with low contraceptive usage, and it is important that

policies which maximize the contraceptive effect of breast feeding should be encouraged.

2. Breast feeding, with its important roles for infant health and fertility control, must be integrated into family planning programmes. Obtaining a major biological impact upon fertility can only be achieved by understanding the mechanisms by which breast feeding affects fertilility.

3. Contraception for nursing mothers requires special consideration because the chosen methods, in addition to providing effective contraception, must not adversely affect the success of lactation or the health of the infant.

Breast feeding and fertility

There are many epidemiological and endocrine studies which have shown that breast feeding delays the return of menstruation, ovulation and conception after childbirth. The delay in return of post-partum fertility in lactating mothers varies enormously from one community to another, depending on the patterns of breast feeding which in turn can be affected by many factors such as local cultural practices. In developed countries, the additional contraceptive protection offered by breast feeding is often very short, whereas, in traditional communities, breast feeding can postpone menstruation and ovulation for many months, contributing to interbirth intervals which are as long as three years or more. Most mothers who do not breast feed have resumed menstruation and ovulation by four months post-partum, and the first ovulation may be as early as six weeks after delivery. In the absence of contraception or sexual abstinence, 50% of non-lactating mothers will have conceived again by about six or seven months post-partum.

The prolonged postponement of fertility by breast feeding has major practical implications for developing countries. In the mid 1970s it was estimated that, in developing countries, breast feeding offered 38 million couple-years of fertility protection per annum compared with 24 million couple-years per annum for all family planning programmes combined. As breast feeding declines and use of contraceptives increases, this ratio will change, but the important contraceptive effect of breast feeding should not be forgotten. It has been estimated that 25% more births would have occurred in the Philippines if breast feeding there was not at its present levels.

Breast feeding, birth spacing and health

Many studies in developing countries have shown that long inter-birth intervals are associated with improved health for mother and preceding child, as well as for the subsequent child. There is evidence that children born both before and after longer birth intervals do better educationally at school and show higher scores in intelligence tests. A study by the World Fertility Survey in Bangladesh in 1982 showed the advantage of longer birth intervals in preventing infant, toddler and child deaths (Fig. 17). Breast feeding has direct benefits for infant and community health, as well as indirect benefits from the increase in length of birth intervals.

Physiology of lactational amenorrhoea

The inhibition of ovarian activity, which is thought to be the result of suckling, plays a key role in controlling the fertility of lactating women (Fig. 18). Within a few hours of delivery, the sensitivity of the nipple to tactile stimuli increases sharply, ensuring a steady stream of suckling-induced nervous impulses to the hypothalamus. These nervous impulses make the hypothalamus of the breast-feeding mother more sensitive to steroid inhibition. This leads to a reduced secretion of gonadotrophins — especially luteinizing hormone — and absent or reduced ovarian activity. It is true that prolactin levels correlate fairly well with ovarian inhibition, but this may be due more to prolactin being a good marker of suckling activity than to a direct inhibitory effect of prolactin itself.

Determinants of lactational infertility

In order to define the best ways of maximizing the contraceptive effect of breast feeding, it is necessary to identify the clinical events which control ovarian activity. The most important single contributor is suckling itself, although other factors may also be involved.

1. Duration of breast feeding

Studies from many parts of the world have shown a positive relationship between the duration of breast feeding and the length of lactational amenorrhoea. Because the phase of amenorrhoea is the

INTERVAL OF YEARS BETWEEN BIRTHS

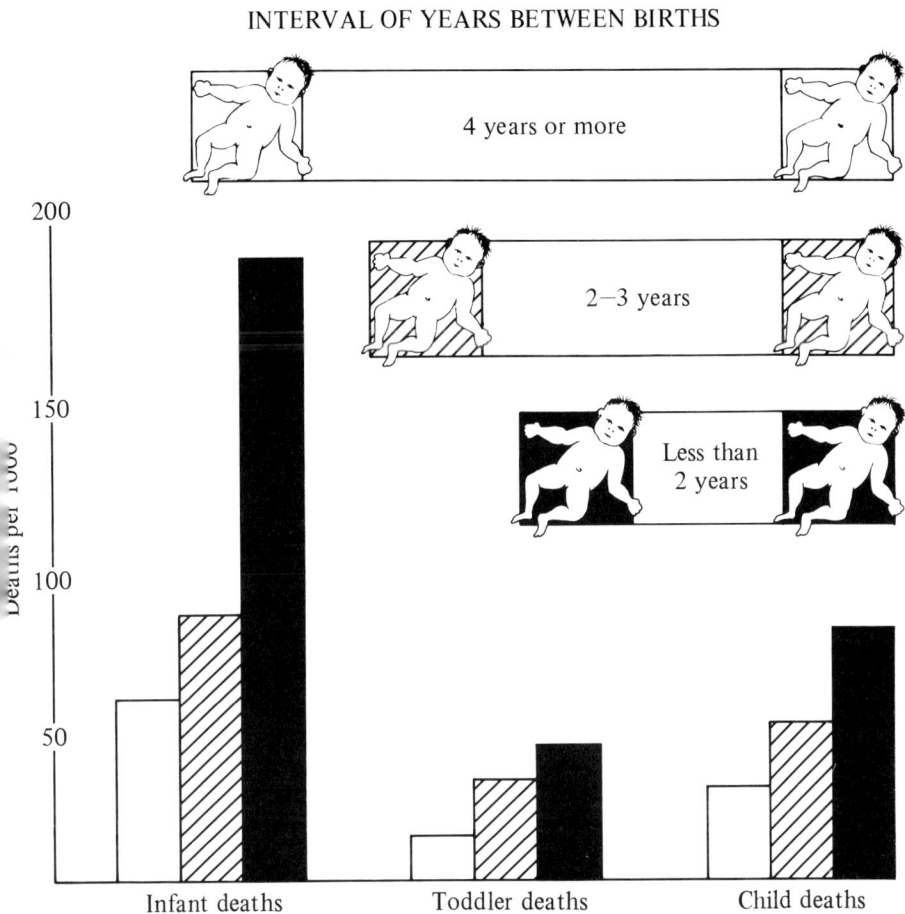

Fig. 17. *This shows the increase in infant, toddler and child deaths when the birth interval is* (a) *less than two years* (black) *and* (b) *two to three years* (hatched), *compared with an interval of four years or more.* (*The information in this graph is based on findings in Bangladesh in 1982*).

time of most profound ovarian suppression, it is a convenient marker for the efficiency of breast feeding as a method of fertility control. Although wide variations occur among populations and individuals, women who practise prolonged breast feeding remain amenorrhœic for about 60% of the duration of breast feeding. Thus, policies which extend the period of breast feeding are likely to extend the duration of amenorrhoea and infertility.

195

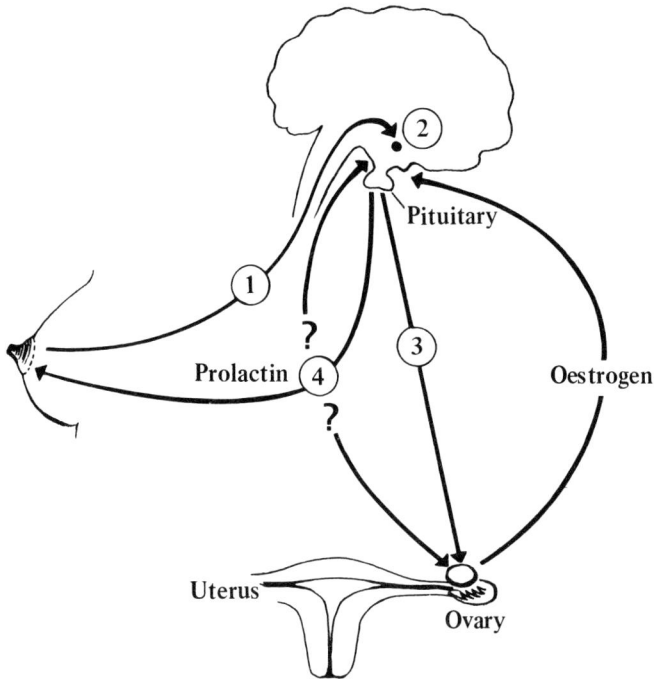

Fig. 18. *Possible mechanisms of lactational amenorrhoea. (1) Nervous impulse from the nipple; (2) changed hypothalamic sensitivity to ovarian steroid feedback; (3) altered gonadotrophin secretion; it is not established if (4) prolactin contributes to the changes in hypothalamic sensitivity or blocks gonadotrophin activity at the ovarian level.*

2. Frequency and duration of suckling

In addition to the duration of breast feeding, the inhibition of ovarian activity is dependent upon the frequency of nursing episodes and the length of time the baby spends at the breast. Detailed studies have been carried out to look at the relationship between suckling patterns and the return of post-partum ovulation. They have shown that the time taken for the return of ovulation is directly related to the suckling frequency, the suckling duration, the gradual introduction of supplementary foods, and the maintenance of night-time suckling.

Extreme contrasts can be drawn between the breast-feeding practices of tribal groups such as the !Kung hunter-gatherers and the

New Guinea Highlanders on the one hand, and those of developed Western societies on the other. In the former, nursing mothers feed their babies for very brief periods (1-2 mins), at frequent intervals (15-90 mins) throughout the day and night, maintain high prolactin levels and achieve prolonged interbirth intervals of three to four years. Western mothers often feed on a regular schedule of four to six times a day, for prescribed periods of 10 minutes on each breast and not at all at night; these mothers have prolactin levels just above the non-pregnant range and commonly find that breast feeding is an unreliable method of fertility control.

3. Sexual abstinence

In some countries, especially in sub-Saharan Africa, there are taboos on sexual intercourse during lactation, and this would clearly reinforce or extend the period of post-partum infertility. In some cultures it is believed that semen, after entering the uterus, can reach the milk and poison it. It would be a pity if, as sometimes happens, mothers prematurely and unnecessarily stop breast feeding in order to resume sexual activity. Education is needed to dispel these unfounded perceptions, but the practice of sexual abstinence during lactation is slowly dying out.

4. Malnutrition

Acute malnutrition, as occurs during famine, can cause an acute but reversible loss of fertility. There is controversy about the effects of chronic malnutrition upon ovarian activity during lactation. Mothers who are poorly nourished generally have longer post-partum amenorrhoea but, having smaller milk volumes, need to suckle more frequently. It may be the increased suckling rather than malnutrition itself which is responsible for the more prolonged inhibition of fertility.

Advice to mothers

From these considerations, guidelines can be given to mothers who wish to maximize the contraceptive effect of breast feeding; these should include the following:

197

(*i*) breast feeds should be given on demand
(*ii*) sleep with the baby and suckle at night
(*iii*) avoid bottle feeds, both of formula milk and sweet fluids
(*iv*) introduce weaning foods gradually, using a spoon and not a
     bottle with a teat
(*v*) avoid the use of teats as comforters

These guidelines obviously place considerable demands upon mothers, but they closely follow the practices which have been established in many traditional communities. It is important that infant feeding practices in developing countries should not be changed without full consideration of how they influence the contraceptive effect of breast feeding.

Breast feeding and family planning programmes

Breast feeding should be seen as an addition to and not a substitute for effective family planning programmes. The close relationship between breast feeding and family planning is illustrated by the dramatic increase in contraceptive usage that would be required to maintain current fertility rates if the contraceptive effect of breast feeding were lost (Table II). As an example, if the average duration of lactational amenorrhoea in Bangladesh fell from 21 to three months, contraceptive usage would have to be increased from the current level of 9% to 52% to maintain the average completed family size unchanged. Failure to recognize the important contribution of breast feeding to fertility control can undermine the effectiveness of family planning programmes.

Inter-birth intervals

In planning contraceptive strategies for nursing mothers, it is useful to consider the components that constitute the inter-birth interval (Fig. 19). These are the lactational amenorrhoea, the menstruating interval (i.e. the time from the return of menses to next conception) and the duration of the pregnancy itself. During the greatest part of lactational amenorrhoea, the nursing mother does not ovulate and is protected against pregnancy. Unfortunately, first menstruation cannot be relied upon as a marker for restarting contraception because a proportion of mothers, variously estimated at between 30% and 75%, will ovulate in the cycle before the first menses, and between

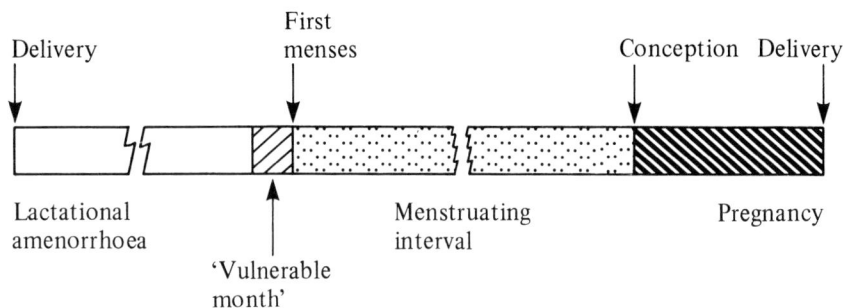

Fig. 19. *Components of the inter-birth interval in a nursing mother.*

TABLE II. Current contraceptive use, breast feeding and amenorrhoea, and projected increase in contraceptive use needed to maintain current fertility if the duration of lactational amenorrhoea declined to three months.

| | **Current Status** | | | **Projected** |
| | Average duration of breast feeding* (months) | Approximate average duration of lactational amenorrhoea* (months) | Married women currently using contraception | increase in contraceptive use required if duration of amenorrhoea dropped to three months |
			%	%
Bangladesh 1976	30.5	21.7	9	52
Indonesia 1976	25.4	18.1	26	57
Pakistan 1975	21.4	14.7	5	39
Thailand 1975	20.4	13.9	33	56
Kenya 1977–78	16.8	10.8	7	32
Philippines 1978	16.1	10.2	36	52
Peru 1977–78	13.8	9.5	31	44
Mexico 1976	11.6	6.9	30	41
Jamaica	7.5	4.5	40	44

*Among mothers with surviving children.

Adapted from: R. Lesthaeghe, *Lactation and lactation related variables, contraception and fertility: An overview of data problems and world trends.* Paper presented at the WHO/NRC Workshop on Breast-feeding and Fertility Regulation, Geneva, February 1982.

199

1% and 10% will conceive. Such mothers will proceed directly from lactational amenorrhoea into the next pregnancy. The longer the duration of lactational amenorrhoea, the greater is the chance of ovulation about two weeks before the first menses. After menstruation returns during lactation, bleeding is often irregular during the menstruating interval, with many cycles being anovular or associated with inadequate luteal phases. This means that, although the protection that breast feeding offers against pregnancy is less after the return of menses, fecundity is not fully restored until complete weaning has taken place.

Starting contraception during lactation

An important practical question is what is the best time to start contraception in breast-feeding mothers. It is important to appreciate that it is impossible to make world-wide generalizations. Each country must set its own policies. In most industrialized countries, prevalent practices of breast feeding make its contraceptive effect unreliable and most mothers are anxious to avoid early conception. In these circumstances, it is wise to start contraception at four weeks post-partum, before the earliest possible ovulation at five to six weeks.

On the other hand, in many developing countries, the early introduction of contraception would add very little to inter-birth intervals and would be a waste of scarce resources. Indeed, we know that combined oral contraceptives reduce milk production and so might shorten lactational amenorrhoea and increase overall fertility. An increase in fertility can occur in those cultures where mothers believe that the end of lactation is the appropriate time to stop contraception and start a new pregnancy. The difficulties of timing contraception for nursing mothers are illustrated in Bangladesh, where a policy of routine introduction of contraception at six months post-partum would mean that, while less than 5% of mothers would have conceived, the remainder would, on average, have 15 months of overlap between contraception and lactational amenorrhoea. In formulating policies for a particular community, it is necessary to know the average duration and range of lactational amenorrhoea. A reasonable aim is to start contraception four weeks before 5% of the population will have reached the 'vulnerable month' (Fig. 19), but policies will be influenced by the availability of resources, opportunities for providing contraception and the cultural beliefs of particular communities.

Methods of contraception during lactation

When counselling nursing mothers about methods of contraception during lactation, it is necessary to consider the effects which the method may have on milk production and on the baby, in addition to the other factors which need to be assessed for any contraceptive method. It is salutary to remember that in many developing countries, up to 40% of married women in the reproductive years may be breast feeding at any one time. Most methods can be used during lactation, but particular care is required in relation to hormonal methods.

Hormonal contraception

The literature concerning the effects of hormonal contraception on breast milk is diverse and difficult to interpret for a number of reasons. Firstly, the studies described, which have examined the effects of the Pill on breast milk, have used many different methods to assess the success of lactation; some studies have used test weighing or milk yield in response to a breast pump, while others have used infant weight gain, duration of breast feeding or even the mothers' subjective evaluation of milk flow. There are arguments for and against all these methods of assessment but, in addition to any effect of a contraceptive method, they can be influenced by other factors, such as the use of supplements or the maternal enthusiasm for breast feeding. These confounding variables inevitably make interpretation difficult. Secondly, a wide variety of preparations is available and it is almost necessary to consider each Pill individually. For example, results for a high-dose preparation of combined Pills started immediately after delivery may not be relevant to a low-dose preparation started after lactation has been established. Finally, because contraception involves personal choice, true randomized trials are difficult to arrange. Most studies which have used controls, have compared 'hormone users' with 'non-hormone users', but mothers who wish to avoid hormones during breast feeding may be more enthusiastic about breast feeding and differ fundamentally from those who are prepared to use hormonal contraception.

Combined oestrogen-progestagen Pill

Despite the difficulties of interpretation discussed above, a broad consensus has emerged that combined oestrogen-progestagen Pills significantly reduce milk volume. In poor countries, where the benefits of breast feeding for infant nutrition and health are so important, it is better to avoid the combined Pill during lactation, if possible. If it is necessary to use a combined Pill, it is wise to use as low a dose as possible and only after breast feeding is well established.

Progestagen-only contraception

If a hormonal method is to be used during lactation, progestagen-only preparations have the advantage that they appear to have little or no adverse effects on milk production, and some studies have reported an increase in milk volume during their use. Similarly, there is no evidence of any adverse effect on the quality of the milk. The progestagen-only Pill is commonly used during lactation and appears to offer effective contraception for the nursing mother. When breast feeding stops, the progestagen-only Pill can be continued, although most women will change to a combined preparation, which is usually more effective.

Artificial as well as natural steroids are transmitted to the milk. For example, the concentration of 19-nor steroids in milk is about one-tenth that in plasma. At present, there are no reports of adverse effects of steroids on breast-feeding infants.

Depot medroxyprogesterone acetate (DMPA) can also be used effectively in nursing mothers, and most studies suggest either no change or an improvement in milk yield. Although the hormone is transmitted in the breast milk after an injection of DMPA, only a minute fraction would be absorbed by the infant. It is best to delay DMPA until at least six weeks post-partum, because any earlier administration can cause irregular and heavy bleeding.

One of the greatest problems with the progestagen-only Pill in non-lactating women is irregular breakthrough vaginal bleeding. Although most breast-feeding mothers are amenorrhœic during a large part of lactation, there is some evidence that the progestagen-only Pill may cause some breakthrough bleeding in nursing mothers. This may be an important drawback in those cultures where breast-feeding mothers expect a prolonged period of amenorrhoea.

In general, the lowest effective dose of progestagen-only contraception is to be preferred to combined oral contraceptives during lactation. However, there is much to be said in favour of non-hormonal methods for breast-feeding mothers, because of the presence of very small quantities of hormones in the milk.

Barrier methods

When used correctly, the barrier methods are reliable methods of contraception. During lactation, fertility is already suppressed, so the failure rates will be even lower, and the methods have the obvious advantage of having no effect on milk production. When couples are prepared to use barrier methods regularly during lactation, they can be recommended as a highly suitable choice.

Intrauterine devices

Intrauterine devices can be used in nursing mothers and no adverse effects on lactation have been shown. Their high efficiency and lack of systemic or metabolic side-effects makes them suitable for use at this time, if they are inserted carefully. Two problems that have been reported, however, are higher expulsion and perforation rates. These may be related to the more complete involution of the uterus brought about by oxytocin secretion during nursing episodes. The higher expulsion rates are mainly encountered after immediate post-partum insertion, and this problem can be reduced by careful fundal placement. Insertion during the first month post-partum, but more than a week after delivery, is associated with a high number of uterine perforations and is not recommended. It is better to delay insertion until six weeks after delivery when the device can be inserted with caution. Because menstruation is suppressed during lactation, the problem of heavy menses induced by intrauterine devices is greatly reduced for nursing mothers, although some bleeding may be encountered at or after the time of insertion.

Spermicides

Vaginal suppositories, aerosol foams, vaginal tablets, spermicidal films and jellies can all be useful for the woman who is lactating and is not sure when ovulation will return. As a method of extending the interval between two pregnancies, they are satisfactory. If the failure rate for a spermicide is 10 per 100 woman-years in non-lactation, the risk of pregnancy during lactational amenorrhoea would be about 1 in 100, since the risk only appears in the last month, when less than 10% of women would conceive. After menstruation returns, a woman who wishes reliable protection should be advised to switch to another method.

Periodic abstinence

Periodic abstinence does not affect lactation adversely, but it does not seem to be a reliable method for nursing mothers. Clearly, the calendar method cannot be used during lactational amenorrhoea and, even after the return of menses, cycles are commonly irregular for a few months until regular ovulation is re-established. Although changes in the cervical mucus can be observed successfully by some breast-feeding mothers, the signs, which are dependent on oestrogen stimulation, can be very difficult to interpret.

During lactational amenorrhoea, ovarian follicles may develop which secrete oestrogen but do not release an ovum, resulting in a 'false-positive' cervical mucus pattern. After the return of menses, unpredictable, irregular patterns of follicle development and oestrogen secretion can continue, making cervical mucus signs so difficult to interpret in some women that prolonged abstinence may be required if pregnancy is to be avoided. Another complicating factor is that the vaginal epithelium can become dry and atrophic from oestrogen deficiency during lactational amenorrhoea, and a prolonged duration of negative results may deter even the most enthusiastic users of this method.

Voluntary sterilization

Post-partum female sterilization is a simple procedure and is commonly performed throughout the world under local or brief general anaesthesia. There is evidence that, if the sterilization is performed immediately post-partum, there is no effect on milk output but that, if the operation is delayed for seven to 14 days, the procedure is associated with a sharp drop in milk volume. Immediate post-partum sterilization, however, gives the ambivalent mother no time to change her decision, and some severe illnesses in the baby may not become manifest until after the first week. Extra care should therefore be taken when counselling women immediately post-partum (see page 184). Special attention should be paid to low-parity women.

An alternative is to delay sterilization until six weeks post-partum, when the uterus will have involuted, and laparoscopic or mini-laparotomy sterilization can be performed. By this time, breast feeding will be well established and the risks of puerperal thrombosis will have diminished. Post-partum sterilization also depends upon logistic factors such as availability of staff and facilities, and each country has to formulate its own policies.

Vasectomy is an alternative to female sterilization which can readily be carried out during lactation, and should be given careful consideration for the couple who feel that their family is complete.

No contraception

The natural birth-spacing effect of breast feeding has been largely discounted in developed countries. There are, however, a small number of mothers who are prepared to breast feed enthusiastically and who wish to space their children. The option of using breast feeding should be explained to such mothers and, provided they understand and accept the possibility of an unexpectedly early conception, some of them will find it attractive to breast feed without the risks and inconvenience of another method of contraception.

IMAP Statement on Breast Feeding, Fertility and Contraception*

Introduction

Breast feeding is an important part of the human reproductive process. It plays an essential role in infant nutrition, and it also protects the infant from exposure to infection, which is more likely with bottle feeding, especially in unhygienic circumstances. Furthermore, antibodies are passed from the mother to the baby conferring protection against certain infections. Breast feeding has an important function in mother-child bonding, and is also associated with prolonged birth intervals which confer major benefits for infant and child health.

Breast feeding plays a major role in the natural regulation of fertility. However, along with urbanization and changes in lifestyle, patterns of breast feeding are altering. These changes are tending towards a shortening of the duration of breast feeding, a reduction in the daily frequency of breast feeding episodes, and an earlier introduction of food

*IPPF reserves the right to amend this statement in the light of further developments in the field of breast feeding, fertility and contraception, when sufficient scientific information becomes available.

supplements. As a result of these changes, the risk of pregnancy during lactation has increased.

Relationship of breast feeding to fertility

Recent reviews indicate great variability in the length of breast feeding and post-partum amenorrhoea and in the duration of lactational infertility among different populations. The return of ovarian activity and fertility is dependent on the time elapsed since delivery. Variables that play a major role in the length of amenorrhoea and infertility include:

1. Duration of breast feeding

Studies from many parts of the world have shown a positive correlation between the duration of breast feeding and the length of lactational amenorrhoea. Although wide variations occur among populations and individuals, it must be remembered that, the longer the woman continues to breast feed, the more likely it is that menses will resume during lactation. The onset of the first post-partum menses is associated with increased risk of pregnancy for lactating women. In women who do not breast feed, menses can occur as early as 35-40 days after delivery.

2. Frequency and duration of suckling

The inhibition of ovarian activity is largely dependent upon the frequency and distribution of nursing episodes day and night and the time the baby spends suckling at the breast. Amenorrhoea lasts longer in women who breast feed more frequently at night as well as during the day, and for a longer time.

3. Administration of supplements to the infant

The provision of supplementary milk or food to the infant reduces considerably the inhibitory influence of breast feeding upon ovarian function and fertility and is associated with a higher risk of pregnancy. Amenorrhoea lasts longer when supplementary foods are introduced gradually, and at a later age of the child. The timing, type and amount of supplementation to breast feeding is subject to wide variations between communities. These variations may, in part, account for corresponding variations in the duration of lactational amenorrhoea in different populations.

4. Nutritional status of the mother

There is controversy about the effect of nutrition upon lactational infertility. Poorly nourished women may experience longer amenorrhoea associated with breast feeding which may be caused by malnutrition itself, or by a more intensive suckling pattern in the presence of inadequate milk output.

5. Geographic, social and cultural factors

The wide variations described for the length of post-partum amenorrhoea in different populations strongly suggests that there are other factors that affect the inhibitory influence of breast feeding upon fertility. Following the same patterns of breast feeding, a higher proportion of women will ovulate and become pregnant in some communities, while in other communities the proportion will be much smaller.

Counselling

Counselling nursing women about potential fertility during lactation should be based on local information about the breast feeding practices and the associated risk of pregnancy. As far as is practicable, all women should be advised and encouraged to breast feed fully. There is no scientific support for the belief in some societies that sexual intercourse while women are still breast feeding is harmful, provided that pregnancy does not occur. Neither should breast feeding be discontinued to start the use of contraception. Women should be informed that it is difficult to predict precisely the duration of lactational infertility of each woman. They should also be informed that:

— Amenorrhoea is associated with a high degree of protection against pregnancy in fully nursing women.
— Breast feeding on demand with a high frequency of nursing episodes through the day and night can defer the onset of fertility.
— Women who wish to rely on lactational infertility should be warned that the risk of pregnancy increases with the first post-partum menses and the introduction of supplementary milk or food to the infant.
— Supplements, and particularly bottle feeding, should not be routinely recommended during the first six post-partum months unless there is earlier indication of inadequate infant growth.
— Contraceptive measures should be recommended as soon as any of the risk factors mentioned is present, or earlier if local experience suggests that this may be necessary.

Relationship of breast feeding to contraception

The timing of the introduction of contraception will depend not only on the risk factors mentioned, but also on some programmatic aspects, such as the possibility that the woman may not return after delivery or after the first post-partum visit as well as the type of contraceptive method chosen.

It is important not to interfere with breast feeding by inappropriate use of certain forms of contraception. Non-hormonal methods should be the method of choice.

Current information on the influence of contraceptive methods upon breast feeding can be summarized as follows:

IUDs

Intrauterine devices have no negative influence upon lactation or infant growth. They are particularly advantageous during lactation because of their high efficacy.

Insertions post-partum and during lactation are appropriate, although special care should be taken to ensure proper placement of the device and to avoid perforation. Immediate post-partum insertions result in more expulsions than those done at other times. The bleeding problems associated with IUD use are greatly reduced in lactating women.

Oral contraception

Both high and low dose combined OCs containing oestrogen adversely affect the quantity and quality of breast milk, and reduce the duration of lactation. Progestagen-only OCs do not have this effect.

The combined OCs should be withheld until six months after delivery or till the infant is weaned, whichever is the earlier. Where they are the only available form of contraception, combined OCs may have to be started earlier, as a pregnancy during early lactation would be more detrimental to the health of the mother and her infant than a decrease in the milk supply. No deleterious effects have been reported so far from the transfer to the infant of small amounts of steroids in the milk. The lowest effective dose of OC should be used.

Injectable contraception

There is no evidence that depot medroxyprogesterone acetate (DMPA) and norethisterone oenanthate (NET-EN) may adversely affect either milk production or the duration of lactation.

The question of possible consequences of the transfer of the steroid to the breast-fed infant has yet to be resolved.

It is known that the amounts of steroid transmitted in the milk and absorbed by the infant are small. Although short-term follow-up studies of children breast fed by mothers using injectable contraceptives have been reassuring, longer-term studies are yet to be evaluated.

Norplant

With the current data available, it is not possible to make a recommendation on the use of Norplant in lactating women.

Barrier methods

When used regularly, barrier methods are reliable contraceptives and the failure rate should be lower when used at a time of reduced fertility, as long as couples do not take the risk of unprotected intercourse, assuming wrongly that they can rely on lactational infertility. Following childbirth, diaphragm size should be checked.

Periodic abstinence

The prediction and recognition of ovulation poses problems during breast feeding. The return of menses is unpredictable, the first cycles post-partum are irregular and the occurrence of oestrogen secretion not associated with ovulation may interfere with the interpretation of the mucus symptom. The efficacy of these methods in nursing women needs further study.

Sterilization

Female sterilization can be performed immediately post-partum. However, the decision to be sterilized should, where possible, be made a reasonable time beforehand, and not at a time of emotional stress, including labour.

(*Statement by the IPPF International Medical Advisory Panel, November 1987. Adopted by the IPPF Central Council, November 1987. It replaces the earlier statement on contraception and lactation.*)

Chapter 13

Contraception for Younger and Older Women

During the reproductive years the need for contraception varies, and this variation may affect the choice of an appropriate method. The age of the woman using contraceptives will affect the medical risks involved in using some methods. It will also produce a change in her fecundity (ability to produce offspring), which will alter the risk of accidental pregnancy when methods fail. These considerations will be outlined for the extremes of the age range in this chapter.

Younger women

Many doubts have been raised on theoretical grounds about the advisability of providing hormonal contraceptives for young women who are relatively close to the menarche. In assessing such risks, the alternatives need to be considered. One of the outstanding features of fertility today is the very high pregnancy rate among women under 20 years of age in countries all over the world, both developed and developing. The only marked exceptions are the Sino-Japanese cultures in the Pacific region. It appears that provision and use of contraceptives has not kept pace with sexual initiation. The resultant high pregnancy rate constitutes a major risk for health and for the social well-being of the younger woman and her child. Maternal mortality and morbidity are higher in adolescent pregnancies compared with those of women in their early twenties. Infant and child mortality and morbidity are also affected adversely.

Regarding the establishment of ovarian cyclical activity, the growth of long bones and the functioning of the reproductive tract generally, very few studies have suggested that any harm has arisen from the use of hormonal contraceptives at a young age.

It is important to protect the young woman from unwanted pregnancy at this time. It has been found that contraceptives are more likely to be used effectively and adolescent pregnancy rates to be lower in those countries (e.g. the Netherlands) which have liberal policies towards sex education and contraceptive availability.

For the young adolescent, there are hazards to health associated with sexuality. For example, the tissues of the cervical epithelium seem more susceptible to dysplasia under the precipitating influence of one or several factors contributed by the male. Relationships tend to be less stable, and if more than one partner is involved there will be an increased risk of sexually transmitted infections. Of these, chlamydia and papilloma virus are less easily detected and treated in good time compared with the more traditional infections, for example gonorrhoea. Gonorrhoea is, however, a serious condition (see page 274) and if not treated early will often lead to pelvic inflammatory disease (as of course does chlamydia too).

Perhaps the most common problem and the most complex in its consequences, however, is the birth of children to inexperienced and immature mothers. This situation is made worse where there is inadequate social support.

Contraceptive services provided for young people can overcome or mitigate some of the difficulties adolescents seem to have in using contraceptives. Contraception clinics should provide an attractive informal setting, staffed by well-trained and caring personnel, who are not likely to prejudge the moral issues or adversely stereotype their clients.

Where possible, counsellors should be available for young people of either sex who may be experiencing problems in their relationships or in their lives generally. Sexual difficulties are not infrequently found in this group, and can contribute to ineffectiveness in the use of contraceptives. Young women may also be suffering from sexual exploitation, harassment or violence, which they need to discuss in confidence with a trained and experienced adviser. Such services need to be provided separately from the general family planning clinics and need rather more resources. The benefits, however, are wide-ranging and economically positive. Parents and teachers can be of great help in this respect, in assisting young people of both sexes to face all manner of adolescent problems, including sexual ones. Their approach, of course, must be tactful.

Contraceptive methods

Combined oral contraceptives (COCs)

Much previous work has demonstrated the thrombotic and cardiovascular risks associated with the use of *combined oral contraceptives*. Mortality and morbidity tends to be concentrated in the older age groups and among women who smoke. The combined Pill is a very safe form of medication for young women. A difficulty which arises fairly often is remembering to take the Pill regularly, in the context of an adolescent's life-style. This may be helped by prescribing an 'everyday' preparation (with seven non-hormonal Pills in the cycle). For some unreliable users it may be unwise to rely on the lowest possible dose level. If they do not remember to take the Pill regularly, blood levels of the hormones will, on average, be lower than when the Pill is taken consistently, so that adverse effects will be less likely. These points need to be fully explained in discussion with the young woman. In addition, as part of general health education and advice, they should be encouraged not to smoke cigarettes and to give attention to healthy food and physical exercise.

Some recent studies have suggested that long-term use of COC may be associated with neoplastic change. There appears to be a dose-relationship with the incidence of cervical intra-epithelial neoplasia, significant after four years' continuous use of COC, but there may be confounding factors not easily accounted for, e.g. the number of sexual partners. An apparently more complex association may exist with the risk of breast cancer occurring before the age of 40. Studies in Sweden, the UK and the USA have suggested about a 2.5 fold increase in relative risk for prolonged use of COC before the first full-term pregnancy by young women. Other studies, particulary a large case-control study in the USA (CASH study) have shown no such relationship. There is at present no clear evidence implicating Pills with certain types or doses of hormones. However, common sense suggests that at present it is best to prescribe the lowest dose COC preparations consistent with effective contraception and good cycle control and emphasize the importance of their consistent use. Overall, it must be remembered that there are considerable health advantages for women in taking the COC Pill, particularly protection against endometrial and ovarian cancers later on and protection against pelvic infection (e.g. acute salpingitis) during the time of taking the Pill, and therefore against ectopic pregnancies.

Progestagen-only Pills (POP)

These are comparatively free of medical risks. There are problems of less effective control of conception and the need to remember to take POP regularly and at the same time each day. This may not suit the needs of young people in most cases. It is the method of choice for those with diabetes mellitus, provided there are no vascular complications or retinopathy, for women who had previous thromboembolism, and for women who are breast feeding (see page 202).

Depot progestagen

Methods of giving progestagens by long-term systemic administration may eventually prove attractive to young people. These methods appear to be free of adverse medical effects but may lead to disordered patterns of menstrual bleeding, which sometimes become scanty and sometimes heavy. There is also the important problem of delayed conception (up to 24 months) in a small proportion of women who have ceased to use the method. All users need careful explanation and warning about these problems.

Intrauterine devices (IUDs)

These may be associated with increased rates of pelvic infection (endometritis and salpingitis) and this is important in women who have never been pregnant. Infection is most commonly seen in women at high risk of a sexually transmitted disease (e.g. women having multiple sexual partners). There appears to be no increase in infection among women in mutually monogamous relationships, particularly those using copper-bearing IUDs. Studies have shown an increased risk of primary tubal infertility in never-pregnant women who have used an IUD, particularly if they have had more than one sexual partner. The IUD is therefore not the method of first choice for young nulliparous women.

213

Barriers

These methods, particularly sheaths or condoms, are widely used contraceptives. It can be argued that all those needing contraceptives should learn to use these methods, which can be applied at any time of unexpected sexual intercourse and have no serious side-effects. Many young women who are concerned about possible risks of IUDs or the Pill, are now turning to vaginal barriers, such as the diaphragm. Regularity of use is very important for success, and the achievement of this may depend on the user's life-style and sense of organization. *Post-coital Pills* should always be available if there is a lapse in use, and it is best if couples know about such possibilities in advance. It may also be necessary for users to consider the possible need for an abortion if barriers fail and to be aware of its availability where it is legal, and their own reaction to such a procedure.

There were hopes that spermicide-impregnated *sponges* might solve some of the contraceptive difficulties for young people, but unfortunately accidental pregnancy rates are high with this method in this very fertile group.

Older women

For women over 35 years of age (regarded obstetrically as 'older women'), there are particular problems with contraception. On the one hand, their fertility (or, to be more precise, their fecundity) decreases and continues to do so until the menopause, so that they may not need as effective a method as women in their twenties. On the other hand, if a woman in her forties with a grown-up family became pregnant accidentally, this would be a most traumatic event for her. So a balance has to be struck.

Women in this age group may be more prone to conditions such as obesity, hypertension and diabetes, which, together with smoking, are risk factors for adverse cardiovascular effects when taking oral contraceptives (see page 53).

Although, as discussed below, sterilization is a suitable option for many women over 35, it must be remembered that many others will not want to give up their potential fertility, even though they have completed their planned family. For them, a reversible contraceptive method will be needed.

For these older women, careful counselling is particularly important, and a contraceptive plan must be devised to suit the particular circumstances of each woman.

Contraceptive methods

Sterilization

This is increasingly being selected as the method of choice in this age group. Female sterilization and vasectomy both have low rates of complications, and are simple operative procedures that can be carried out under local anaesthesia (see page 162). Neither should be regarded as easily reversible when the decision is first made, although costly and technically difficult techniques for reversal give good anatomical results, without necessarily ending in pregnancies. Sterilization procedures, in particular vasectomy, are cost-effective methods of fertility control in family planning programmes. However, a woman nearing the menopause may not be the best candidate for sterilization — the operation may be carried out for only a short time of protection before ovulation ceases.

Combined oral contraceptives (COCs)

These can be used for some older women. However, as mentioned above, age and smoking and other risk factors enhance the possibility of cardiovascular complications for users of COCs. It therefore becomes necessary for COC users to review their contraceptive strategy at a certain stage. The accepted age for review is between 30 and 35 years for those who smoke significantly (15 or more cigarettes daily) and between 35 and 40 years for those who do not smoke. However, women over 40 who have no risk factors, may, with appropriate informed consent, still consider using COCs.

The progestagen-only Pill (POP)

POPs are suitable for women until the menopause even if they smoke or in certain associated medical conditions for which COCs would be contra-indicated, e.g. a history of thromboembolism, uncomplicated diabetes mellitus, essential hypertension and some types of hepatic disorder. If there is a previous history of COC-induced hypertension, POP should be given with caution. Equally, depot injections of progestagen or other progestagen-only applications may be used, e.g. subdermal implants or vaginal rings. There is at present no evidence of adverse medical effects enhanced by age with these contraceptives.

Intrauterine devices (IUDs)

These are often most acceptable to older multiparous women, by whom they are well tolerated. Menstrual loss may be increased and, with long-term use, monitoring of haemoglobin levels may be advisable to detect iron deficiency in its early stages. Other disturbances of the menstrual pattern are relatively common in the forties, and if symptoms arise for the first time late in the use of an IUD, uterine pathology should be considered as a cause rather than attributing the problem entirely to the IUD. Devices should be removed about a year after the menopause; otherwise, cervical stenosis may make removal difficult or impossible without general anaesthesia.

Barriers

These methods are often found acceptable for older women, either *condoms, vaginal diaphragms* or *cervical caps.* The reduction in the older woman's fertility implies that accidental pregnancy rates will be low. Spermicide-impregnated *sponges* are also suitable for older women for the same reason. Although vaginal sponges are available without medical prescription, it is advisable to ensure that women place them correctly in the vagina. Sponges or *spermicides* alone are reasonable contraceptives for women over the age of 50 who are still menstruating.

Hormone replacement therapy (HRT)

This is frequently prescribed for women around the time of the menopause to prevent the occurrence of symptoms associated with reduction in endogenous oestrogen production, e.g. vaginal dryness, vulval mucosal atrophy and inflammation, and hot flushes and sweating attacks. There is also an argument for providing HRT to prevent loss of bone calcium with increasing age (osteoporosis). It seems certain that women whose ovarian function has been reduced prematurely owing to essential surgery, should be given HRT to prevent osteoporosis as well as other discomforts. In all these cases, contraception is not effectively achieved with routine HRT preparations if the woman is still ovulating. It is probably advisable to give additional progestagen throughout the cycle, for example as a progestagen-only Pill, to ensure effective contraception. If, however, oestrogen subdermal implants are used, together with complementary intermittent low-dose progestagen medication, ovulation is usually inhibited and contraceptive cover is automatically provided as well.

IMAP Statement on Choice of Contraception for Adolescents*

Introduction

No single method of contraception can be considered satisfactory for adolescents as a group, and the following factors need to be considered carefully in assisting the individual adolescent to make a choice:

— personal, cultural and environmental factors
— age
— parity — including previous history of unplanned pregnancy
— sexual habits — both frequency of sexual intercourse and number of partners
— the risk of infection on the basis of past history and the number of partners
— the risk associated with pregnancy
— medical contraindications
— the availability or non-availability of abortion as back-up.

A full examination of various contraceptive methods is contained in the International Medical Advisory Panel statements on these methods. The specific advantages and disadvantages of different methods of contraception for adolescents are the following:

Steroidal contraceptives

Oral contraceptives may be prescribed for adolescents, although caution in prescribing for very young girls is recommended and other methods of contraception are to be preferred until regular menstruation is established. However, if sexually active adolescents are not able to use other methods,

---

*The statements on choice of contraception are valid for the contraceptives currently distributed by IPPF. The Federation reserves the right to amend the statements in the light of further developments on new methods and improvements to existing ones when sufficient scientific information becomes available for objective assessment.

the Pill may be prescribed, since the social, medical and psychological consequences of pregnancy and abortion in this age group outweigh any physiological reservations that may exist. The effects of suppression of the hypothalamic mechanism on sexual development remain uncertain. The possible long-term effects of oral contraceptives still need further attention.

Oral contraceptives have a protective effect against pelvic inflammatory disease (PID) which may be a consideration for some adolescents; in addition, cardiovascular complications are rare in this age group. A low-dose combined Pill should be chosen. The progestagen-only Pill is another possible choice, although the need for scrupulous regularity in its use, and the incidence of breakthrough bleeding, may make it less acceptable.

Injectables are subject to the same warning as oral steroids. When they are prescribed, the adolescent should be fully informed about possible delay in the return of fertility. This makes injectables less desirable for nulliparous adolescents planning to start a family.

Post-coital steroidal contraception should be made available and used only as an emergency procedure. However, its availability should be widely publicized. It is important that the adolescent should be aware of the importance of a follow-up visit to check that no pregnancy has occurred. This opportunity offers a suitable occasion for counselling about future contraceptive needs.

Intrauterine devices (IUDs)

There is a need for caution in offering an IUD to an adolescent who has never had a child, or who is likely to have more than one partner and is therefore more likely to be exposed to PID. Age is in any case a significant factor in the incidence of PID, and younger adolescents are at greater risk. On the other hand, for the parous adolescent an IUD may be the method of choice.

Copper IUDs may also be offered as a post-coital contraceptive within five days of unprotected sexual intercourse. They have the advantage of ensuring future contraceptive protection but should only be offered subject to the considerations already described, and when the adolescent is willing to consider the IUD as a contraceptive method.

Diaphragms

These can be a good method for the highly motivated adolescent who is adequately trained in their use. However, storage and washing may create problems if the adolescent wishes to maintain secrecy. Their effective use requires detailed instruction which may demand considerable time on the part of family planning personnel. Since spermicide use with the

218

diaphragm is recommended, there may be a protective effect against STDs and PID.

Condoms

Condoms, when properly used, constitute one of the most suitable methods of contraception for this age group. They have no medical side-effects, do not require prescriptions, and are generally widely available. They also provide some protection against STDs and PID. Their effective use requires motivation and adequate knowledge.

Spermicides

When used with diaphragms or condoms, these ensure high effectiveness. Used alone they are less effective, but for adolescents they are usually easy to obtain and use. They may have a protective effect against some forms of STDs and even PID.

Withdrawal

Sexual control in adolescence may be low, leading to a higher failure rate with this method. However, in some circumstances it may be the only method available, and adolescents should be fully informed about the technique.

Periodic abstinence

This method, which relies on attempts to identify the time of ovulation, is heavily dependent on regular menstrual cycles. It is also likely to be difficult to use by those who only have occasional sexual intercourse.

Sterilization

This is very rarely indicated in this age group, and should be considered only in exceptional medically dictated circumstances.

Which method?

Contraceptives for the adolescent cannot be ranked in a single order of preference. The home circumstances of the adolescent; the attitude of partner, parents or family; the existence of health-care facilities and their use by the adolescent; as well as the factors mentioned earlier, will all be important considerations in making such a choice. Above all, the adolescent's own preferences after full counselling will be crucial in ensuring effective, regular contraception. It is clear that all currently available methods of contraception have shortcomings, especially for this age group.

(*This statement is part of a policy statement and guidelines on meeting the needs of young people, drawn up jointly in 1983 by the IPPF International Medical Advisory Panel and the IPPF Programme Committee.*)

IMAP Statement on Contraception for Women Over 35*

Introduction

Women over the age of 35 constitute at least 20% of candidates for contraceptive use. They need special consideration concerning contraception because pregnancy for these women can carry increased health hazards for both the mother and her baby. This group of women have certain characteristics which may affect their choice and use of contraceptive methods. While fertility is declining in these women and it could be argued that a less effective method may be appropriate, it is important to recognize that an unwanted pregnancy may be especially traumatic for women in this group. The sexual behaviour of older couples is another factor which should be considered; available evidence suggests that they are more likely to be monogamous and that sexual intercourse takes place relatively less frequently. Diseases more common in older women, such as obesity, diabetes and hypertension, as well as genital tract disorders, should influence the type of contraception chosen. The hazards caused by smoking are also more serious for these women. Because of the likelihood of the presence of these pre-existing conditions, it is good medical practice to screen these women when providing contraception. The choice of a particular method may be affected by a woman's prior experience of it. Advisability of methods may also be different for women considering contraceptives new to them at this stage of their lives.

Choice of methods

Surgical contraception (sterilization)

Surgical contraception may be considered to be the best method of contraception for informed, adequately counselled couples, since

---

*This statement is valid for currently available methods of contraception, as they apply to women aged over 35. IPPF reserves the right to amend this statement in the light of further developments in the field, when sufficient scientific information becomes available.

termination of fertility, rather than pregnancy spacing, is the usual fertility regulation objective at this time. As a general rule, vasectomy is a safer procedure than female sterilization. For older women, it may be important to weigh the risk of the surgical procedure against the number of years for which the contraceptive protection will be needed. Recent studies do not support the clinically held impression that women who have undergone sterilization are more likely to experience heavy bleeding. It should, however, be borne in mind that women in this age group may be prone to heavy bleeding. Service providers should exclude the possibility of uterine pathology and other gynaecological problems that may necessitate additional gynaecological surgery before carrying out any procedure, in order to minimize the likelihood of women being subjected to further surgery. Hysterectomy should not be considered as a method of contraception in the absence of pelvic pathology.

Intrauterine devices

The IUD is a good method for older women. It is a long-acting, effective method with no systemic effects. Particular contra-indications to its use which are found more often in this group are the presence of uterine pathology, such as undiagnosed irregular vaginal bleeding, and the presence of fibroids distorting the uterine cavity. Pelvic inflammatory disease may be less frequent with the use of IUDs at this age, because women are more likely to be in a monogamous relationship. The IUD should be removed one year after the last menstrual period.

Barrier methods and spermicides

Barrier methods and spermicides have no known significant side-effects, but the relatively high failure rates associated with their use are a particular drawback at this age. Where national laws permit, the availability of back-up abortion may increase the acceptability of these methods. Older couples may be better motivated to use barrier methods effectively. Advantages of barrier methods for this age group may include the lubricating effect of spermicides where dryness of the vagina is a problem. However, laxity of the vaginal muscles may rule out the use of the diaphragm, while the acceptability of the condom may be reduced where male erectile problems are present.

Periodic abstinence

Periodic abstinence may be a more acceptable method for older couples, since they may be more likely to follow the instructions for identifying the fertile phase of the cycle and to comply with the practice of abstinence. However, information on the effectiveness of the method among this age group is insufficient. In pre-menopausal women with irregular cycles, the method may be unsuitable. Interpretation of changes in cervical mucus may be difficult in the older woman; when the basal body temperature method is used there may be many anovulatory cycles with no biphasic changes in temperature, making the periods of abstinence prolonged.

Hormonal contraception

Combined oral contraception

Although it appears established that OCs are not the method of first choice for women in this age group, low-dose OCs may be considered as a contraceptive option for women who have been suitably screened. If OCs are chosen, it is particularly important that the woman be kept under medical supervision.

There is suggestive evidence that the increased risk of cardiovascular hazards are minimal in these women if they do not smoke, have no other risk factors, such as hypertension, obesity, or a poor family history of cardiovascular disease, and use low-dose OCs. Further data on this are being collected. One factor needing further attention is the potential effect on lipoproteins.

Progestagen-only contraception

There is insufficient scientific information available about the use of progestagen-only contraception — minipill, injectables and Norplant — in this age group to establish their suitability for women over age 35. They offer the advantage of freedom from oestrogen-related side-effects which may occur with combined OC use. Progestagen-only contraception may be associated with irregular bleeding, which may be of concern. The inter-menstrual bleeding that can occur with these methods may be confused with bleeding caused by possible gynaecological pathology. However, the long term and high effectiveness of injectables and implants may be especially attractive to this group.

(*Statement by the IPPF International Medical Advisory Panel, April 1987. Adopted by the IPPF Central Council, November 1987.*)

Chapter 14

Infertility

Introduction

Although this chapter is entitled 'Infertility', and discusses in some detail the causes, diagnosis and treatment of infertility in men and women, this is only one of several conditions all classified under the general heading of childlessness, involuntary or voluntary. The many possible causes of infertility are discussed in some detail in this chapter and need not be listed here. Other conditions ending in childlessness include pregnancy wastage, early child loss and voluntary childlessness.

Pregnancy wastage covers spontaneous abortions or miscarriages, and stillbirths. Causes include endemic infections such as syphilis and malaria, malnutrition in the mother, inadequate ante-natal care and obstetric complications.

Early child loss, which includes neonatal deaths and deaths in the first year of life, may be associated with low birth weight, poor breast feeding, poor nutrition of the baby, unsanitary conditions in the home leading to severe infections, a hostile environment in which the child is being brought up, and inadequate medical care, which is experienced in some developing countries where medical facilities are immensely overstretched.

Another cause of childlessness which must not be forgotten is voluntary childlessness in which the man, woman or couple decide for one of a number of reasons not to become parents. In many cases this is for economic reasons, while some women do not want to interrupt their careers with child bearing. Sometimes the presence of a hereditary disease in one or other family line (see page 304) makes couples want to avoid possibly passing this trait on, and occasionally what is seen as a bleak future for mankind contributes to a couple's unwillingness to bring up children in the modern world.

This chapter discusses the basic physiology of reproduction in relation to the major causes of infertility, the management of the infertile couple and methods of treatment available. Although specialized facilities are needed for some of these, even without them much can be achieved in treating infertility and its psychological effects. Simpler methods of treatment and investigation are considered in detail, but more specialized methods are also mentioned as knowledge of what is available elsewhere will allow appropriate referral by the doctor or health worker concerned.

Counselling and consultation

Infertility itself affects 10-20% of couples in the UK. The incidence in other populations may be higher, being influenced by socio-economic conditions, general health and nutrition. The anxiety and the feeling of failure that follows, especially when family and social pressures are great, often lead to marital disharmony and breakdown. These factors have led to increasing requests for investigation and treatment, which are as important, particularly to the individual couple, as is fertility control. Thus the IPPF believes that family planning includes help for infertile couples just as much as helping fertile couples to space or limit their families.

A sympathetic approach, an appreciation of cultural and social customs (and taboos), and an understanding of the physiology and pathology of reproduction are the major requirements in the management of this complex problem.

Conception occurs in only 15-20% of fertile cycles, and fecundity declines with increasing age of the female partner. Thus, approximately 85% of couples in whom the woman is 20-25 years of age will achieve a pregnancy within 12 months of starting regular unprotected sexual intercourse, whereas only 60% will do so in the female age group of 30-34 years, and 50% of women aged 35-40 years will conceive in this time. For these reasons deferment of investigation until the couple have been 'trying' for 12 months is often advocated. However, earlier consultation is an index of the couple's anxiety. A simple but comprehensive programme of investigation enables a diagnosis to be reached and a prognosis given without undue delay, and also enables early referral of those couples needing more specialized investigation and/or treatment.

Early consultation with the couple gives an opportunity for the assessment of general health and of fitness for pregnancy, including establishment of immunity to rubella, and enables advice to be given about nutrition and alcohol or tobacco consumption. If no obvious

224

cause for infertility is found, explanation and reassurance can be given and further investigation deferred, although in older couples, further investigation or referral to a specialist clinic should not be delayed. The extent to which the couple wish to have investigations and treatment should be established after careful explanation of what may have to be done, and the couple's wishes in this matter should be respected. It may not be possible for the couple to make this decision until after several visits and after embarking upon investigations, but it is essential that the couple's needs and desires direct both investigation and treatment.

The infertile couple

The couple should be seen together in a quiet and relaxed atmosphere with adequate time for discussion. A full and detailed history is taken from each partner, with particular attention to symptomatology, past and present, which may indicate one of the causes discussed below. Each partner is examined separately, enabling further factors in their histories unknown to the other partner (e.g. previous pregnancy or sexually transmitted infection) to be discovered. The examination should be detailed, assessing general health as well as sexual development, genital anatomy and signs of reproductive pathology.

Following this a simple explanation of the basic physiology of reproduction and factors which may affect fertility is given and the proposed investigations discussed. The couple should be reassured that they have not failed and that feelings of guilt or blame, which are common, are unfounded. It should also be stressed that infertility is a shared problem and not that of an individual. Counselling along these lines goes a long way towards alleviating the anxiety brought about by infertility.

Physiology and pathology of conception

Conception requires, in the female partner, regular ovulation, pick-up and transport of the oocyte to the site of fertilization in the uterine tube, transport of the fertilized ovum to the uterus, endometrial development appropriate for implantation, and the production at mid-cycle of cervical mucus which is receptive to sperm. In the male, the essential factors for fertility are the production, transport and nutrition of sperm and intra-vaginal ejaculation of semen, so that it comes in contact with the cervical os near the time of ovulation.

Disturbance of any of these factors leads to sub-fertility. Regular sexual intercourse (two to three times a week) should be taking place.

Approximately one third of infertility is due to male factors, one third to female factors, and the remaining third to a combination of these. In 10-20% no cause will be identified, although development of new methods of investigation is reducing this figure as knowledge of reproductive physiology and pathology increases.

Psychosexual disorders account for less than 1% of infertility in developed countries, but may be more common, or present more commonly in the guise of infertility, in other cultures. Lack of understanding of reproductive and sexual physiology, and anxiety (or guilt) may cause impotence, premature ejaculation or ejaculatory failure in the male, and vaginismus or dyspareunia in the female. Occasionally a marriage may not have been consummated or the couple may have discontinued regular intercourse because of dyspareunia secondary to pelvic pathology. Careful and tactful enquiry about how the couple's sexual intercourse takes place is, therefore, an essential part of the history. Where possible, any difficulties should be resolved before embarking upon further investigation. This resolution, following careful counselling, may be all that is needed for a successful pregnancy.

Anatomical abnormalities such as hypospadias in the male or vaginal septum in the female may prevent ejaculation of semen in the upper vagina or preclude seminal contact with cervical mucus.

The major causes of infertility may be classified as follows:

Male causes

Abnormal spermatogenesis
Disorders of secretory function of accessory organs
Obstruction of the genital tract
Abnormal sperm function

Female causes

Ovulatory disorders
Tubal occlusion
Peritoneal factors, e.g. pelvic inflammatory disease, endometriosis
Cervical factors
Failure of implantation

Male factors

Disorders of spermatogenesis or of the accessory glands account for 35-40% of male infertility. Hypogonadism is uncommon and is suggested by absent or under-developed secondary sexual characteristics and small soft testes. Elevated concentrations of gonadotrophins in the serum will differentiate primary from secondary testicular failure, in which gonadotrophin concentrations are low. Other male factors to bear in mind include physical or psychological inability to deposit semen in the vagina. These include inability to produce or maintain erection, and physical anomalies such as hypospadias.

The usual initial investigation of the male is by semen analysis. The sample is produced by masturbation and collected into a clean dry container, after 2-3 days without sexual intercourse. Samples collected by coitus interruptus or into contraceptive condoms are unsuitable. When religious doctrine forbids masturbation, special non-spermicidal condoms may be used.

A sperm density of less than 20×10^6 per ml (oligozoospermia) and progressive motility in less than 50% (asthenozoospermia) are associated with sub-fertility, although 12% of these couples achieve a pregnancy within 4-5 years. The sperm density and/or motility just mentioned are found in 75-80% of infertile men, and no definite cause can be identified in half of them.

Spermatogenesis may be suppressed by acute or chronic illness (e.g. coeliac disease), by drugs (e.g. cytotoxic agents) and by irradiation. Azoospermia (no sperm in the ejaculate) or severe oligozoospermia (less than 5×10^6 per ml) is rarely the result of hypogonadism, but is commonly due to ductal obstruction, frequently post-infective, and is occasionally associated with fibrocystic disease or bronchiectasis.

Genital-tract infection may be suggested by a history of penile discharge or episodes of dysuria and by the finding of thickening of the epididymis and/or of tenderness of the prostate on rectal examination. Liquefaction of the ejaculate is often delayed beyond the normal interval of 20 minutes, and seminal viscosity remains high. Bacteria and leucocytes may be seen on microscopy. Cultures of semen, expressed prostatic fluid and urethral swabs are indicated. *Chlamydia trachomatis* is a common infective agent, and where facilities allow, titres of serum antibodies to chlamydia should be measured.

Sperm motility is assessed subjectively by light microscopy, but objective measurements can be made by laser scattering or multiple exposure photomicroscopy where these are obtainable. Motility may be inhibited in ejaculates of high viscosity, by drugs such as sulphathalazine and alcohol, by smoking, or by raised scrotal temperature from tight underclothing or testicular reflux associated with a varicocele.

Sperm morphology has little prognostic value, although multiple immature forms indicate spermatogenic arrest. Similarly, biochemical analyses of seminal fluid are generally of little clinical value, but the fructose concentration may be reduced in the presence of infection. Sperm agglutination occurs in association with infection or in the presence of antibodies to sperm. The latter, which are identified by specific immunological tests, are secreted into the genital tract, impair sperm motility and inhibit sperm penetration of cervical mucus, accounting for 5-10% of infertility. Antibodies may be specific for sperm or be anti-bacterial, cross-reacting with sperm components.

Female factors

Ovulatory disorders

Chronic anovulation resulting in amenorrhoea or severe oligomenorrhoea requires specialist investigation and management, and women with these complaints should be appropriately referred. Only women with fairly regular menstrual cycles are considered here.

The potentially fertile cycle is characterized by a phase of follicular development, increasing secretion of oestradiol and endometrial proliferation, a mid-cycle phase in which the luteinizing hormone surge invokes ovulation and initiates luteinization of the follicle and the luteal phase of at least 11 days, during which progesterone secretion induces secretory transformation of the endometrium. During the pre-ovulatory phase, cervical mucus becomes profuse and watery as a result of oestrogen stimulation, and changes its fibrillar structure, making sperm penetration and migration easy.

Ovulatory cycles last for 26-35 days and ovulation is often associated with transitory mid-cycle pain (Mittelschmerz), bleeding (Kleine

Infertility

Regel) or mucoid discharge (ovulation cascade) and mild spasmodic dysmenorrhoea. Progesterone secretion increases at mid-cycle and raises the basal body temperature (BBT) by 0.4°C (see pp 149). Daily recording of the BBT gives some indication of whether ovulation has occurred, although many women are unable to take or record their temperature, and some with regular ovulation do not show a temperature change. Furthermore, the recording of BBT serves as a daily reminder of infertility.

Ovulation is often inferred from a plasma concentration of progesterone in the mid-luteal phase greater than 30 nmol/l, but this does not exclude a defect of luteal function, and two or three estimations during the luteal phase are preferable. Recent development of radio-immuno assay (RIA) methods of measuring free progesterone in saliva (where available) enables daily measurements to be made and samples can be stored in a domestic refrigerator. Defects of luteal function account for 3-10% of conception failures and may occasionally be associated with luteinization of an unruptured follicle (the LUF syndrome).

Hyperprolactinaemia and hypothyroidism also cause luteal dysfunction, and thyroid hormone and prolactin levels should be measured in all infertile women where facilities exist, although a single estimation of prolactin may be misleading owing to the circadian and cyclical variation in its secretion. Suprasellar tumours of the pituitary or of the hypothalamus need to be excluded by CAT scan before treatment of hyperprolactinaemia, and patients suspected of having these conditions should be referred to an endocrinology unit for this specialist investigation and treatment.

A luteal phase of less than 11 days or reduced progesterone secretion lead to inappropriate endometrial development and failure of implantation. The BBT may reveal the short luteal phase, but rarely reflects inadequate progesterone secretion, since the thermogenic response is not quantitative. Histological examination of the pre-menstrual endometrium assesses the biological response to progesterone, but cannot be repeated frequently. In conjunction with measurements of progesterone concentrations, an inappropriate endometrial response to progesterone can be detected.

Most of the investigations discussed in this section are specialized ones, and will not be available in all centres. They are mentioned here to show what can be done, where facilities exist, to discover the causes of ovulatory disorders.

229

Tubal and peritoneal factors

Tubo-peritoneal dysfunction is mainly due to chronic pelvic inflammatory disease (PID) or endometriosis. Occasionally a cornual fibroid or polyp or surgical adhesions may cause tubal occlusion.

Chronic PID

This is usually the result of infection with *Chlamydia trachomatis*. Gonorrhoea accounts for 7% of PID in the UK, but may have a greater incidence in some populations where chlamydial infection is less common. Both are sexually transmitted, and other less common sexually transmitted diseases may also be a cause of PID. Ascent from the cervical reservoir frequently follows abortion or insertion of an intrauterine device (IUD). Bacteroides, coliforms and peptococci may also be isolated and often gain access to the genital tract in the post-abortal or puerperal phase. Tuberculous salpingitis is uncommon in developed countries, but more common in the developing world. One episode of salpingitis causes infertility in 15-20%, and three episodes in 75% of women. Fibrosis of the oviduct, formation of intraluminal, peritubular and peri-ovarian adhesions and loss of endo-salpingeal rugae and cilia result in failure of oocyte pick-up and transport.

Chronic PID causes pelvic pain, congestive dysmenorrhoea, deep dyspareunia and menorrhagia, together with tenderness and fixity of pelvic organs on examination. Microbiological examination of the cervix, including chlamydial culture when possible, is indicated in all infertile women, together with assays for chlamydial antibodies in serum.

Endometriosis

The presence of endometrial tissue in extra-uterine sites occurs in approximately 15-30% of women with otherwise unexplained infertility. This is known as endometriosis. Major degrees cause reactive fibrosis and pelvic adhesions, giving rise to secondary dysmenorrhoea, pelvic pain and deep dyspareunia. Tender nodules may be felt in the utero-sacral ligaments, together with generalized pelvic tenderness and organ fixity, particularly when examination is made in the pre-menstrual phase. The effects of minor degrees are obscure. Abnormalities of luteal function often co-exist, and the release of abnormal amounts of prostaglandins into the peritoneal fluid may alter tubal motility, prevent oocyte release and/or inhibit sperm motility.

Other factors

Hysterosalpingography (HSG), with appropriate antibiotic cover, can demonstrate fibroids, polyps or even a forgotten IUD, and outlines the lumen and rugal pattern of the endosalpinx in patent tubes. The site of tubal occlusion may be seen, although tubal spasm may prevent the passage of contrast medium. Peri-tubular adhesions prevent 'smearing' of the abdominal viscera and cause loculation of dye around the fimbriae.

Laparoscopy is an essential adjunct to HSG, since unexpected adhesions or endometriosis are found in 20-40% of patients. This examination requires general anaesthesia and an experienced operator and anaesthetist to avoid complications such as perforation of a viscus or cardio-respiratory arrest. Laparoscopy is preferably undertaken in the pre-menstrual phase when endometriotic tissue is most prominent, a corpus luteum can be sought and an endometrial biopsy taken at the same time for histology and tuberculosis culture. Aspiration of peritoneal fluid is necessary to enable examination of the depths of the pelvis to be made. The mobility and relative anatomy of the fimbriae and ovaries are assessed, and tubal patency tested by instillation of a dye into the cervical canal. The need for and feasibility of tubal surgery or *in-vitro* fertilization (IVF) can also be determined.

Tubal insufflation of gas is unreliable and carries a risk of tubal rupture in the presence of obstruction. It is now an obsolete investigation.

Combined factors

Sperm-mucus interaction

Abnormalities of either semen or mucus reduce sperm penetration and account for up to 15% of infertility. Reduced secretion or persistent viscosity of mucus result from inadequate oestrogen secretion, resistance of the cervical cells to oestrogen stimulation, loss of cervical cells following surgery or chronic infection. Infection may give rise to a muco-purulent discharge, and evidence of chronic cervicitis may be seen on speculum examination. The most frequently occurring causative organism is *Chlamydia trachomatis*, and thus swabs for chlamydial culture and blood for chlamydial serology should be taken when facilities allow.

The post-coital test

This test assesses the mucus and survival of sperm within it. Pre-ovulatory mucus is aspirated 6-18 hours after intercourse. Correct timing and interpretation in relation to menstrual dates, the semen analysis and ovarian function are critical. The couple should be advised to avoid the use of lubricants and post-coital douches. Mucus is aspirated with a small narrow bore (e.g. tuberculin) syringe. The important characteristics are the volume, elasticity (Spinnbarkeit – assessed by measurement of the distance to which the mucus may be pulled out in a thread) and cellularity of the mucus. These, and the dilatation of the cervical os and the degree of 'ferning' which develops with drying of the mucus (Fig. 20), are scored numerically (the Insler score).

The number of progressively motile sperm in 10 high-power fields is

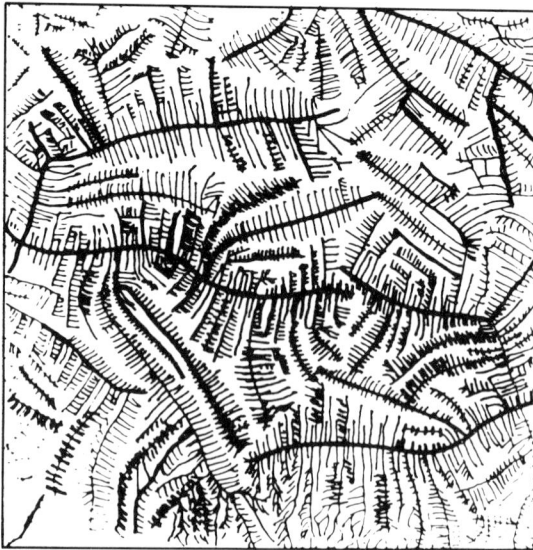

Fig. 20. *Fern-like pattern of cervical mucus crystallization (arborization) on Day 13 of an ovulatory cycle.*

counted. A high Insler score for the mucus, with at least five progressively motile sperm per high-power field implies adequate coital technique, folliculogenesis and semen quality, the absence of cervical 'hostility' and a good prognosis for fertility. Repeatedly unsatisfactory results with well-developed mucus and a normal semen analysis require further investigation.

Sperm-mucus interaction can be assessed *in vitro*. After 2-3 days of coital abstinence, pre-ovulatory mucus is drawn up into a capillary tube, one end of which dips into a reservoir of fresh semen. Sperm normally penetrate at least 2 cm up the mucus column and remain progressively motile for two hours or more. Immobilization or poor penetration of ductile mucus is associated with poor quality semen, acute cervicitis or the presence of immobilizing or agglutinating antibodies, but for the most part is unexplained. Antisperm or antibacterial immunoglobulins immobilize sperm in apparently normal mucus, and can be identified by specific immunological investigations. Cross-testing with fertile mucus and semen identifies the source of the abnormality.

Defective capacitation and fertilization

Sperm actively migrate through the cervical mucus but are transported to the site of fertilization in the ampulla by uterine and tubal contractions. Decapacitation factors are gradually removed in the uterine fluid and sperm become capable of the acrosome reaction. This occurs in the oviduct, releasing enzymes which enable sperm to pass between the cumulus cells and bind to and penetrate the zona pellucida and plasma membrane of the oocyte. Disorders of these processes result in failure of fertilization.

The *fertilizing capacity* of sperm can be assessed *in vitro* using immature human oocytes or zonae pellucidae or zona-free hamster eggs. This correlates with sperm motility, movement patterns and their ability to penetrate cervical mucus *in vivo* and *in vitro* and to migrate through the female genital tract. Reduced fertilizing capacity of sperm may be a factor in up to one third of couples with otherwise unexplained infertility, and may be the result of supra-optimal levels of decapacitation factors in semen, antibodies against sperm or, as preliminary studies suggest, of auto-antibodies to the zona pellucida which may prevent sperm binding to and penetrating the oocyte.

Implantation failure

The factors controlling implantation are largely unknown. This complex interaction between blastocyst and endometrium is progesterone-dependent, but may involve embryonic steroids. Inadequate endometrial development leads to failure of nidation. Genetic abnormalities contribute to a high conceptual loss in normal women, and may be greater in 'unexplained' infertility.

Treatment

Male factors

Little can be offered for the treatment of male factors in infertility. General measures such as avoidance of hot baths, tight underwear and excess tobacco and alcohol consumption may improve sperm motility.

Eradication of infection rarely improves semen quality, but may prevent further damage to the genital tract. Occasionally ligation of a varicocele may improve sperm motility.

Primary hypogonadism is irreversible, but may require hormone replacement. Secondary hypogonadism may be amenable to treatment with gonadotrophin or pulsatile GnRH therapy. For this reason, and to exclude serious endocrine disease, hypogonadal men need to be referred to a specialist clinic.

Although serum levels of antisperm antibodies can be reduced by high doses of corticosteroids, the effect of this treatment upon local immunosecretion has not been established. Severe and serious side-effects (e.g. peptic ulceration, ischaemic necrosis of the femoral head) can occur, and this treatment should be used only in highly specialized centres.

Artificial insemination using the husband's or partner's semen (AIH) is ineffective with poor quality semen and in cases of sperm immunity. However, in selected cases concentration of semen can be achieved *in vitro* and without compromise of motility, and semen thus treated may be used for AIH or even IVF. Highly viscous semen may respond to enzymatic digestion *in vitro* and can afterwards be used for AIH.

Female factors

Ovulation is rapidly restored in hypothyroid women by thyroxine replacement therapy. Dopamine agonists (e.g. bromocriptine) inhibit prolactin secretion and rapidly restore ovulation in women with prolactin-secreting pituitary microadenoma or with functional hyperprolactinaemia. Suprasellar extension of a pituitary tumour needs to be excluded or dealt with surgically before therapy, as expansion of the tumour during pregnancy can cause visual defects.

Oral administration of clomiphene citrate, 50-100 mg daily for five days during the early part of the cycle, results in regular and apparently ovulatory cycles in 80% of cases, but conception in only 40-50%. The response to treatment is monitored by serum progesterone measurements during the luteal phase. Clomiphene may induce follicular maturation without ovulation which can be effected by injection of human chorionic gonadotrophin. The timing of this is critical if premature luteinization is to be avoided, and daily oestradiol measurements and/or ultrasonic follicular scans are required. Other ways of inducing ovulation (gonadotrophin and GnRH therapy) require specialist facilities.

Treatment of cervical factors is dictated by the underlying cause. Cryocautery and antibiotic therapy may reverse hostility caused by infection, and improvement of follicular development will enhance the quality of mucus. There is no effective treatment for unexplained or immunological abnormalities of sperm-mucus interaction. AIH is stressful and ineffective for these couples and is only useful when coital abnormalities prevent contact between semen and mucus, or when mucus is absent or scanty as a result of previous cone biopsy. However, if sperm have normal fertilizing capacity, *in-vitro* fertilization may be appropriate.

Chronic pelvic sepsis requires vigorous antibiotic therapy. Erythromycin or tetracycline, with metronidazole, is given in rotation with trimethoprim/sulphamethoxazole for 3-4 months to prevent further pelvic damage. The freeing of adhesions and, if necessary, fimbrioplasty using microsurgical techniques, may restore tubal patency, but if the tubal mucosa has been damaged, the prognosis for conception will be poor and the risk of ectopic implantation high. *In-vitro* fertilization may have a better prognosis for some of these women. Division of adhesions resulting from previous surgery carries a better prognosis, as the endosalpinx is usually undamaged.

235

Endometriosis regresses during pregnancy and after the menopause. Induction of a state of pseudo-pregnancy by continuous administration of oestrogen/progestagen therapy, or of pseudo-menopause with danazol or GnRH analogue, are equally effective in eradicating minor degrees of the disease, although endocrine abnormalities may persist. Treatment needs to be continued for 6-9 months and dose regimens adjusted to maintain amenorrhoea. Side-effects are common, though rarely severe. Endometriosis complicated by adhesions or large endometriomata requires surgical treatment. Pre-operative medical treatment makes dissection easier and improves the prognosis for subsequent conception.

In 10-20% of infertile couples, infertility remains unexplained, but up to 80% of these will achieve pregnancy within two years. *In-vitro* fertilization is being more frequently employed for this group, but is probably more appropriate for those with prolonged infertility.

Artificial insemination by donor (AID)

AID is the most effective method of treatment of childlessness due to factors which cause the husband or male partner to remain infertile. The major indications are azoospermia and severe oligozoospermia. The success rate for AID is comparable with that of normal fecundity rates.

At present, in the UK, the resulting child is illegitimate in law and registration of the child as the husband's is a criminal offence. This is not the case in all countries, however. Careful selection and sensitive and thorough counselling in AID are essential, and secrecy may be of paramount importance if the couple opts not to inform the child of its origins. The couple are usually seen by the clinician responsible for treatment and, in ideal circumstances, a counsellor. The latter helps with further discussion to ensure that the couple understand and are able to cope with the difficulties involved, and is also able to offer ongoing emotional support. Contact is maintained during treatment and for some time afterwards.

Donors, selected from healthy men of proven fertility and with high sperm density and motility, should be screened for sexually transmitted diseases (including the presence of the HIV virus), hepatitis B, cytomegalovirus and hereditary diseases. Personal features such as hair and eye colour, height and build are noted so that these can be matched with those of the husband as far as possible. Anonymity of the donor is ensured by use of a coding system, and by screening being undertaken by a clinician not involved in the treatment of the infertile couple. Relinquishing all rights and responsibilities in relation to the resulting child by the donor is essential.

Donated semen is kept frozen for three months or, in some countries, for six months, until a second or third HIV screening test is carried out to eliminate any donor showing sero-conversion in that time. Where freezing of semen cannot be carried out, the woman must be warned of the possible dangers of receiving fresh semen. She should be allowed to decide for herself whether to proceed with the insemination.

In-vitro fertilization

This method of treatment of infertility is becoming increasingly available, primarily for irreparable tubal damage, but also for oligozoospermia, cervical hostility and unexplained infertility. The success in terms of clinical pregnancies is up to 20% per treatment, but 50% of these may end in early abortion. In addition to the vast resources required, this treatment can be stressful, and selection of couples for this therapy has to be done very carefully. Many will not return for further cycles of treatment.

A similar procedure is becoming quite common. In this, by laparoscope, gametes mixed outside the body are inserted directly into the fimbrial end of the uterine tube to encourage normal fertilization there. This technique is known as gamete intra-fallopian transfer (GIFT). Where at least one tube is patent, the pregnancy rates with GIFT are higher than with *in-vitro* fertilization.

Adoption

The social and legal position in relation to adoption varies from country to country, and clinicians advising infertile couples should familiarize themselves with their local situation. Few children are available for adoption, either because of social acceptance of single mothers, a liberal abortion law or because children are rarely born out of wedlock in the society in question. Thus waiting lists are long, and criteria for selection of prospective parents stringent. This can be very frustrating for couples already distressed by their infertility. They will need considerable support from those with whom they have shared their problems—the clinician, social worker and nursing staff involved in the investigation of their infertility.

237

Childlessness

Many couples with involuntary infertility will eventually have to come to terms with their childlessness. Some do this during the course of their investigations or treatment and may choose not to continue with these. With careful counselling and the building of a relationship upon mutual respect and goodwill, the number unable to give up and requiring long-term support should be small. However, there will always be those who cannot accept a childless future, and the role of the doctor, social worker and nursing staff in helping these people to come to terms with their situation is as important as, if not more so than, restoring fertility to others.

IMAP Statement on Infertility*

Introduction

IPPF has always recognized that 'planned parenthood' includes concern for individuals and couples who are unable to have children when they desire them. Impaired fertility may be due to a relative or absolute inability to conceive, or to repeated pregnancy wastage. Some cases of impaired fertility can be corrected by simple measures, including counselling. Many require complicated diagnostic procedures and treatment. Even in expert and multi-disciplinary clinics, success canot be guaranteed, although progress is constantly being made. In addition, the impaired fertility of many couples remains unexplained. Counselling, with particular sensitivity to the psycho-social implications of infertility, is an important part of any service provided for infertile couples.

Prevalence and aetiology

The incidence of impaired fertility, variously described as infertility or sub-fertility, varies from region to region, and, in some, may affect such a high proportion of couples as to constitute a major public health problem. Although the magnitude of the problem and its causes are still the subject of intensive study in many regions, certain facts are now known. Many conditions leading to the impairment of fertility are preventable. These

---

*IPPF reserves the right to amend this statement in the light of further developments in the field of infertility when sufficient scientific information becomes available.

include sexually transmitted diseases (STDs), and infections following childbirth or abortion. Where common, tuberculosis may also cause some infertility.

Social conditions may be a factor in infertility, and are likely to influence the perceptions of and about couples suffering from infertility. No relationship between contraceptive use and permanent impairment of future fertility has been convincingly established in studies of populations. There is evidence that IUDs carry an added risk of pelvic inflammatory disease (PID), but there is no statistically proven direct link between IUD use and subsequent impairment of fertility. Though depot medroxyprogesterone acetate (DMPA) may cause delay in the return of fertility, this does not extend beyond 18 months after cessation of use. On the other hand, barrier methods of contraception are known to protect against STDs, and there is now sufficient evidence showing the protective effect of oral contraceptives against PID.

Diagnosis and management

FPAs have a responsibility to educate clients with regard to the prevention of infertility and to be responsive to their questions on this difficult and sensitive problem. However, the investigation and diagnosis of infertility is a complex process, requiring facilities and expertise not readily available within most FPAs' programmes.

With properly trained personnel (not necessarily doctors) some screening may be conducted by FPAs, including the taking of a detailed sexual history, instruction on timing of sexual intercourse, and recording of basal body temperature. When laboratory facilities are available, post-coital testing, semen analysis and endometrial biopsy can also be carried out. However, it is usually in the best interests of the couple that diagnostic procedures and management are performed in a centre where systematic and comprehensive services are available. FPAs can play a useful role in helping infertile and sub-fertile couples by establishing a link with such a well-equipped centre for infertility diagnosis and management.

At present, results of treatment of infertility are often disappointing. It is therefore important not to build up false hopes in those seeking assistance for infertility. FPAs have a legitimate role to counsel individuals and couples in an effort to help them to come to terms with infertility if treatment fails, and to provide advice and assistance where adoption can be seen as a desirable alternative.

It is important to recognize the burden placed on couples seeking infertility treatment by many of the diagnostic and therapeutic procedures. Time should be allowed to elapse between instituting different procedures. Involvement of the male partner should be encouraged. Health professionals should avoid a paternalistic attitude towards female patients, and make every effort to understand the real needs of the couple. This is particularly important in cases where only one partner is keen to have a child. Health professionals need to investigate carefully issues such as this, and should involve couples fully in decision-making about referral and treatment.

Prevention

FPAs should be aware of the prevalence and major causes of infertility in their areas. Since several of the major causes of infertility are preventable, FPAs can play an important advocacy role in reducing these preventable causes, and thus help to diminish the magnitude of the problem in the community.

This role could be fulfilled by promoting: programmes for the control of sexually transmitted diseases; better obstetric care at the primary health care level, including adequate training of traditional birth attendants; improved access to effective contraceptive services to reduce the incidence of illegal abortion; the availability of reproductive health services (including information and education) for adolescents; and programmes for the control of certain diseases which may have a definite causative relationship to infertility in certain areas, e.g. tuberculosis. Co-operation, where possible, with other international organizations such as the World Health Organization, in assessing the problem, and in the prevention and treatment of infertility is encouraged.

(Statement by the IPPF International Medical Advisory Panel, October 1984; approved by the IPPF Central Council, November 1984. Statement amended by IMAP, April 1987.)

Chapter 15

Menstrual Regulation

Introduction

Menstrual regulation is commonly defined as evacuation of the uterus in a woman who has missed her menstrual period by 14 days or less, who previously had regular periods and who has been at risk of conception. It may be performed before proof of pregnancy. The procedure most commonly used is that of uterine evacuation using a small flexible plastic cannula (Karman cannula) in association with a hand-held gynaecological syringe as a source of negative pressure.

The use of the gynaecological aspiration syringe spread around the world with great rapidity after it was described by Karman and Potts in 1972. It can be used for: (1) diagnostic or therapeutic curettage; (2) the treatment of incomplete abortion; (3) uterine evacuation to ensure that no early pregnancy is present at the time of tubal ligation if this is done in the second half of the menstrual cycle; and (4) uterine evacuation in cases of suspected pregnancy.

Uterine aspiration with a syringe, but using metal equipment, was experimented with in the 19th century, although it was only with the advent of plastic syringes and cannulas that the method became widely used. Detailed research on many thousand consecutive women who have undergone menstrual regulation has been conducted in several countries. Menstrual regulation has been carried out by a range of trained personnel, from specialist gynaecologists to paramedical workers.

In some countries, menstrual regulation has proved remarkably popular, and individual practitioners sometimes perform several thousand operations a year. In certain countries menstrual regulation is legal, even when therapeutic abortion is illegal, as in many Latin American countries, where prosecution for abortion requires proof that a pregnancy was terminated. However, in other jurisdictions, influenced by British and French law, the intention to perform an abortion, whether the woman is pregnant or not, is a criminal act, thus causing menstrual regulation to fall under the same provisions as abortion (see page 347).

Every month many women fear the possibility that their menstrual period may not appear. Among those who think they may be pregnant, many are eager to seek an immediate procedure which will either end the pregnancy or confirm that they are not pregnant. Menstrual regulation is quick, effective and acceptable in many cultures. It avoids much of the emotional concern which normally accompanies uterine evacuation at a later stage.

Counselling and contraceptive advice

The woman undergoing menstrual regulation should understand the nature and consequences of the operation and the operator should be sure she is making a voluntary, informed, unpressured choice, if a pregnancy is suspected. Often the woman seeking menstrual regulation has used no effective method of contraception, although this is not always the case. It is wise to discuss a firm plan for future fertility regulation during the initial interview, and implement it at the time of operation or immediately afterwards.

Experience from clinics using menstrual regulation in many parts of the world shows a marked improvement in contraceptive practice after the procedure has become available. Menstrual regulation has become an integral part of family planning advice in a number of situations, in adding to the acceptability of contraceptives. It also provides a useful starting point for contraception.

An intrauterine device can be inserted at the time of the procedure, and excellent results have been obtained in a number of countries. In some situations it is the contraceptive method of choice at the time of menstrual regulation. Oral contraceptives can be started on the evening of the operation, and any problems arising from their use discussed at follow-up. Sterilization has been performed by laparoscopy or minilaparotomy at the time of menstrual regulation, or a short time afterwards. Conversely, menstrual regulation has been performed at the time of routine sterilizing operations, to ensure the non-pregnant state.

Examination

The woman's history is important, and attention should be paid to the previous pattern of menstruation, to whether the woman has taken oral contraceptives recently, and to the symptoms of early pregnancy such as nausea or sore breasts. Both combined and progestagen-only oral contraceptives may cause delay or absence of monthly withdrawal bleeding. Following cessation of either type there may be a delay of several weeks before the first spontaneous menstrual period.

Careful bimanual examination of the uterus is essential to exclude pregnancies which exceed six weeks' maturity. The woman's memory of the last menstrual period may be inaccurate or she may falsify the date. When assessing uterine size, previous parity and the possibility of fibroids must be taken into account.

The simplicity of menstrual regulation can encourage over-confidence. The most serious complications can arise, not in the performance of the routine procedure, but in cases where the operator embarks on what is expected to be a simple procedure but turns out to involve a more advanced pregnancy than was expected. The responsible way to act in every case of doubt about the length of gestation is to refer the woman to a hospital or clinic which is fully equipped and staffed to carry out first-trimester operations.

Operative procedure

A trained operator can readily use the gynaecological syringe in the simplest of clinical settings, and successful services have been established in primary health centres, and in unsophisticated premises belonging to practitioners, sometimes without running water. A clean, well-lit room, of the sort where a vasectomy can be performed, is adequate. Menstrual regulation has also been adopted by some traditional practitioners and, without doubt, represents a significant step forward in safety relative to older, traditional techniques of abortion.

Equipment

The minimum equipment needed is a vaginal speculum to expose the cervix, a tenaculum to stabilize the cervix, the plastic syringe and cannulas, and a sterilizer for the metal equipment. The syringe should be kept clean and the piston adequately lubricated. The cannula has a sealed rounded end and two oval apertures on opposite sides with a small overhanging lip which, when in contact with the endometrium, acts as a curette (Fig. 21). The 50 ml syringe has an adapter to hold the cannula, catcher arms to hold the plunger at full extension, and a stop to prevent total withdrawal of the piston (Fig. 22). The syringe is easy

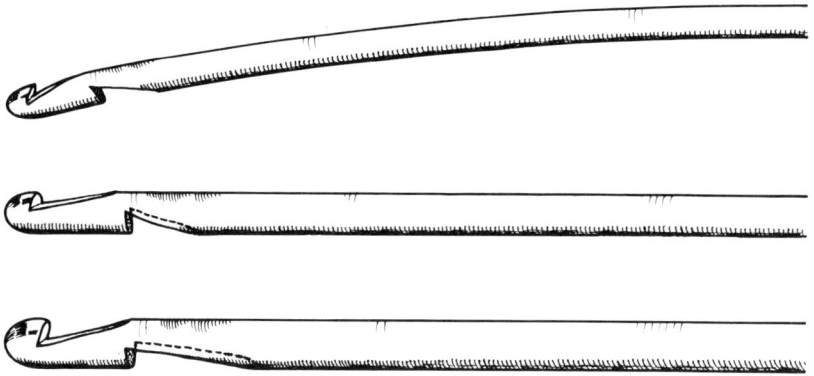

Fig. 21. *Cannulas in 4, 5 and 6 mm sizes.*

Thumb-operated valve   Catcher arm

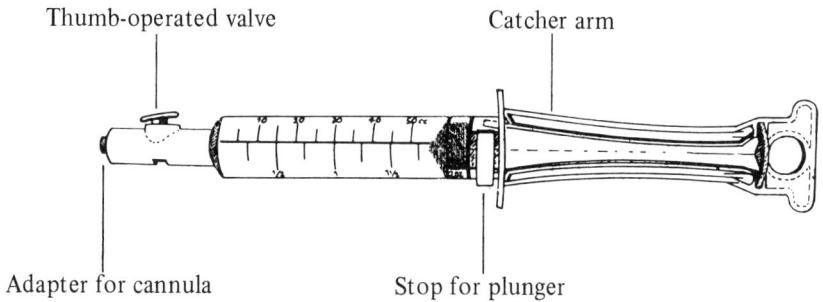

Adapter for cannula   Stop for plunger

Fig. 22. *Hand-held 50 ml vacuum syringe.*

to take apart and clean, and this should be done after each operation. A properly maintained syringe is capable of performing at least 40 operations, and some syringes have been used many hundreds of times.

The cannulas should be disinfected by immersion in a solution of 1 : 2,500 aqueous iodine (a definite orange colour, not yellow or brown) or other suitable disinfecting solution for at least 20 minutes before use. They can be dipped in boiling water, but should not be left in a hot-water sterilizer for more than a minute or so, as the plastic will suffer.

Most menstrual regulations around the world are performed without any form of local or general anaesthesia. Cramping uterine pains, of varying severity, are felt during the operation, especially as the uterus begins to empty. The operation is more painful in women who prove not to be pregnant than in those who are.

In order to decrease pain, a local anaesthetic can be given, as for first-trimester abortion. General anaesthesia is not usually indicated, since cervical dilatation is not performed. Neither oxytocin nor ergometrine are administered routinely.

Technique

The woman is asked to empty her bladder, and after the bimanual examination the vulva is cleaned in whatever way is normal practice for the locality concerned. Shaving is unnecessary. Adequate explanation should be given to the woman as the procedure takes place.

With the woman in the dorsal lithotomy position, a speculum is inserted. A Cuscoe's or short bivalve speculum can be used.

The cervix should be cleaned with any appropriate aqueous antiseptic and stabilized with a tenaculum. A local anaesthetic, if it is to be used, is injected at this stage.

There is no need to sound the uterus with a metal instrument. A technique of 'soft abortion' depends on the use of plastic instruments, and the cannulas themselves can be used as uterine sounds. Cannulas can be used 10 times or more providing they are properly sterilized each time, but the tip should be inspected and a cannula rejected if the plastic near the apertures is beginning to crack.

The largest cannula which can be passed without any force and without great discomfort for the woman should be used. This will usually be 5 mm diameter in primigravidae and 6 mm in parous women. If the cannula fits too tightly in the cervical canal, sensitivity of touch is lost by the operator. The cannula should be passed gently and left in place in the cervix. The vacuum is then created by withdrawing the plunger of the syringe until the catcher arms hold the piston at its fullest extent. The syringe is then attached to the proximal end of the cannula, commonly with a slight twist to ensure a good seal. When the valves are open the vacuum is transmitted to the uterine cavity, but there is no significant loss of pressure since the cannula fits firmly in the cervix.

The cannula is pushed gently in and out and rotated until a grating sensation is felt on all surfaces of the uterine cavity, and aspirate ceases to flow along the cannula. Aspiration takes about two minutes on average, although it may be as little as 45 seconds or as long as six minutes. The difference between the smooth feeling of the cannula passing over the embryonic membranes or endometrial surface, and the rough grating sensation once the uterus is evacuated, is easy to distinguish with experience, and is an important sign of the completeness of the operation.

If the cannula becomes blocked it should be withdrawn until the apertures have passed the external os of the cervix, without removing the whole cannula; any material blocking the cannula should be removed with sterile instruments. Then the cannula can be pushed gently forwards into the uterus again and the vacuum re-established. If it is uncertain whether the cannula remains uncontaminated, it is better to use a new sterile one. It is a sound surgical principle not to introduce any instrument into the cervix on more than one occasion, as it is impossible to sterilize the cervix, and the possibility of infection arises whenever a foreign body is passed along the cervical canal. An operator should have a number of correctly sterilized cannulas of different sizes available, and may use several during any single procedure.

During the evacuation the operator or another counsellor should re-assure the woman and explain what is happening.

When the procedure is complete the cannula is withdrawn and the cervix can be swabbed with antiseptic. The volume of aspirate should be noted and the material floated in water. If the woman is pregnant at the time of operation, the conceptus (placenta and embryo) is only a few millimetres in diameter, and most of the growing tissue is devoted to the development of the placenta. If the aspirate is floated in water, villi can usually be seen. Microscopic examination is not obligatory. If the symptoms of pregnancy are present but the volume of material is small and/or villi are absent, then ectopic pregnancy, septate uterus or failure to aspirate the small pregnancy sac should be suspected and a follow-up maintained.

Women are usually fit to leave the place where the operation was performed within an hour or less of having the procedure. Before leaving they should be told what symptoms to expect in the following week and should be given advice about how to contact the operator or some other responsible person. If the menstrual regulation was carried out to treat an incomplete abortion or in the case of a suspected pregnancy, they should know that they must return if the signs and symptoms of pregnancy persist. Future contraception must be discussed both before and after the operation. The woman must be told to return if she feels unwell in any way.

The symptoms experienced in the postoperative week are similar to those of normal menstruation for the majority of women. A number of women report a transient pyrexia in the week following the procedure.

Possible problems

At the time when most menstrual regulations are performed and a pregnancy is present, the embryo is so small that it is possible for it not to be evacuated at the initial curettage. Up to 1 in 50 first aspirations fail, and then a repeat procedure is necessary. Women should be informed at the initial counselling that this is possible. They should know they must return if the signs and symptoms of pregnancy persist.

Sometimes, it is impossible to pass even the smallest cannula through the cervix, and in this case the end of the cannula should be grasped with an appropriate forceps (such as Kelly's) and the tip introduced into the cervix, gently but firmly.

Occasionally, the cannula will pass with no apparent resistance, and if perforation is suspected the procedure should be stopped. If necessary, advice should be obtained from an experienced gynaecologist. The woman should be observed for four hours, and the pulse and blood pressure taken half-hourly. The procedure should be rescheduled for another occasion in an adequately equipped operating theatre.

When the cannula is removed, the cervix should be inspected for bleeding. If excessive bleeding continues it may come from damage caused by the tenaculum or from the cervical canal. If from the latter, a cannula should be re-inserted to check that all products of gestation have been removed. If bleeding still continues, the operator should bimanually massage the uterus for two minutes. If bleeding persists, oxytocin, 2-5 units intramuscularly, or ergometrine 0.5 mg intravenously, should be injected. If bleeding still persists despite all these measures (and this is exceedingly rare), then experienced advice should be sought and arrangements made to transfer the woman to a properly equipped centre.

Convulsions have been observed during menstrual regulation, either owing to a sensitivity reaction to a local anaesthetic, or to fright and pain from manipulation of the cervix. The woman should be observed, and protected from accidentally hurting herself, and when the attack has subsided the procedure should be completed under general anaesthesia in a properly equipped operating room.

Occasionally the tip of a Karman cannula breaks off and remains in the uterus. If this happens, a larger cannula should be used, and usually the tip will appear in the aspirate. If this does not happen, the uterine cavity should be explored with a small sterile clamp or curette. A detached tip can be left in place and will usually be passed, in the same way as an intrauterine device is sometimes expelled.

If the woman feels faint, she may need to lie on a bed for 15-20 minutes. If the pulse is rapid and/or there is abdominal pain for more than half an hour, which is not relieved by a mild analgesic, then bleeding should be suspected. A pelvic examination is performed and if the uterus is enlarged and tense, especially if blood clots are passed when the uterus is squeezed gently, then it should be re-evacuated and ergometrine given.

Infection is a risk of all intrauterine operations, and the symptoms generally appear on the second or third day after the procedure, but can be delayed for up to 10 days. The signs of infection are fever with uterine tenderness, and should be treated with antibiotics and with re-evacuation if there is evidence of retained products.

No serious long-term complications of menstrual regulation have been demonstrated, although it should be accepted that infection at the time of the operation could threaten future fertility. It is debatable whether Rhesus sensitization occurs in the first six weeks of pregnancy, but without proof to the contrary, some centres administer gamma globulin to Rhesus negative women. Where this is the case, a blood sample should be taken at the first interview and examined to discover the woman's blood group and Rhesus factor. Anti-D gamma globulin should be given within 72 hours of the procedure when applicable. In countries where this is not possible, menstrual regulation would appear to present much less risk of sensitization than a later abortion.

Many women feel a considerable emotional relief when the operation is completed, and long-term depression has not been reported. The majority believe themselves to have been among those who were not pregnant.

Perhaps the most controversial aspect of menstrual regulation has been the possibility of performing redundant operations on women who feared they were pregnant, but proved not to have been. In early series of cases, a considerable number of women proved not to be pregnant, but by taking simple administrative steps, the number of unnecessary operations can be greatly reduced.

The probability of pregnancy being the cause of menstrual delay increases with the number of days of amenorrhoea. Of women requesting menstrual regulation within 14 days of the expected period, 50% will have a positive pregnancy test, and this group should be offered an immediate menstrual regulation. Of the remainder, more than half will prove to be pregnant, but if the woman is within one week of a period, it may, in certain circumstances, be reasonable to ask her to return one week later. In recent series only about 10% of women have proved not to have been pregnant at the time of operation.

Pregnancy testing can be carried out where facilities exist, but easily available tests are not positive until some days after the first missed period. Even more sensitive tests have been developed which can indicate a pregnancy within a few days of fertilization. However, these are not universally available as yet.

All pregnancy diagnosis tests depend on the the detection in urine or blood of chorionic gonadotrophin which the placenta produces in increasing amounts from approximately 10 days after fertilization. The sensitivity and specificity of immunological tests have been greatly enhanced by the use of antibodies which react with the β-sub-unit of chorionic gonadotrophin alone, thereby eliminating previous cross reaction with pituitary luteinizing hormone which could pro-duce false-positive results in climacteric women. The widely available and relatively cheap agglutination test performed in three minutes on a slide at room temperature gives reliable results within 14 days of the first missed menstrual period. A more expensive enzyme-linked anti-body kit test takes five minutes at room temperature, but gives accurate positive and negative results by the time of the first missed period.

Radio-immune assays are very expensive and require use of a Geiger-type counter. In addition, each kit contains a minimum of 20 tests, and is uneconomic unless one is performing that number of tests per day. These tests are used only in research laboratories.

The currently available immunological tests are undergoing con-tinuous improvement. When the tests mentioned above, which indi-cate pregnancy a few days after fertilization, become routine they will remove any controversial aspects of menstrual regulation in countries where abortion is legal. However, the implications of the use of pregnancy tests are different in countries where evacuation of the uterus is a criminal offence if pregnancy can be proved, but legal where it cannot be proved (see page 347).

During the early stages of pregnancy, when gonadotrophins are low, an early morning specimen of urine (EMU) will be relatively more concentrated. Where urine specimens are used, an EMU is more likely to be positive than one collected at another time of the day. If collection of an EMU is not feasible for the first visit, the woman should at least be given a container to bring an EMU with her, if a re-test is thought necessary.

When the pregnancy test is positive, but the aspirate obtained by menstrual regulation is small, the operator should be alerted to the possibility of the presence of an ectopic pregnancy. If facilities exist, the aspirate should be examined histologically for signs of an intrauterine pregnancy, and if these are absent, an ectopic pregnancy should be seriously considered.

Chapter 16

Management of Unwanted Pregnancy

The reaction to an unwanted pregnancy

The difference between an unplanned and an unwanted pregnancy is not always obvious. The recognition, by a woman, of early unwanted pregnancy may be followed by conflicting emotions; triumph, fear, anger, excitement and despair following in rapid succession, depending on her social circumstances. Even the attitude to a planned and wanted pregnancy may change dramatically if it is rejected by her partner or parents. For some women, pleasure at becoming pregnant may give way to morbid fear of childbirth or to the realization of the practical difficulties of bringing up the child. Pre-natal diagnosis may reveal an unexpected fetal abnormality, but the fear of abnormality, even when unjustified, may be equally distressing. Such reactions are often manifest as psychiatric illness, such as depression or an anxiety state.

While few would disagree that effective contraception is preferable to abortion, cultural and religious attitudes to induced abortion vary enormously, and in some East European communities, abortion is preferred to contraception as a method of fertility regulation. On the other hand, in some Roman Catholic and Muslim communities, any interference with the embryo or fetus is abhorrent and even contraception is frowned on. If this is coupled with a strong disapproval of illegitimacy, the conflict for the woman is increased and the temptation to use illegal abortion becomes overwhelming.

Any doctor or nurse who deals with pregnant women should therefore be sensitive to early expressions of rejection. It is easy to ignore the situation because it may involve uncomfortable discussions about abortion and personal relationships, but the problem will not go away and delay usually makes matters worse.

The options

Faced with an unwanted pregnancy, a woman has to choose between the following options:
1. Continue the pregnancy and keep the baby.
2. Continue the pregnancy and give the baby for adoption.
3. Seek legal abortion, where that is permitted.
4. Seek illegal abortion.

Keeping the baby

A woman's decision to keep a baby will be influenced largely by the support offered by her partner and family or by some social agency. Within a marriage, the rejection of a pregnancy is often caused by financial and social problems made worse by inadequate contraception; the offer of post-partum sterilization may provide a reassuring solution to uncontrolled fertility.

For the single girl much depends on the attitude of society to illegitimacy. In some countries, e.g. Sweden, the term is meaningless and housing and financial help for the single parent is readily available. Even where having an illegitimate child is frowned on, religious organizations, like the Catholic Rescue Society or 'pro-life' groups like LIFELINE, may give considerable practical help, especially when it avoids an abortion.

Even among women who did not seek abortion, the attitude to the pregnancy has been shown to affect outcome. In a study of more than 12,000 married women in California, those who admitted negative feelings towards the pregnancy had a higher perinatal mortality, a higher incidence of congenital malformations and more anxiety symptoms than those who were ambivalent or very positive.

Adoption

Adoption used to be seen as a neat solution to the problem of unwanted pregnancy, which avoided the difficult issue of abortion and the social stigma of illegitimacy. A number of events have contributed to its declining popularity. The availability of safe, legal abortion and the increased acceptance by society of single parenthood have brought about a complete change in the meaning of 'illegitimacy'. New laws in the USA and the UK now make it possible for adopted children to seek out their biological mother and have removed the guarantee of secrecy from a girl who gives away her baby in the expectation of concealing from the world the fact that she was ever pregnant. The combination of social change and the availability of abortion and contraception has resulted in a sharp fall in the number of babies available in Western countries for adoption. The laws which govern adoption in most European countries are very strict, but in some developing countries there are disturbing reports of abuse in the use of adoption. Infertile couples from the West, desperate for a baby, may seek to adopt from countries where uncontrolled fertility and poverty make the mothers of large families vulnerable to exploitation. Even more worrying is the possibility that unwanted babies may be bought as potential cheap labour.

Although a good deal has been written about the fate of the children who are adopted, remarkably little attention has been paid to the natural parents. Many such parents grieve for the child they have relinquished, and an organization called Concerned United Birth-parents has been formed in the USA. A questionnaire was sent to members, and most respondents reported that the adoption had affected their relationships, but not always for the worse. Some, who had married the father, felt that the sense of guilt united them, but for others the loss of the child was a source of friction. Often, the experience of surrendering a baby for adoption left an emotional scar which took a long time to heal. Occasionally, a woman who decides, on becoming pregnant, to have the baby and then offer it for adoption, changes her mind after the birth. The months of pregnancy, plus the experience of labour, prevent her from handing over the baby to a stranger.

Legal induced abortion

Legal abortion is now widely available throughout the world, but nowhere is it available unconditionally. The minimum requirement is agreement with the doctor who is to do the operation, but in practice it is much more complicated than that. The wider availability of abortion has occurred alongside improvements in the medical care of diseases complicating pregnancy, so that in industrialized countries there are now very few purely medical indications for abortion. Indeed it is not uncommon for women with serious illnesses, like renal failure treated with a kidney transplant, to expect medical science to nurse them through pregnancy in spite of the risks. The determining factor is overwhelmingly the attitude of the pregnant woman, but there are still many doctors who fail to recognize this fact.

Most abortion laws seek to ensure that abortion is done as safely as possible, and only after careful thought. Restrictions may be minimal, such as the compulsory delay between decision and operation, which is the law in the Netherlands. More usually, two or more doctors have been involved in certification, with more stringent rules for abortion after 12 weeks' gestation. It follows that women who are denied abortion will include those who cannot negotiate the legal system (especially the very young and socially disadvantaged) or those who are ambivalent.

In Britain, the provisions of the Abortion Act require that two doctors must sign a certificate in advance of the operation. The limit of gestation is governed by the Infant Life Preservation Act which protects the fetus after it is considered to be 'viable', defined as 28 weeks. There is no legal restriction on second-trimester abortion, but there has recently been voluntary agreement to limit abortion to less than 24 weeks.

When more than one doctor is involved in the decision, as in Britain, Canada and some states of the USA, the woman may be dissuaded, at the first consultation, from proceeding further. Granted that gynaecologists differ in their attitude to abortion, the medical decision is not easy. In advising surgical treatment for any other condition, the doctor requires a knowledge of the pathology and natural history of the disease, the benefits and the value of alternative management. In the case of abortion the views of the woman are paramount, and this is an uncomfortable situation for many doctors.

Illegal abortion

Reliable information about the extent of illegal abortion is understandably hard to find. The Lane Committee, which reviewed the working of the Abortion Act in Britain, estimated that about 30% of those first refused eventually obtained an abortion. Del Campo, from a study of the American experience of those denied abortion, concluded that between 10% and 20% of them later obtained an abortion elsewhere, possibly illegally. Experience in Romania and the USA suggests that restricting legal abortion is followed by an increase in illegal abortion. In the USA, the Hyde amendment reduced the use of Federal money to assist poor women to obtain a legal abortion, and there were reports of individual cases of death and of mutilation from attempts at self-induced abortion. In Romania, the law on abortion was severely restricted in 1974, and this was followed by an increase, not only in the birth rate, but also in deaths attributed to abortion. Certainly deaths attributed to abortion in Britain and the USA have continually declined since the liberalization of the laws on abortion (Fig. 23). Nevertheless, illegal abortion continues to represent a major health hazard, and in some countries of Latin America, the complications of abortion still account for up to a third of maternal deaths. To

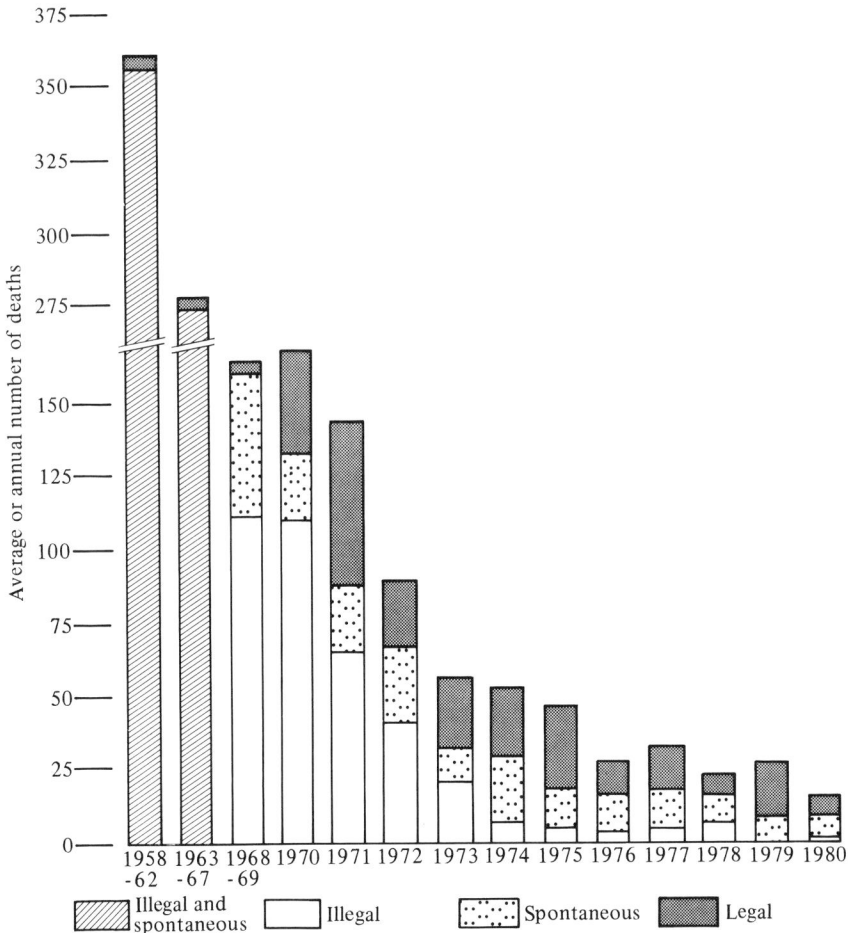

Fig. 23. *Number of deaths associated with abortion, by type of abortion: United States, 1958-80.*

make matters worse there is often an ambivalent attitude to the use of contraception, so that societies which prohibit legal abortion, sexual intercourse outside marriage and contraception, will turn a blind eye to illicit abortion under such guises as 'regulation of the periods'.

Incomplete abortion

The problem of incomplete abortion (septic or otherwise) is greatest in countries with a high birth rate but with poor family planning services. The consequences are a high maternal morbidity and mortality, with infertility as a serious long-term sequel in the survivors.

The management of incomplete abortion is not difficult in countries with good medical facilities. But much can be done to reduce morbidity in developing countries with limited resources. The vacuum curette, devised for induced abortion, is also very effective for incomplete abortion, and where the cervical os is already dilated, the procedure can be performed without a general anaesthetic. Suction pumps which are hand operated obviate the need for mains electricity, and the technique can be learned by a trained nurse or midwife.

The importance of counselling

The sooner the conflict over a pregnancy is resolved, the better the chance of limiting the psychological and physical harm. It is important that the woman has the opportunity to talk to someone who is sympathetic, emotionally neutral and well informed. Not only should all the options be considered, but practical help offered. To agree to abortion without question is no better than to reject it automatically or condemn it. The request for an abortion should be regarded as evidence of some sort of crisis, and provides an opportunity to mitigate the effects and perhaps to deal with the underlying cause, whether it is a failure of contraception or a breakdown of human relationships. Counselling is an extremely helpful exercise in assisting the woman to reach a decision, and is incumbent on all doctors dealing with such problems, whether or not assistance is available from paramedical staff, such as social workers.

Above all, contact with a woman with an unwanted pregnancy (whatever the eventual outcome) provides an important opportunity to offer help with future contraception. An intrauterine device can be inserted immediately after an evacuation of an incomplete or induced abortion, or arrangements can be made to provide practical help after the baby is born. Vague promises to attend a clinic sometime are not good enough: 'sometime' may be too late.

Methods of induced abortion

Medical

Abortifacient drugs have been used since ancient times, but most were both toxic and relatively ineffective. An important advance came with the discovery of the oxytocic properties of two naturally occurring prostaglandins, E_2 and F_{2_a} (and some of their derivatives) which are powerful smooth-muscle stimulants. When given by mouth, vaginal pessary or intravenous or intramuscular injection, they cause regular uterine contractions at all stages of pregnancy and can therefore be used to induce abortion. By these routes, however, the doses which are needed cause unacceptable side-effects, such as diarrhoea, vomiting and rigors, and prostaglandins are now rarely used in the first trimester except by local application in order to ripen the cervix.

A new progesterone antagonist, RU 486 (mifepristone), binds to receptors in the corpus luteum and has been shown to be effective in producing abortion very early in pregnancy. Combined with a low dose of prostaglandins, it seems a most promising technique for inducing early abortion.

Instillation techniques

In order to minimize the side-effects of prostaglandins, the drug is administered directly into the uterus, either into the amniotic sac (intra-amniotic) or into the potential space between the membranes and the uterine wall (extra-amniotic). However, newer analogues of prostaglandins can be administered parenterally. Hypertonic saline and urea solution are sometimes instilled into the amniotic sac.

Surgical methods

Evacuation of the uterus via the cervix

Conventional dilatation and curettage and vacuum aspiration can be used from about six to 14 weeks of gestation. Dilatation and evacuation are suitable from 12 to about 16 weeks of gestation.

Hysterotomy and hysterectomy

These procedures carry the risks associated with abdominal surgery and are not advised for abortion as such. Hysterectomy may be needed if there is uterine pathology severe enough for its employment apart from the question of abortion.

Choice of anaesthesia

Local anaesthesia

Local anaesthesia has the following advantages:
— it does not require stay overnight, either before or after operation
— it does not inhibit uterine contractility
— it has fewer respiratory or cardiac complications than general anaesthesia.

General anaesthesia

The main advantages are the excellent operating conditions and the fact that the procedure is free of pain or discomfort. Against this must be set the increased cost and inconvenience and the need for a trained anaesthetist and the provision of recovery facilities.

Induced abortion before 12 weeks

The method of choice, widely used throughout the world, is *suction curettage*. Following dilatation of the cervix, a specially designed plastic cannula is introduced into the uterine cavity. This is connected to a suction pump capable of inducing rapid vacuum and the uterine contents are aspirated into a reservoir jar. The cannulas are made in a variety of sizes, and the usual formula is to choose a diameter in millimetres equivalent to the gestation in weeks, although with practice it is not necessary to go beyond 10 mm. Using this technique, blood loss is less than 200 ml and damage to the cervix is minimal.

The method of *conventional dilatation and curettage* is still being used in some countries (e.g. Hungary and Poland), although suction curettage is replacing it. The contents of the uterus are removed using ovum forceps, and so it is necessary to dilate the cervix sufficiently wide to accept the instrument, which usually means 12 mm. Blood loss is greater and the risk of damage to the cervix increased, compared with suction curettage.

The use of cervical pre-dilatation

In order to reduce the amount of cervical damage from the use of dilators, two methods may be used to prepare the cervix. Their use is more popular in the USA than in the UK and they are particularly useful when dilatation above 10 mm is likely (e.g. in a 12 to 14 week abortion) or in a very young girl where the cervix is firm and the cervical canal is narrow. The method also has the advantage of reducing the discomfort when dilatation is carried out under local anaesthesia.

The first method involves the insertion of a pessary containing 2 mg of prostaglandin E_2 about four hours before the operation. This has the effect of softening the cervix.

The second method is a revival of the laminaria tent, made from the compressed seaweed *Laminaria norvegicus*. In the dehydrated form the tent looks like a short stick, but in contact with water it swells to more than twice its diameter. The tent is placed into the cervical canal and the slow stretching makes subsequent dilatation much less traumatic, even up to 14 mm. Laminaria tents are expensive, and synthetic substitutes such as the 'Lamicell' or 'Dilapan' are now available.

Induced abortion after 12 weeks

After 12 weeks of pregnancy, abortion becomes technically more difficult. In the UK there is a tendency to use instillation techniques, but there is evidence that such methods are less safe, at any rate up to 16 weeks, than the methods which have become known as 'D & E' (dilatation and evacuation).

Dilatation and evacuation

In the *one stage D & E*, the method is an extension of suction curettage. Where the uterine contents are too formed to enter the curette, a pair of strengthened ovum forceps (Sopher or van Lith) are introduced into the uterine cavity and the uterine contents broken up so that they can enter the curette. The method requires skill and experience, and it is claimed that it can be done through only 10 mm dilatation. A variation of the technique is to prepare the cervix before dilatation by inserting a vaginal pessary containing prostaglandin E_2, which softens the cervix and facilitates dilatation.

There is more than one *'two-stage D & E'*. The term may be used to describe the preliminary use of a prostaglandin pessary or a tent (see above), but it is more usually applied to the method described by Davis. The first stage consists of vacuum aspiration through a 10 or 12 mm cannula. Amniotic fluid is aspirated and the fetal umbilical cord brought down; the cord is cut and the ends left in the vagina. Death of the fetus follows and evacuation of the uterus is performed 24 hours later, usually without difficulty. The method has been used as late as 24 weeks, and is claimed to have a low morbidity, compared to other methods of late abortion.

Intra-amniotic injection

The substances used are hypertonic saline, urea solution or prostaglandins $F_{2\alpha}$ and E_2. The solution to be used is introduced into the amniotic sac via the abdominal wall and the fundus must therefore be easily palpable. The site is chosen, if possible, with the aid of ultrasound to avoid the placenta, and after anaesthetizing the abdominal wall, a needle is introduced into the amniotic sac and about 20 ml of liquor is aspirated. The chosen solution is then injected. Prostaglandins are the most effective, and urea is sometimes added to the solution to increase its effect.

Uterine contractions usually start within two hours, but the whole process takes up to 24 hours and resembles a miniature labour. Retention of the placenta is common and it is often necessary to remove the retained uterine contents under anaesthesia.

Extra-amniotic injection

While popular in the UK, this is not favoured in the USA because of the fear of introducing infection. With the woman in the lithotomy position, a Foley catheter is introduced through the cervix, a surprisingly easy manœuvre, and the bag inflated. A solution of prostaglandin E_2 is then injected at the rate of 100 mg per hour, using a continuous infusion pump or syringe. The interval between induction and abortion is about 18 hours, longer in primiparae than multiparae. As with intra-amniotic injection, retention of the placenta is common.

Abdominal hysterotomy

This is a caesarean section in miniature and therefore a major abdominal operation. At this stage of pregnancy, the lower uterine segment is not yet formed and the muscle wall is very thick. Apart from the fact that the operation has a much higher morbidity than the other methods described above, it also leaves behind a uterine scar which may cause problems in a subsequent pregnancy. For these reasons, it is often combined with sterilization. Hysterotomy is seldom indicated except when other methods go wrong.

Hysterectomy

Hysterectomy is very rarely used unless there is another condition such as carcinoma of the cervix which coincides with the pregnancy. Occasionally it has to be used as a life-saving measure to deal with complications such as injury or haemorrhage.

Risks of abortion

These can be divided into immediate risks, delayed risks and long-term risks. They are also related to the length of gestation at the time of the abortion.

Immediate (within 48 hours)

Haemorrhage related to abortion can be due to failure of uterine contraction or to incomplete evacuation of the uterus. Injury occurs when the cervix is torn or if an instrument perforates the body of the uterus, and such injury can in turn be complicated by bleeding or infection. Pharmacological complications can occur from reactions to local or general anaesthetic agents or to the substances, such as prostaglandins, injected into the uterus.

Delayed (within four weeks)

Delayed complications include prolonged bleeding from retained contents, with or without infection. Damage to other organs may also show up as peritonitis several days after the damage occurred. An important complication which is sometimes overlooked is failure to

261

terminate the pregnancy. This can happen when a second twin is missed or when the curette has unknowingly perforated the uterus. More serious is the occurrence of an early, unruptured ectopic pregnancy which comes to light several days or weeks after the apparent termination of a pregnancy.

Long-term complications (months or years later)

A number of conditions, such as infertility, cervical incompetence, second-trimester bleeding and abortion, and premature labour have all been reported as late complications following induced abortion. The true relationship is difficult to judge because many of these sequelae, such as premature delivery and spontaneous abortion, are themselves correlated with the social circumstances which preceded the abortion.

On the whole, evidence about the morbidity of abortion is reassuring. Abortion carried out early in pregnancy and in ideal conditions carries a very small risk. The possibility of later infertility, which worries many women, is increased where abortion is complicated by pelvic infection; that risk is very much increased in illegal operations.

Long-term psychological sequelae are also very difficult to assess. Most of the studies that have been carried out in the UK suggest that nearly all women suffer transient guilt, but that the incidence of depressive illness or of prolonged feelings of guilt is increased where there is a past history of emotional disturbance or where the abortion was advised on medical grounds rather than at the instigation of the woman herself.

Endogenous depression can be a particularly difficult problem, because the feeling of rejection of the pregnancy can be due to the depressive illness itself rather than its cause; treatment of the depressive illness is therefore sometimes more appropriate than abortion, but extra psychiatric help should be sought before making a decision.

Rhesus iso-immunization can occur as a result of abortion (spontaneous or induced), and rhesus-negative women should be offered anti-D immunoglobulin within 72 hours of abortion.

Risk of abortion and the duration of pregnancy

The risk of post-operative complications following abortion is very much related to the length of gestation. There is a sharp rise between the first and second trimesters, and to some extent this reflects the

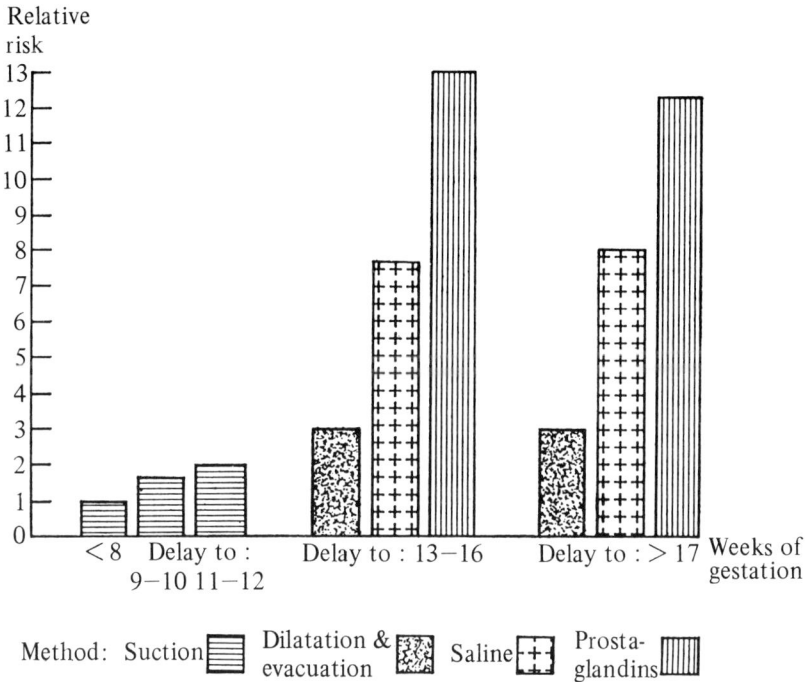

Fig. 24. *Relative risk of major abortion-related morbidity by length of gestation and choice of method, compared with risk associated with suction up to and including eight weeks gestation.*
Source: *Cates, W. et al. (1977) The effect of delay and method choice on the risk of abortion morbidity.* Family Planning Perspectives, **9**, *266-269.*

methods which are used (Fig. 24). Even within the same method, the morbidity following suction curettage rises with increasing gestation. In general, the mortality from induced abortion carried out after 16 weeks' gestation exceeds that of childbirth (Fig. 25). Late abortion has other disadvantages. It is also more unpleasant for the woman and the medical and nursing staff who are involved. For all these reasons, gynaecologists are reluctant to carry out late abortions without a reason strong enough to outweigh these disadvantages.

Choice of procedure

For abortion in the first trimester, few would disagree that vacuum curettage (aspiration) is the method of choice, but in the second trimester there is more uncertainty. Hysterectomy is now discredited

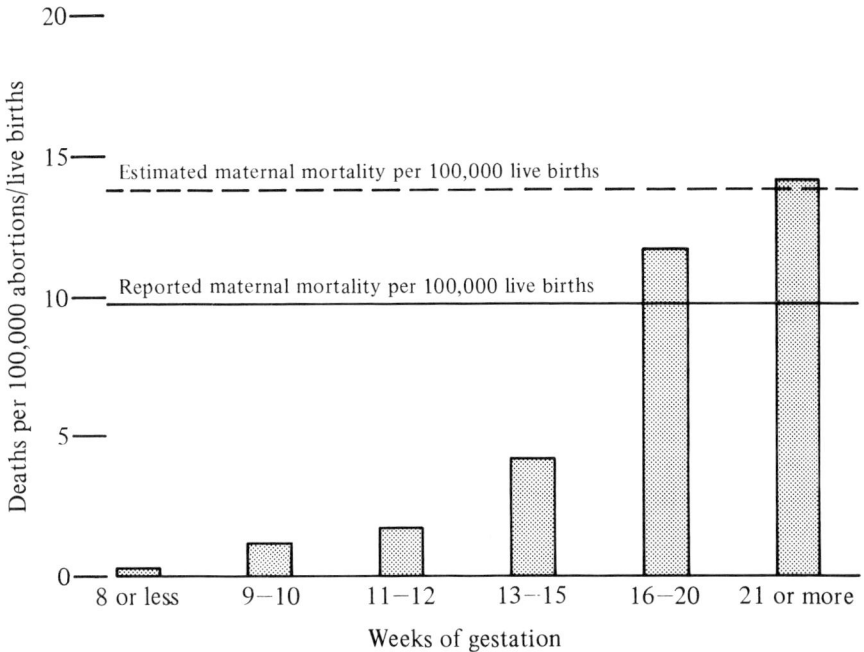

Fig. 25. *Deaths per 100,000 legal abortions, by weeks of gestation and maternal mortality per 100,000 live births: United States, 1972-80.*

(except as a last resort) and in the UK most gynaecologists favour the use of intrauterine injection. There is, however, growing evidence that 'D & E' (dilatation and evacuation) in one or two stages, is much safer than intra- or extra-amniotic injection, especially in that grey area between 12 and 15 weeks (Fig. 24). These methods are unpopular because they are distasteful, but of course intrauterine injection with its miniature labour is unpleasant for the woman and for the nursing staff in the wards, who have to deliver the fetus.

Extent of induced abortion

Induced abortion is now available legally to more than 60% of the world's population. There is a wide variation in the use made of induced abortion, the best index being the number of abortions per 1,000 women aged 15-44. In Cuba and Hungary, where abortion has been in use for many decades, the numbers have declined over the past 12 years. In the USA, England and Wales, Singapore and Tunisia, where the law was liberalized between 1965 and 1970, there was a steep rise for the first 10 years, and rates are now almost level.

Unfortunately, it is unlikely that contraception could ever prevent the need for all induced abortion, but it can contribute a great deal to reducing the large numbers that are carried out.

IMAP Statement on Abortion*

Introduction

Contraception is the first line of defence against unwanted pregnancy, as stated by the IPPF Governing Body, October 1971. The International Planned Parenthood Federation (IPPF) hopes that with increased provision and use of contraceptive services, the need for abortion will decrease. However, at least 30 to 55 million induced abortions are estimated to take place annually throughout the world. More than half are thought to be performed by unskilled persons mainly in the developing world, and mostly in settings where abortion is legally restricted. There is no way to determine the accuracy of these figures because of the many difficulties involved in reporting abortions by unskilled persons.

It is generally recognized that the numbers of maternal deaths attributable to abortion are much higher following abortions done by untrained persons than those done by trained practitioners. In some situations, where abortions are performed by unskilled persons, deaths may reach or exceed 1,000 per 100,000. The level of mortality reflects not only the skill of persons performing or initiating the procedure and the conditions under which it is done, but also the availability, utilization and quality of subsequent medical services if life-threatening complications develop. The drain on scarce health resources resulting from the treatment of such complications is excessive.

First-trimester abortion procedures carried out by well-trained practitioners carry a very low risk of complications for the woman. Beyond 10 weeks of gestation the health risks of abortion rise with each week of pregnancy, the risks of second-trimester abortion being 3-4 times greater than those of the first trimester. For this reason, where abortion services are offered, every effort should be made to provide them as early in pregnancy as possible.

In countries where abortion is legal, FPAs should be encouraged to ensure its provision as part of health and fertility regulation services: also

---

*This statement incorporates an earlier policy adopted in 1971 and reaffirmed in 1979, and is valid for currently available methods of abortion. The Panel reserves the right to amend this statement in the light of further developments in this field.

265

FPAs should seek to maximize the provision of contraceptive services immediately after abortion. Since the skill of the provider is a key variable in the safety of the procedure, FPAs should make certain that there are health personnel adequately trained to provide abortion services.

In countries where the legal status of abortion is unclear or restricted, some FPAs have demonstrated that a close examination of the law can reveal a margin of flexibility in its interpretation. In such countries FPAs should seek, where appropriate, to bring their influence to bear towards ensuring that adequate and socially humane services are available to treat incomplete abortions and other complications and that such services be linked with the provision of contraceptive advice. In those countries in which abortion is illegal, legislation which punishes a woman who has had an abortion may deter her from seeking medical advice if she is ill after such an abortion, and may inhibit her from obtaining immediate contraceptive advice.

Counselling

Every woman seeking abortion should receive supportive and sympathetic counselling responsive to her circumstances. Every effort should be made to encourage the woman's partner to be present at counselling sessions. Such counselling should include the different options open to her, including carrying the pregnancy to term and keeping the child, or having it adopted, and the opportunities which exist in the society for assistance.

The woman should be fully informed of the procedures to be performed, including anaesthesia. Their safety and their possible immediate and future side-effects and complications should be discussed. It may be necessary to explain that an early termination of pregnancy (in the first trimester) is very safe in skilled hands — and is significantly safer than carrying a pregnancy to term. The risks associated with a second-trimester abortion should be explained without exaggeration and should not be stated in such a way as to deter the woman from opting for abortion. It may be advantageous to allow, wherever possible, an interval of at least 24 hours to elapse between counselling and the performance of the abortion.

Contraceptive counselling both before and after the abortion should be comprehensive and include information about all the various contraceptive methods available, and their advantages and disadvantages. With adequate counselling before the procedure, IUD insertion immediately after abortion has proven to be acceptable and effective.

Abortion procedures can be conveniently and safely combined with laparoscopy or minilaparotomy sterilization operations. Where concurrent sterilization is contemplated, counselling should include stressing the essentially irreversible nature of sterilization. The need for a period of reflection is even more important under these circumstances. Practitioners, operators and counsellors should ensure that abortion is not being provided or considered as being conditional on the acceptance of sterilization.

Pregnant adolescents seeking abortion require special care and attention during counselling. The proportion of second-trimester abortion in this group is high, as teenagers tend to present later. Their feelings of anxiety and even guilt are often stronger. They may be concerned about their future fertility. These matters should be understood and appropriate counselling given. It may be necessary to provide for longer follow-up to deal with residual feelings of guilt, anxiety or fear. Adolescents should receive intensive contraceptive counselling as part of any comprehensive abortion service delivery programme.

During counselling, special care should be taken with women having any of the following conditions:

— women with a gestational age of over 12 weeks
— young adolescents (15 years or younger)
— women over the age of 40
— women with significant pre-existing medical conditions or complications
— women having had a previous operation on the uterus
— women requesting concurrent sterilization

First-trimester procedures

(A) *Less than 6 weeks*

Very early pregnancy, that is, in the first two weeks after a missed period, provides the clinician with two options:
1. To wait until the duration of pregnancy is 6–8 weeks and perform a procedure as outlined below under (*B*)
2. To perform an endometrial aspiration. This can be done without anaesthesia and cervical dilatation.

In carrying out the latter course of action, the following should be kept in mind:
(*a*) The possibility that the woman was not pregnant and therefore had a procedure which may be considered unnecessary.
(*b*) The likelihood of missing the products of conception altogether or carrying out an incomplete evacuation.
(*c*) The possibility of missing an ectopic pregnancy.

If a decision is taken to carry out an aspiration procedure, then the woman should be carefully followed up to exclude the possibility of (*b*) and (*c*) above. In addition to vacuum aspiration, the newer techniques currently being developed (such as prostaglandins used vaginally or orally) may provide further options for use at this stage.

(B) 6-8 weeks

Vacuum aspiration is the preferred technique at this stage of pregnancy. Cervical dilatation may not be needed, but if it is, either paracervical block or a general anaesthetic can be used. The procedure is done on an out-patient basis.

The possibility of missing an ectopic pregnancy at this stage can be decreased by examining the aspirated material.

(C) 9-12 weeks

Cervical dilatation and vacuum aspiration is the preferred technique, but dilatation and curettage may still have a place in some centres. Laminaria tents or prostaglandin analogues should be used, where available, for cervical dilatation. Paracervical block or general anaesthesia can be used for vacuum aspiration or curettage. At this stage, the operation can be done in an out-patient setting.

Second-trimester abortion

Second-trimester abortions should be performed only by appropriately trained medical personnel and preferably in hospital facilities.

Dilatation and evacuation is the recommended method of abortion at 13-16 weeks of gestation, the dilatation ideally being carried out by the use of laminaria tents or prostaglandin analogues. Practitioners experienced in dealing with late second-trimester abortions may use this procedure up to 18 weeks. The most commonly used method to induce abortion after 16 weeks is the intrauterine instillation of hypertonic saline, ethacridine lactate, urea, or prostaglandins. This can be done by intra-amniotic or extra-amniotic instillation techniques. Oxytocin can be given by intravenous infusion if there is a need to shorten the time interval between the instillation and the abortion.

Vaginal hysterectomy does not have a place in second-trimester abortions.

Complications

Complications of abortion are related to many factors. The most important of these factors are the period of gestation, the state of the woman's health and the skill and training of the operator. In the first trimester, if the procedure is carried out by a well-trained person, the mortality and morbidity risks associated with abortion are significantly less than those of continuing pregnancy. However, the morbidity and mortality risks associated with second-trimester abortion may be greater than those for continuing pregnancy. Early complications of abortion include trauma, haemorrhage, sepsis and retained products of conception. Anaesthetic complications may occur. These are 3-5 times more frequent after second-trimester abortions than after first-trimester abortions, and are particularly common and more serious when the procedures are carried out by unskilled persons. Psychological problems may also occur.

Late sequelae

1. Rh sensitization — wherever possible the woman's Rh factor should be checked. If the woman having the abortion is Rh(D) negative she should be given anti-D gammaglobulin within 72 hours of the procedure. The dose given should be in keeping with the length of gestation.
2. Infertility — pelvic infection resulting from abortion by unskilled persons, if untreated, may lead to relative or complete infertility.
3. The risk of low birth weight, premature delivery or mid-trimester spontaneous abortion in a subsequent pregnancy in a woman who has previously had a vacuum aspiration abortion is minimal. This risk is not significantly higher than the risk of an adverse outcome of a first pregnancy carried to term.

Prophylactic antibiotics

When the procedure is performed by trained personnel, there is no evidence that the use of prophylactic antibiotics is indicated to reduce the incidence of sepsis.

Repeated abortions

There have been reports that repeated induced abortions may affect future fertility or the outcome of future pregnancies, predisposing women to complications such as spontaneous abortion, premature labour, or babies of low birth weight. The data are equivocal and currently are not considered to be statistically significant where the abortion has been carried out by skilled practitioners. When repeated mechanical dilatation of the cervix takes place, as in the older D & C procedures, there may be an increase in the risk of adverse outcome of subsequent pregnancies.

(*Statement by the IPPF International Medical Advisory Panel, October 1983; approved and adopted by the IPPF Central Council, November 1983.*)

Chapter 17

Sexually Transmitted Diseases

Introduction

The range of diseases spread by sexual activity continues to increase. The types of diseases spread by sexual contact will vary in their incidence and clinical manifestations throughout the world. Despite this, all clinicians realize that the three traditional venereal diseases, chancroid, syphilis and gonorrhoea, only account for part of their practice and that more and more diseases are being recognized as spread by sexual intercourse or contact. Thus, non-specific and chlamydial infections are now common conditions with profound morbidity. Other sexually transmitted conditions such as trichomoniasis, scabies, pediculosis pubis and genital warts are increasingly diagnosed. Also commonly diagnosed is vaginal candidosis which is rarely spread by the sexual route. In the last few years some of the new generation of diseases are being seen more frequently. The incidence of herpes genitalis is rising, more sexually transmitted hepatitis B as well as A is seen, and even more recently doctors have become aware of enteric pathogens (*Entamoeba histolytica* and *Giardia lamblia*) being spread by sexual contact. The acquired immune deficiency syndrome (AIDS) with accompanying opportunistic infections and Kaposi's sarcoma is the most recent condition found to be spread by the sexual route.

It is difficult to estimate the size of the problem represented by sexually transmitted diseases (STDs) throughout the world, since some countries do not report to the World Health Organization (WHO), and within some countries there are inadequacies in the reporting systems. However, from returns made to the WHO it is estimated that about 200 million new cases of gonorrhoea and 40 million new cases of syphilis occur in the world each year.

The reason for the increase in the STDs is probably multifactorial. The age of sexual maturity has decreased, the age at which people have sexual intercourse for the first time is lower, and more people have premarital sexual intercourse than previously. Obviously, none of these indicate promiscuity, but as such it must be a factor. Also, the increasing use of oral contraceptives and intrauterine devices has removed the protective effect of barrier techniques such as condoms. Since populations are now more mobile, nationally and internationally, the behaviour of certain individuals puts them at risk. They are separated from their families and social restraints, and are more likely to have sexual contact outside a stable relationship.

Over the years the partial resistance of the gonococcus to penicillin has increased in many countries so that higher and higher curative doses have to be used. More worrying than this is the recent emergence of completely penicillin-resistant strains of *Neisseria gonorrhoeae*.

Finally, it has to be realized that throughout the world services for the STDs have never received the resources required for their adequate control. It is only through good health education and the availability of good treatment facilities and co-ordinated research that control of these diseases will ever be achieved. It is particularly important that those practising family planning are well aware of the STDs, since the age group of those coming forward for contraception is exactly the same as the age group of the great majority of those suffering from such diseases. Also, doctors working in family planning clinics are often able to take good sexual histories, perform examinations and offer appropriate health education.

Presenting symptoms

The three commonest symptoms of the STDs are a urethral discharge, a vaginal discharge and genital ulceration.

1. Urethral discharge

A urethral discharge is the commonest presenting symptom of an STD in men. Such discharges are usually pathological. A common cause is gonococcal infection, but many other organisms can be involved. The commonest cause of a non-gonococcal urethritis is

Chlamydia trachomatis, but the urethritis can also be due to other organisms such as *Ureaplasma urealyticum* or *Trichomonas vaginalis.* Local lesions within the urethra such as herpes, warts or a primary syphilitic chancre can also occasionally give rise to a urethral discharge.

Urethral discharge tends to be more purulent in gonococcal than non-gonococcal infections. The discharge associated with chlamydia and other non-gonococcal infections may not be so noticeable by the man. However, burning on urination is an important and frequent symptomatic complaint. If the individual has received some antibiotic treatment before the collection of the urethral discharge specimen, both the smear and the culture may be negative.

A specimen of urethral discharge should be collected for Gram-staining and microscopic examination. The slides can be stained immediately and a presumptive diagnosis for gonococcal or non-gonococcal urethritis can be made on this initial test. Gonorrhoea is confirmed by the presence of Gram-negative intracellular diplococci, whereas a non-gonococcal urethritis is confirmed by their absence and the presence of five or more polymorphonuclear leucocytes per high-power field (× 1,000 magnification). *Chlamydia trachomatis* cannot, however, be identified by direct microscopy. In the male up to 10% of cases of gonorrhoea may be missed if microscopy alone forms the basis of diagnosis. In ideal situations a specimen of discharge should be cultured for *Neisseria gonorrhoeae.* The material taken from the discharge can be plated onto a selective medium, for example Thayer Martin or modified New York City Medium, which contains antibiotics to suppress over-growth by other micro-organisms. If direct plating is not possible, a transport medium can be used, such as Stuart's or Amies', as long as the specimens reach the laboratory for plating out within 24-48 hours.

The treatment of a gonococcal urethritis in the male is penicillin, either intramuscularly or orally; for example, three grams of ampicillin plus one gram of probenecid. A non-gonococcal urethritis should be treated with a tetracycline, 250-500 mg four times a day for one week. This treatment is also adequate for an infection caused by *Chlamydia trachomatis.* It is preferable to follow up the patient at least once with one test of cure to see that the condition has resolved. Treatment of a urethral discharge includes carrying out contact tracing, not only of the partners who could have infected the patient, but also of sexual partners that the patient may have infected during the incubation period of his urethritis.

2. Vaginal discharge

Vaginal discharge is a common presenting symptom seen by general practitioners, gynaecologists and those working in family planning clinics. As with a urethral discharge, a vaginal discharge may be either physiological or pathological in origin. The common causes of a pathological (infective) vaginal discharge are *Candida albicans*, *Chlamydia trachomatis*, *Neisseria gonorrhoeae*, *Trichomonas vaginalis* and *Gardnerella vaginalis*. Lesions on the cervix, caused by herpes, warts or syphilitic chancre, can also cause discharge. Non-infective lesions on the cervix such as ectropion, polyps and neoplasm can also give rise to a discharge. Symptoms associated with a vaginal discharge are a burning feeling on urination and sometimes dyspareunia.

As with urethral discharge, a careful history, physical examination and microbiological tests are essential to establish an accurate diagnosis and to confirm or exclude a sexually acquired infection. Certain points in the clinical history are suggestive of such an aetiology. For example, the development of symptoms after a recent change of sexual partner, or recent multiple sexual contacts. If an STD is suspected from the clinical and sexual history, the patient should be examined fully to exclude possible complications and coincidental abnormalities. Neither the patient's symptoms nor a description of the colour and quality of the discharge are of much value in reaching an accurate aetiological diagnosis. The macroscopic appearance of a vaginal discharge does not help in making a diagnosis. For example, to rely on the suggestion that the discharge for vaginal candidiasis is thick, curdy and white will result in the wrong diagnosis in most instances. Similarly, no reliance should be placed on the supposed association between a frothy, greenish discharge and trichomoniasis.

Infection can be diagnosed accurately only after microbiological tests have been carried out on samples taken from the appropriate anatomical sites. The normal procedure to exclude an STD is to take specimens for gonorrhoea from the endocervix and urethra, for *Trichomonas vaginalis* and *Gardnerella vaginalis* from the posterior fornix, and *Candida albicans* from the lateral vaginal wall. If facilities for testing for *Chlamydia trachomatis* are available then a specimen should be taken from the endocervix. The reason for taking specimens from all these sites is that many of the STDs occur concurrently. For example, *Trichomonas vaginalis* is associated in approximately 20% of instances with concurrent gonorrhoea.

273

Candida albicans can be excluded by microscopy of a Gram-stain smear and culture of material from the vaginal wall. Both spores and mycelia will stain Gram-positive. Some cases can be missed by microscopy alone, and if possible cultures should also be performed using a traditional Sabaraud's medium. Failing this, Stuart's or Amies' transport medium, as described earlier, can be used.

Trichomonas vaginalis is usually best isolated from the posterior fornix and a wet preparation, using a drop of saline, can be examined immediately under a dark-ground microscope. Where this is not available, a 'hanging drop' technique can be used. Here the wet preparation is placed on a cover glass and positioned over the depression on a special slide made for wet-drop preparations. Microscopy alone with either technique is extremely reliable. If cultures are to be used, a sample of the discharge should be placed in a Feinberg-Whittington medium and incubated for 48 hours or sent to the laboratories in Stuart's or Amies' transport medium.

Gonorrhoea is an infection of mucous membrane surfaces, and this is the reason why specimens should be taken from the endocervix and urethra and not the vagina. Specimens taken from these two sites should be Gram-stained and cultured, as in the male. If direct plating cannot be carried out, transport medium can be used. Gram-stain microscopy for *Neisseria gonorrhoeae* in women is unreliable. Reliance on this test alone results in approximately half the cases being missed, therefore ideally all women in whom gonorrhoea is suspected should have cultures performed in addition to microscopy. In fact, one set of smears and cultures usually detects 90-95% of cases. This figure may be increased by repeat testing and sampling other sites (for example, the rectum). The gonococcus can be isolated from the rectum in women with gonorrhoea in about 6% of those cases in which it is not found in the conventional site of the cervix and urethra. This proctitis does not necessarily arise from anal intercourse but may be caused by auto-inoculation.

Chlamydia trachomatis is an important infection in women, and may be asymptomatic, unlike the situation in men. In addition, facilities for isolating this micro-organism are not readily available in most centres.

The final agent that should be looked for is *Gardnerella vaginalis*. Certain clinical and diagnostic features are associated with this infection. For example, a fishy smelling discharge which is particularly noticeable after sexual intercourse, the presence of clue cells (these are bacteria attached to vaginal epithelial cells), pH of the vaginal discharge of 5 or greater, and a positive result on the Ames test. This test is performed by adding one or two drops of discharge to 5-10% potassium hydroxide on a glass slide. A typical fishy ammoniacal odour is released when the result is positive. However, a similar smell can be obtained when *Trichomonas vaginalis* or sperm are present in the vaginal discharge in the absence of gardnerella. The organism may be cultured using Stuart's or Amies' transport medium.

All patients who present with either urethral or vaginal discharge should have serological tests for syphilis carried out to exclude this as a concurrent infection if there is any possibility that their symptoms could be due to a sexually acquired condition. Other common STD organisms should also be looked for, since there is often multiple infection.

The treatment of *Candida albicans* is by the use of vaginal pessaries containing nystatin, clotrimazole, miconazole or econazole. The treatment of *Trichomonas vaginalis* is with metronidazole 400 mg twice daily for five days, or a single dose of this at a level of two grams. The treatment of uncomplicated gonorrhoea in the female is the same as for the male. When the condition is sexually acquired, sexual contacts should be seen.

Pelvic inflammatory disease

The major complication associated with chlamydial and gonococcal infections in women is pelvic inflammatory disease (PID). Approximately 10% of patients develop this complication. PID is associated with long-term morbidity, such as chronic abdominal pain, menstrual disturbances, dyspareunia, tubal pregnancy, psychological sequelae, and, most unfortunate for many women, infertility. The proportion of patients with salpingitis who develop complete tubal occlusion following a first attack of gonorrhoea is 5%, and 16% after a first attack of chlamydia. After three or more attacks the chances of complete occlusion of the uterine tubes rise to 75% (see page 230).

The diagnosis of PID is often extremely difficult. Clinically the symptoms are of lower abdominal pain, malaise, vaginal discharge, dyspareunia and dysmenorrhoea. The signs of fever, abdominal tenderness, adnexal tenderness and cervical motion tenderness in association with a purulent cervical discharge are indications of PID. However, even when these symptoms and signs are correlated with laparoscopic findings, the clinical diagnosis is correct in only 65% of patients. The condition is often confused with appendicitis, endometriosis and ectopic pregnancy. Full microbiological tests should be carried out to detect infection with *Chlamydia trachomatis* or *Neisseria gonorrhoeae*. The former condition should be treated with tetracycline at a dose of 500 mg four times a day for at least 10 days, in association with metronidazole, provided the woman is not pregnant. Ideally she should rest in bed during the treatment. A gonococcal salpingitis should be treated with ampicillin 500 mg four times a day, again for a period of about 10 days. Contact tracing should be performed.

3. Genital ulceration

There are many causes of genital ulceration, and the commonest causes depend on the part of the world in which patients live. For example, the commonest cause of genital ulceration in the United Kingdom will be *Herpes genitalis*, with syphilis being a rare cause. However, in tropical environments granuloma inguinale, lymphogranuloma venereum, chancroid and syphilis would be common causes of ulceration, but *Herpes genitalis* would be rare.

Multiple painful ulcers are most commonly due to an infection with herpes simplex virus. If this is the patient's first attack the ulcers occur within one to two weeks of exposure to infection. The patient feels ill and the inguinal lymph nodes are large, discrete and usually painful. Recurrent attacks are less severe, bear no relation to sexual intercourse, and can sometimes be preceded by prodromal symptoms.

The commonest cause of painless genital ulceration is primary syphilis. The incubation period of this disease is usually 21 days, but the lesions may appear from nine to 90 days after sexual intercourse with an infected person. Inguinal lymph nodes are moderately enlarged, painless and usually discrete. Other stages of syphilis may also result in genital ulceration; for example, ulcers of the secondary stage which are evident as multiple, painless eroded papules or mucous patches.

Other causes of solitary, painless ulcers are carcinoma, circinate balanitis, balanitis xerotica obliterans, lymphogranuloma venereum and granuloma inguinale. The doctor should not forget that self-inflicted trauma or dermatitis artefacta can give rise to genital ulceration with rather atypical lesions.

Herpes is diagnosed by culture of the virus and the clinical story and appearance. To exclude primary or secondary syphilis, specimens should be taken from the ulcer and examined for treponemes by dark-ground microscopy. Serological tests for syphilis are not always positive when primary syphilitic lesions are present. The tests do not become positive for about 3-4 weeks after infection, whereas a primary lesion or chancre may be evident as soon as 9-10 days after exposure.

Pregnancy and the neonate

There are a number of STDs which can affect the unborn or newly born child. Most of these diseases that occur in the mother, affecting the fetus or neonate, can be prevented or are usually not serious if recognized and treated early on. Some problems that may arise if STDs in the mother are not treated include low birthweight in the infant, premature rupture of the membranes and premature delivery. Neonatal sepsis may also occur.

Both gonococcal and chlamydial infections can be transmitted by direct inoculation into the neonate's eye and additionally, in the case of chlamydia, by inhalation of infected material during birth, and neonatal pneumonia may occur. Likewise, herpes is contracted at the time of birth by direct inoculation of infected material. There is no good evidence to suggest that the herpes virus can cross the placenta. Cytomegalovirus can also be transmitted causing congenital defects.

Unlike infections with herpes, chlamydia and gonorrhoea which are acquired at birth, syphilis is a prenatal infection. Fetal infection with syphilis may occur at any time during pregnancy, leading to fetal death, neonatal death or congenital syphilis. Infection is more likely to occur if the mother has primary, secondary or early latent syphilis, since this is the time that large numbers of organisms are present in the circulation. Congenital syphilis still remains a large public health problem in developing countries and can only be controlled both by screening mothers during antenatal care, and also having good facilities to treat syphilis in women when they are not pregnant.

The Acquired Immune Deficiency Syndrome

Five cases of *Pneumocystis carinii* pneumonia and 26 of Kaposi's sarcoma were reported in homosexual men in Los Angeles, New York and California in mid-1981. This was the first indication of a new disease complex which was subsequently defined and given the name

277

of the acquired immune deficiency syndrome (AIDS). To date (October 1988), 76,670 cases have occurred in the USA, 15,340 in Europe and 1,794 in the United Kingdom. In Africa the epidemiology is different from that in the UK and the USA, where the majority of cases occur in homosexual men and intravenous drug abusers. In the African setting the disease is heterosexually acquired by those with multiple partners.

AIDS is caused by the Human Immunodeficiency Virus (HIV). However, infection with this virus only results in this condition in a proportion of instances of infection. Currently, this is thought to be up to 40% of individuals infected. The spectrum of infection is wide-ranging, from asymptomatic infection and full recovery to AIDS.

Acute infection with HIV can result in the minority of instances in an overt sero-conversion illness. This can take the form of an acute infectious mononucleosis-like picture or, occasionally, an acute encephalopathy. The majority of people who are infected acutely probably recover, but it is prudent to assume that they are infectious to others. A proportion who are acutely infected and do not recover go on to develop chronic infection with the virus. This can take many forms including a totally asymptomatic illness, cytopaenia, constitutional symptoms and minor opportunistic infections. The best documented state is that of the persistent generalized lymphadenopathy syndrome (PGL). It is currently thought that up to 20% of the people with PGL progress to develop AIDS. The major prognostic factors in the progression of PGL to AIDS are oral candida, a raised erythrocyte sedimentation rate, cytopaenia, herpes zoster and an involution and decrease in the size of lymph nodes. Again, it is only a proportion of people who are chronically infected with the virus who progress to 'end stage' AIDS. AIDS manifests itself in two major ways, either with tumours such as Kaposi's sarcoma or with various opportunistic infections.

The median survival varies, depending on the original presentation of AIDS. The median survival for people presenting with Kaposi's sarcoma is about 31 months, for *Pneumocystis carinii* 9 months, and for other opportunistic infections 4.5 months. Kaposi's sarcoma can be localized or widely disseminated and the opportunistic infections that occur can involve any system within the body. Other clinical phenomena are now being seen as manifestations of AIDS; for example, central nervous system involvement manifest in a variety of neurological signs and symptoms and also dementia.

Currently, there is no effective cure for HIV infection even though antiviral agents are being developed and tested, as are immune modulatory drugs. In view of this, the current cornerstone of control and prevention is health education.

Both sexes are at risk of acquiring AIDS, although in Europe and the USA males are mainly involved. In the USA, 7% of cases of AIDS occur in females, and 3% in the UK. In the USA 30% of all female cases appear to have occurred through heterosexual intercourse, the largest proportion (49%) occurring in intravenous drug users. However, the fact that in Africa equal numbers of men and women suffer from AIDS should be a warning that heterosexual transmission can occur and that maybe soon it will be seen more commonly in countries currently experiencing homosexual transmission.

Control of sexually transmitted diseases

No one disputes that STDs represent a major public health problem in the world today. Control can be achieved through the availability of good facilities for diagnosis and treatment, tracing and treatment of sexual contacts, health education of the public at large, but also of groups such as nurses and doctors, and teaching patients about personal prophylaxis. For example, health education material can point out that the risk of developing an STD increases with the number of partners that one has, and that if a person is monogamous with a monogamous partner, there is no chance of contracting an STD. Once the number of contacts increases, the probability of an STD increases, and it is worth pointing out to potential patients the usefulness of using a barrier form of contraception which will reduce the risk of certain diseases, and is a wise prophylactic measure when changing sexual partners. However, the condom can give a false sense of security, since it does not prevent the spread of all infections.

Throughout the discussion of clinical syndromes it has been assumed that laboratory facilities would be available. Clearly, in most parts of the world this is not so, and a more pragmatic approach has to be adopted. Such approaches are outlined in a WHO publication (1985) entitled *Control of Sexually Transmitted Diseases.*

IMAP Statement on Acquired Immune Deficiency Syndrome (AIDS)*

Introduction

The disease referred to as AIDS occurs in the majority of persons infected with a virus currently termed Human Immunodeficiency Virus (HIV). This virus attacks, in particular, the lymphocytes which are responsible for part of the body's defences against infection. The virus, however, may remain in a state of latency for varying lengths of time in the lymph cells without producing clinical symptoms. On the basis of current information, in the first five-year period, it appears that 10-30% of HIV-infected persons will develop AIDS, and 25-50% more will develop the AIDS-related syndrome. Current data suggest that the majority of HIV-infected persons may develop AIDS during the first 10 years after HIV infection and that the remainder may have AIDS-related syndromes. The virus has been detected in blood, semen, breast milk, saliva and tears of patients with clinical AIDS, and in those who are infected but have no clinical symptoms.

Since the first recognition of AIDS in 1981, more than 59,000 cases from 144 countries have been reported to the World Health Organization (WHO). Additional human retroviruses have been identified, principally in West Africa.

Epidemiology

In the USA and Western Europe, the major risk groups for AIDS are homosexual or bisexual men, prostitutes, persons who have ever been intravenous drug abusers (possibly sharing contaminated needles, syringes, etc.) and recipients of infected blood or blood products. In Africa, the risk groups are different in that the majority of cases appear to be in heterosexual men and women who are neither abusers of intravenous drugs nor recipients of blood or blood products.

No effective treatment is available either for the immune defect caused by the virus, or for the virus itself. However, many of the manifestations of AIDS can be treated, but they tend to recur.

With regard to outcome, it is important to differentiate between persons with HIV infection and no disease, and those with AIDS. Why some

---

*IPPF reserves the right to modify or change this statement in the light of further developments in the field of AIDS, when sufficient scientific information becomes available.

persons with HIV infection develop disease and others do not is presently unknown. Infected persons who do not develop disease may have a normal life span, whereas the mortality rate of those with AIDS is approximately 50% within one year of diagnosis. The five-year survival rate of AIDS patients approaches zero.

Transmission

HIV can be transmitted from an infected person with no symptoms as well as from AIDS patients. Transmission of HIV occurs through sexual intercourse (vaginal or anal) with an infected person, either from man to woman, from woman to man or from man to man. It can also be transmitted by transfusion of infected blood or blood products, injection with a needle contaminated with the virus, or artificial insemination with infected semen. Also it can occur perinatally from an infected mother to her newborn, and possibly by transplantation of infected organs or tissues. At the present time, it is not known whether perinatal transmission occurs transplacentally, or during or immediately after birth. There is a theoretical concern about transmission of HIV from infected mothers to children through breast feeding. Current breast-feeding policies should be maintained pending research underway to clarify the respective roles of intrauterine, peripartum and breast-feeding periods in perinatal HIV transmission.

Large studies of family members living with AIDS patients in the USA show that those who were not sexual partners and who had daily close contact with the patient did not develop infection. Likewise, a study of health care workers has shown that those caring for patients with HIV infection have no increased risk of infection. Infection has occurred in health workers through the accidental stick of a needle previously used on a patient with AIDS, though this is extremely rare. It is clear that transmission of the virus does not occur during non-sexual direct contact with an infected person.

Diagnosis

Diagnosis of HIV infection can be made by culture of the virus from the patient or by detection of serum antibody to HIV. Cultures are only available in a few highly sophisticated research centres, and are reserved for special studies. Several tests for the detection of antibody are commercially available. In many developed countries, all donors of blood, semen, or organs or tissue for transplantation are screened for HIV antibody. At present, persons who have antibody to HIV are believed to harbour the virus, and therefore are considered to be infectious.

Diagnosis of AIDS is made on the clinical presentation of the patient.

The presence of unusual infections such as *Pneumocystis carinii* lung infection, or unusually severe presentations of other infections in persons who have no known cause for immunosuppression may be indicative of AIDS, but the infections which are predictive of AIDS vary between geographic areas. Tumours such as Kaposi's sarcoma are also an indication of AIDS in western countries, but in tropical Africa this condition often exists in the absence of AIDS. HIV is neurotropic. It affects the neuraxis at all levels, resulting in clinical disorders involving the central and peripheral nervous systems. Approximately one-third of AIDS patients have clinical neurological findings attributable to HIV infection itself, rather than to opportunistic infections affecting the nervous system. Other manifestations of AIDS include severe candidiasis of the mouth and throat, and cytomegalovirus infection.

Symptoms

The symptoms of AIDS are variable and depend on the particular manifestations of the disease. For example AIDS patients with lung infection may have fever and night sweats, whereas those with skin tumours will have skin lesions. Non-specific symptoms in AIDS patients include profound fatigue, swollen glands in the neck, armpits and groin, unexplained weight loss and prolonged diarrhoea. Since these latter symptoms can be found in many other conditions, only when these conditions have been ruled out and the symptoms persist should the diagnosis of AIDS be considered, especially in persons not in high risk groups.

Prevention

For the prevention of HIV infection or AIDS, the following information is provided:

1. Prevention of sexual acquisition or transmission

(a) Monogamous relationships are safe, providing that neither partner is infected.

(b) Casual sexual intercourse and multiple partners increase the risk.

(c) Risk is decreased by avoiding sexual intercourse with partners who may have been exposed to HIV infection.

(d) Since the virus is transmitted during sexual intercourse, proper use of condoms reduces the risk of transmission for both male and female partners. Evidence of a possible protective effect of spermicidal preparations is inconclusive. There is *in-vitro* evidence that suggests that the addition of spermicides containing nonoxynol-9 to condoms may provide additional protection.

2. Prevention of transmission by non-sexual means

(*a*) Persons in high-risk groups are unacceptable as donors of blood, semen, or organs or tissue for transplantation.

(*b*) Use of contaminated needles among intravenous drug abusers increases the risk.

(*c*) As always, use of non-sterile needles for injection is unacceptable.

(*d*) Health workers involved in providing artificial insemination services, or blood or blood products, should be aware of the risk of HIV infection.

(*e*) Blood and semen donors should be screened for antibody at the time of donation and semen donors be retested after three months. The semen should be frozen and not used until the results of the second test are known.

(See also section for health workers.)

3. Prevention of perinatal transmission

(*a*) Women with HIV infection who become pregnant have an increased risk of developing AIDS compared with those who do not become pregnant. Further epidemiological studies need to be carried out.

(*b*) Women with HIV infection who become pregnant may transmit the infection to their newborn in about 50% of cases. Therapeutic abortion should be offered, where national laws permit, and the woman requests it.

(*c*) Newborns who develop AIDS have a particularly severe course and shorter life span than adults.

(*d*) In counselling for contraception, women with infection should be advised that apart from the need for a highly effective form of contraception, such as oral contraceptives or sterilization to prevent pregnancy, use of a condom reduces the risk of transmission to their partners.

Information for health care workers

Family planning workers, while being aware of HIV and AIDS, should not overestimate the risk of the infection in the course of their professional duties. It is important to remember that AIDS is still an uncommon disease of low infectivity. Even prolonged non-sexual contact with an AIDS patient has not resulted in transmission.

The risk to health care workers is the same as that for the general population. Gloves should be worn when handling body fluids to avoid direct contact. Handwashing after caring for a patient is a usual hygienic procedure which should be emphasized. The risk of transmission of HIV by accidental needle sticks is much lower than that for hepatitis B: however, it can occur. Therefore, the usual precautions for preventing needle sticks should be observed, and reinforced. Services should observe proper practices in sterilization and disinfection. The virus is sensitive to heat and chemical agents. Therefore, controlled heating of blood products or breast milk can be carried out to inactivate the virus. Chemical agents such as sodium hypochlorite can be used to disinfect contaminated surfaces. Hygienic precautions, including non-re-use of disposable syringes, and adequate disinfection of equipment between clients are not only important for the protection of health workers — they can also play a vital role in preventing transmission from one client to another.

It is recommended that WHO guidelines in sterilization and disinfection be observed.

(Statement by the International Medical Advisory Panel February, 1986. It has been under constant review and was updated the last time in November 1987. Adopted by Central Council, November 1987.)

IMAP Additional Statement on Acquired Immune Deficiency Syndrome (AIDS)*

Since IMAP last reviewed this topic, in February 1986, the alarming worldwide dimension of the public health problem posed by the spread of AIDS has become increasingly apparent. IMAP drew up the following recommendations to assist FPAs to play a more active role in helping to control the spread of AIDS.

Information and education

Of primary importance is an effective programme of Information and Education so that the following basic information about AIDS is understood.

1. AIDS is a fatal disease for which there is, as yet, no cure.
2. AIDS is spread by sexual intercourse, by contaminated blood, and by contaminated hypodermic needles.
3. An infected woman can give AIDS to her fetus during pregnancy.

---

*IMAP reserves the right to modify or change this statement in the light of further developments in the field of AIDS, when sufficient scientific information becomes available.

4. A stable, faithful relationship with another uninfected person is safest. In any case, reducing the number of sexual partners reduces the chances of getting AIDS.
5. For the sexually active, always using condoms is good protection against AIDS.
6. An infected person can look and feel well and still be able to transmit the virus that causes AIDS.
7. AIDS is not spread by ordinary day-to-day human contact with an infected person. This should be emphasized to health workers, families, co-workers and employers.

Among the target audience for information and education activities are family planning workers, family planning clients and the general public including youth, teachers, parents, employers and community and national leaders.

Special attention should be given to high risk groups which include homosexual and bisexual men, haemophiliacs, male and female prostitutes, clients of sexually transmitted disease clinics, people with many sexual partners, illegal users of intravenous drugs, and the sexual partners of those in any of these groups.

In addition, health workers and traditional practitioners who administer drugs by injection, should be aware of the importance of only using sterile needles and syringes.

Those working in the media need to be kept fully informed in order that they publish accurate information on this problem.

Family Planning Associations should take every opportunity to include information on AIDS in all their existing information and education projects. In addition, special educational material may be developed and/or adapted from existing ones.

Services

(a) Contraceptive advice

FPAs have a special role to play in the prevention of AIDS. Wide promotion of the use of the condom, particularly among high-risk groups is a priority. In the management of clients who have either been identified as carriers or have the active disease, it is essential that they understand that:

1. the disease can be transmitted to sexual partners, and
2. if pregnancy ensues, there is a strong likelihood that the fetus will be infected.

Even where other methods of contraception are chosen, condom use is still essential to prevent transmission of viruses.

(b) Diagnostic tests

Some clients will request diagnostic assistance. Since currently available inexpensive screening tests have a high false-positive rate, they should not be used for diagnostic purposes unless a more definitive confirmation test with a very low false-positive failure rate is available. FPAs, however, should know what referral services are available and use them.

Chapter 18

Cervical and Vaginal Cytology

Introduction

Family planning clinics have a role in the wider aspects of medical care. One such role, where facilities and manpower permit, is in the area of cervical and vaginal cytology. This is not a primary role of family planning clinics, and taking cytological smears should only be included in their work if it does not overstrain their facilities and deny some women the family planning they are looking for.

Exfoliative cytology

During life, cells in the body which are old and worn out are constantly replaced by newly-formed ones. Exfoliative cytology is the study of cells that have been exfoliated (shed) by various membranes or epithelia (surface coverings). The cells which are shed or dislodged may be collected and spread on to slides and the resulting smears stained and examined under the microscope. In clinical practice, surfaces are usually scraped to provide cells for study, e.g. a cervical scrape.

The examination of the exfoliated or the dislodged cells serves two main purposes:

1. To find out if the lining membranes (epithelia) are healthy or diseased, and to determine the type and severity of the epithelial abnormality, e.g. inflammation, dysplasia, or some form of carcinoma.

2. In the case of vaginal smears to study hormonal changes.

Collection of material for preparing smears

Material for cytological examination may be collected from various sites. These include the posterior, anterior or lateral fornix of the vagina, the ectocervix and squamo-columnar junction, the endocervical canal, the endometrial cavity or the upper third of the lateral vaginal wall. Most smears from the female genital tract are, in practice, intended to detect cervical lesions. The choice of site and technique depends largely on the available facilities and the purpose of the examination, e.g. material from the lateral vaginal wall is eminently suitable for estimating hormonal effects, but useless for the detection of cervical cancer; similarly, material from the ectocervix is hardly appropriate in the search for an endometrial carcinoma. Each of these methods has its merits and limitations. It is often advantageous to obtain smears from several sites to increase the scope of the examination.

Several methods, depending on the site and the circumstances of the collection, are used to obtain material for preparing the smears. They include aspiration from the posterior fornix (a simple but not particularly reliable method); a scrape of the ectocervix and squamo-columnar junction (the most useful method for detecting cervical lesions); and scraping the lateral vaginal wall (this method is only suitable for studying hormonal effects). Although there is as yet no entirely satisfactory method available for detecting early stages of endometrial cancer, various washing techniques carried out under negative pressure are recommended. The cytologist must be informed by which method the material has been collected. This chapter will concentrate on the cervical scrape method.

The cervical scrape smear

This method has been described by Ayre and collects cells directly from the ectocervix and the squamo-columnar junction.

Instruments required:

A vaginal speculum and an adjustable light, a wooden or plastic Ayre spatula*, slides, fixing jar or spray fixative, and hard pencil (Fig. 26).

It is advisable to get ready the essential equipment for making and fixing the smear, preferably laying it out on a tray, before collecting

---

*After 40 years of domination, the Ayre spatula has been largely superseded by better designed devices, all intended to gain a sample of cells from the endocervix, where the Ayre device falls short. Experience with the Aylesbury and Cervex devices leaves little doubt as to their superiority, with final preference for the Cervex (Fig. 27) for its superb harvest from the endocervical canal as well as from the ectocervix.

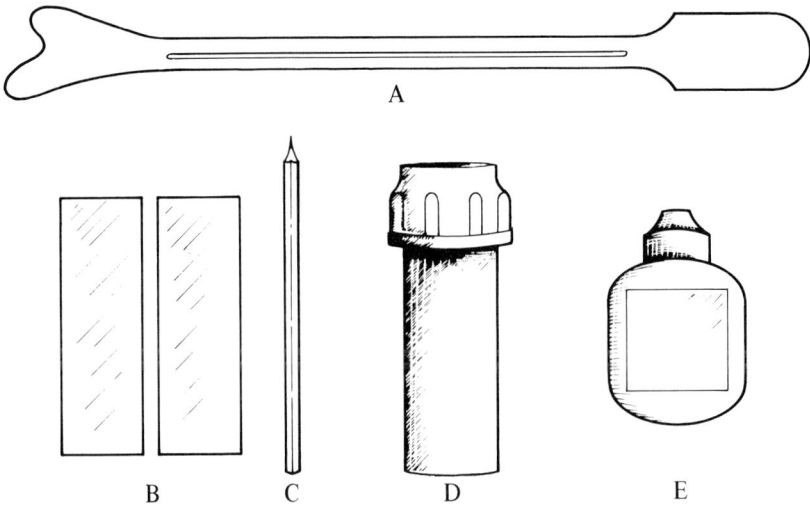

Fig. 26. *Requirements for cervical scrape smear: A. Ayre spatula; B. Glass slides; C. Hard pencil; D. Fixing jar; E. Spray fixative.*

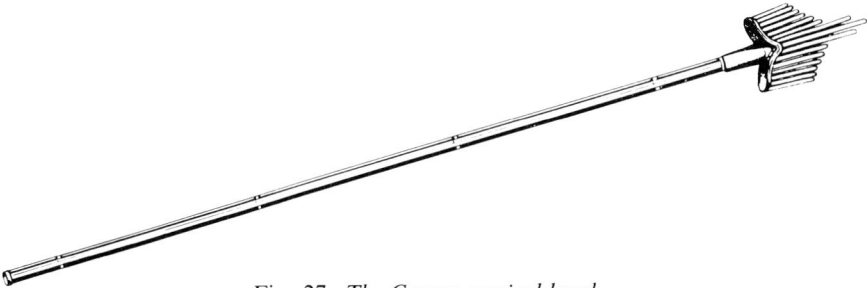

Fig. 27. *The Cervex cervical brush.*

the material. Identification marks must be put on each slide, e.g. numbers may be scratched on with a diamond or, if slides with ground glass ends are used, the name of the woman should be noted with a hard pencil (not with a ball-point pen, as the ink may dissolve).

The following information about the woman should be available and entered on the form: first name and surname of the woman; her age; clinic registration number; date of last menstrual period; length of menstrual cycle and whether the woman is pregnant; number of previous pregnancies; dates of previous gynaecological operations; if she has had radiotherapy; results of any previous smears; whether she is symptom-free or not; whether she has an intrauterine device fitted;

whether she is taking oral contraceptives or other hormones; and if she has a history of administration of hormones or antibiotics in the past. Optional information includes the woman's complaints and clinical findings.

Method

The woman lies on her back or side with her knees drawn up. No bimanual examination should be carried out before the smear is taken. An unlubricated vaginal speculum is introduced and the cervix exposed. The ectocervix, and especially any areas which appear abnormal (e.g. an erosion), and more importantly the squamo-columnar junction, are lightly scraped with the shaped end of the spatula (Fig. 28). The full circumference of the squamo-columnar

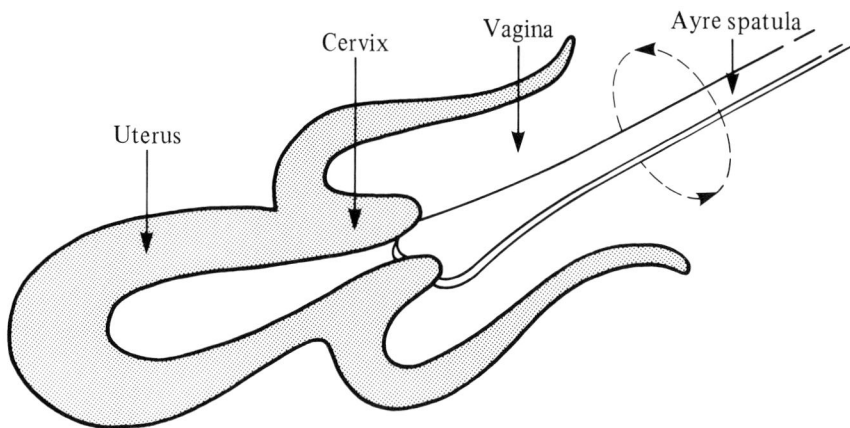

Fig. 28. *Scraping the squamo-columnar junction with the shaped end of the Ayre spatula.*

junction should always be scraped. In multiparous women better results are obtained with a larger spatula or by using the broad instead of the shaped end for scraping.

The spatula is carefully withdrawn from the vagina, the speculum still holding the walls apart, and the scrapings are immediately placed on one or two slides kept in readiness. Using the shaped end of the spatula, the scrapings are evenly spread over the slide (Fig. 29). Fixing and staining are as described below. It is essential, while they are still wet, to immerse the slides immediately in the fixative, or to cover the smears with spray fixative, in order to avoid their drying in the air.

After the smears have been put in fixative or sprayed with it, the speculum should be removed from the vagina.

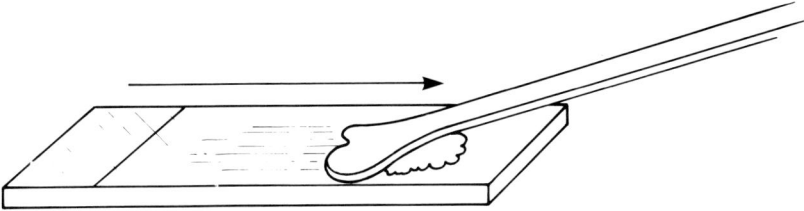

Fig. 29. *Spreading the scrapings on to the glass slide with the Ayre spatula.*

Scope of the method

Cells of the ectocervix and squamo-columnar junction are removed directly by the spatula, and will not be contaminated by cells from other sites.

Atypical cells arising from sites other than the cervix cannot be detected in cervical scrapes. Adenocarcinoma cells from the endometrium or endocervix may occasionally be caught in the cervical mucus and seen on the films; this, however, is the exception rather than the rule, and the majority of glandular cancers remain undetected by this method. Furthermore, the material obtained by scraping the cervix is unsuitable for the evaluation of hormonal effects.

Fixing the smears

Once material is collected it must be spread on to a glass slide and the resultant smear fixed and suitably stained before it can be examined under the microscope.

It is important that the secretions have been spread evenly over a previously prepared and labelled glass slide (see page 289). Lumps must be avoided and should be broken up by exerting a little pressure with the Ayre spatula. Speed is an essential factor in preparing the slides because air drying damages the cells and interferes with their staining properties. Cytological interpretation of air-dried cellular samples may give rise to false diagnoses. Fixation of the slides must be carried out quickly while the smears are still wet to prevent their drying in the air. This may be achieved by immersing the slides in jars filled with fixing fluid or by spraying them with commercially available spray fixative. Spraying is more modern and is probably better

291

and simpler, but sprays are expensive and not always easily available in outlying areas. Therefore, the method for fixing in fluid is given as well since this is still likely to be used extensively.

Fixing in fluid

Suitable containers for fixing fluids are clean jam or honey jars and commercially available Coplin jars made of glass or plastic material (Fig. 30). When jam or honey jars are used, not more than one pair of

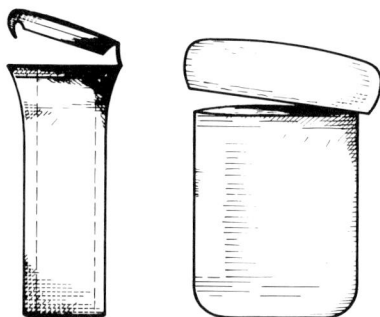

Fig. 30. *Jars or containers with fixing fluid for taking slides.*

slides should be immersed in each. Coplin jars can take up to five pairs of slides. The slides should be placed back to back (smear-carrying sides outwards) into the grooves of the fixing jar.

Fixing fluids in common use are various alcohols, e.g. 95% ethyl alcohol, methyl alcohol, isopropyl alcohol; or mixtures of different alcohols such as three parts of 95% ethyl alcohol and seven parts of tertiary butyl alcohol.

The slides should remain in fixative for at least 15 minutes, but may be left there for as long as seven or even 10 days without deterioration. After adequate fixation the slides are ready for staining. The staining procedure requires laboratory facilities and should be carried out by a trained technician. It may, therefore, be necessary, when such facilities are not available, to dispatch the slides to a laboratory for further processing. This can be done quite easily by removing the slides from the fixing jars after adequate fixation, allowing them to dry in the air, and posting them in flat cardboard or wooden boxes. On arrival in the laboratory they will be re-suspended in fixative and stained.

Spray fixation

Spray fixation gives excellent results, and overall is much simpler, more economical and saves time and equipment, compared with fixing in fluid. Care must be taken to ensure an even spread of the spray fixative over the whole of the smeared area on the slide (Fig. 31).

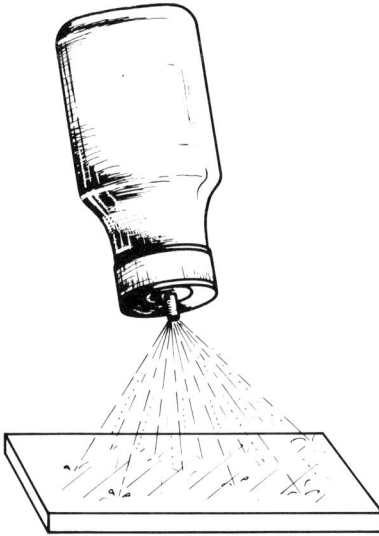

Fig. 31. *Spraying slide to fix the smear.*

The spray can must not be held closer than 15 cm from the slide or it may tend to wash the specimen away. There are various spray fixatives on the market containing an aerosol agent and different mixtures of alcohol, acetic acid, ethylene or propylene glycol. Spray-fixed slides, once they are dry (usually within 10 minutes) may be dispatched to the laboratory for staining directly without additional measures. The commercially available spray fixatives are relatively expensive; it has been shown recently that ordinary hair sprays are as effective and are considerably cheaper.

Common errors in smear preparation and processing

1. Insufficient material in the scrape.
2. Thick films with inadequate spread of the material.
3. Material collected from the wrong site, e.g. scraping the posterior vaginal wall instead of the cervix.
4. Use of slides which are insufficiently cleaned or degreased.
5. Air drying before fixation or during the staining procedure.
6. Insufficient fixation for too short a time or use of too weak alcohols.
7. Incorrect staining (incorrect staining times and insufficient dehydration or mistakes in the preparation of the stains).

Any one of these mistakes may seriously interfere with the correct interpretation of the slides. Correct preparation, fixation and staining of the specimens are fundamental steps in the cytological investigation of a woman. Even the most experienced cytologist cannot achieve a correct diagnosis when a faulty specimen is submitted to him.

Who needs testing?

Who needs testing? The answer is, every sexually active woman, regularly, at least every three years, and some more often than others. An extraordinary variety of excuses by various health authorities has been raised to show why comprehensive screening programmes are impossible, usually on financial grounds, it must be said. The cost of not testing, in terms of morbidity and mortality, is never given equal consideration.

Recently, irrefutable evidence has come to light, showing that cancer of the cervix in young women is a different disease to that found in older women — more rapidly growing, aggressive, with a transiently short pre-invasive stage, making the old guidelines as to who is and who is not at risk, quite out-dated. Such women should ideally be tested at yearly intervals from the age of 20 years onwards. Indeed, annual cytotesting of all women until the age of the menopause, as practised in British Columbia, Canada, is very difficult to argue against — where else has mortality from cancer of the cervix been reduced to a mere 25% of what it was only 20 years ago?

However, bearing in mind the limited resources generally available, the following recommendation would seem both practical and effective: all women should be tested, from the age of 20 years, every two years — annually if resources permit — until the age of 40 years. Then the highest risk period will have passed, and five-yearly testing until the age of 60 years would be adequate. With consistently negative tests, no further examination would then be necessary.

Chapter 19

Genetics and Family Planning

Introduction

Anxieties about reproduction are often presented to doctors working in family planning. A substantial proportion of couples have grounds for concern about risks of abnormality of their offspring. They may already have had a miscarriage or an abnormal baby or there may be a family history of a serious condition that they fear is inherited.

The aims of genetic counselling are to assess the risks as accurately as possible, to present all the relevant available information to the couple in an understandable form, and to help them to reach their own reproductive decisions.

Risk assessment requires a precise diagnosis and a carefully-taken family history. Specialized investigations and medical library facilities may be needed, together with the help of a trained specialist. In many countries such facilities are non-existent, and far more pressing medical problems remain to be solved. As many of the infections and nutritional disorders come under control, however, the proportion of disease which is genetic in origin will rise. At the same time the improving survival and health of children will encourage parents to have smaller families and to be more concerned for the welfare of each individual child. All doctors should be equipped with an understanding of genetic mechanisms to help them give sensible advice when they encounter genetic disorders in their practice.

There are three main categories of genetic disorders:

1. Those caused by microscopically-visible chromosome abnormalities.

2. Those caused by defects of individual genes.

3. Those caused by contributions from multiple genes, often associated with environmental factors (multifactorial).

Chromosomal abnormalities

There are normally 46 chromosomes in each nucleated cell: 22 pairs of autosomes and 2 sex chromosomes. The sex chromosomes are the X chromosome, which is paired in the female (46, XX) and the Y chromosome, present only in the male, who also carries a single X chromosome (46, XY).

The chromosome number is halved by meiosis, which takes place during gamete formation. Thus, egg cells contain a complement of 23, X, and sperm are of 2 types, 23, X and 23, Y.

Chromosome analysis is most conveniently carried out by culturing lymphocytes from a blood sample for three days, followed by fixing and staining. The chromosomes can be seen in those cells which are undergoing division (mitosis) at the time of fixation. Special staining methods ('banding') in use since 1971 produce the characteristic striped appearances seen in Fig. 32.

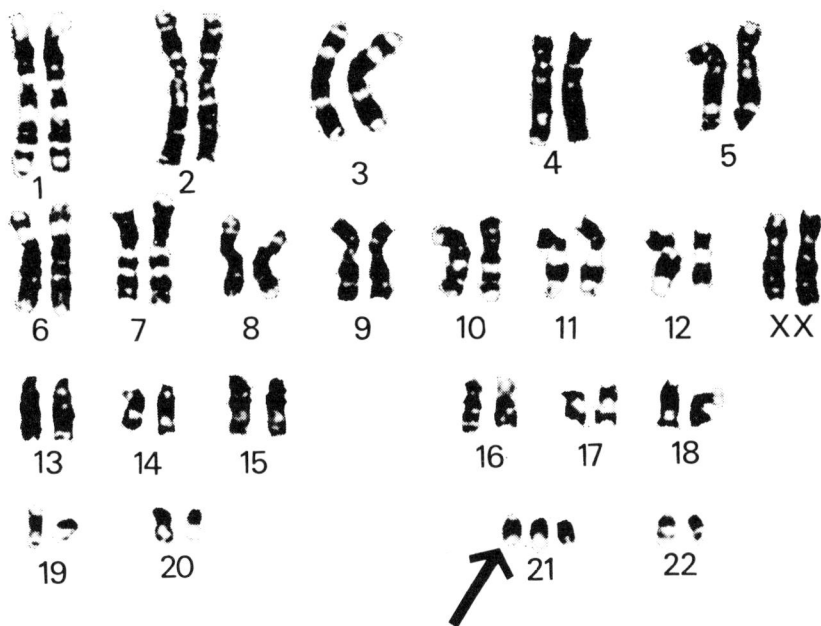

Fig. 32. *Karyotype of female with Down syndrome, showing trisomy 21 (arrowed).*

The staining of buccal smears for sex chromatin gives limited information on an individual's sex chromosome constitution, and should now be regarded as an obsolete procedure.

Numerical abnormalities

The commonest abnormalities are those of chromosome number. Extra chromosomes are far commoner than missing chromosomes; the latter, except for the missing sex chromosome condition, Turner syndrome (45, X), are too severe to produce a viable fetus. The same applies to most of the trisomies (where a particular chromosome is present in 3 instead of 2 copies). Those listed in Table III are, relatively speaking, the mildest. Up to a half of all first-trimester miscarriages are of chromosomally abnormal fetuses. Even trisomy 21, the mildest of the autosomal trisomies, is commoner in spontaneous abortions than in live births.

The numerical chromosome abnormalities mostly arise as meiotic errors in egg or sperm formation. Such errors are usually sporadic, with no clear evidence of a familial tendency, but they become more common in the ovaries of older women. The most important risk is that of Down syndrome, which behaves as shown in Table IV.

Structural chromosome abnormalities

These are the result of chromosome breakage, sometimes followed by rejoining in new combinations. The commonest types are as follows:

Deletion: A segment of chromosome breaks off and is lost. This is always *unbalanced* in that it produces a deficiency of genetic material with clinical effects.

Translocation: Breaks occur in two chromosomes simultaneously, and rejoin in such a way that material is exchanged between the two chromosomes. A translocation may be *balanced*, with no effect on the carrier's health if there is no gain or loss of material.

Inversion: Two breaks occur in a chromosome and the segment rejoins in reversed orientation. Like translocations, inversions may be *balanced*.

The importance of balanced structural rearrangements is that they interfere with the normal orderly segregation of chromosomes at meiosis, increasing the risk of unbalanced gametes which may lead to miscarriage, perinatal death, or a surviving mentally handicapped child.

The parents of any child with a structural chromosome anomaly

TABLE III. Numerical chromosome abnormalities: prevalence at birth (per 1,000 births)

Down syndrome (trisomy 21)	1.4
Edwards syndrome (trisomy 18)	0.2
Patau syndrome (trisomy 13)	0.1
Klinefelter syndrome (46, XXY)	1.0 (males)
47, XYY	1.0 (males)
47, XXX (triple X female)	1.0 (females)
Turner syndrome (45, X and variants)	0.3 (females)

should have their chromosomes checked. It is less important to check the parents' chromosomes in a numerical abnormality, as the only relevant high-risk situation is mosaicism, where a parent has a mixture of normal and abnormal cell lines, but it is rare.

Down syndrome

The great majority (97%) of cases have a numerical chromosome abnormality, trisomy 21 (47, XX or XY, +21), which arose at the time of gamete formation (in testis or ovary, more commonly in the latter), and which has a low recurrence risk (1%).

In around 2% of cases, there is a normal cell line as well as the trisomy 21 cell line (mosaicism). On average, the mosaic cases are milder, but this is not a reliable prognostic factor.

Occasionally, mosaicism is found in an apparently normal parent of a trisomy 21 child. This is the main justification for checking parental chromosomes in such cases, but it is not a strong indication. If parental mosaicism is found, recurrence risks will be somewhat higher.

About 3% of Down syndrome cases are found to carry a translocation involving chromosome 21. Usually one chromosome 21 is joined to a 13, 14, 15, 21 or 22 chromosome. The importance of these rare translocation cases lies in the fact that one or other parent may carry the translocation chromosome, and be at increased risk of another affected child. The balanced carrier parent will have 45 chromosomes and the affected child 46.

Males with Down syndrome are not usually fertile, but some females have reproduced; there is a high risk of affected offspring.

Whenever possible, chromosome analysis should be performed on patients with Down syndrome and, if indicated, on the parents, in order to confirm the diagnosis and give the appropriate recurrence risk.

TABLE IV. The risk of Down syndrome and other chromosome abnormalities by maternal age (at time of delivery).*

Maternal age (years)	Risk of Down syndrome in live births	Risk of any unbalanced chromosome abnormality at amniocentesis
20–24	1 in 1700	
25–29	1 in 1100	
30–34	1 in 770	
35	1 in 380	1 in 78
36	1 in 300	1 in 71
37	1 in 230	1 in 67
38	1 in 180	1 in 61
39	1 in 140	1 in 48
40	1 in 100	1 in 42
41	1 in 90	1 in 35
42	1 in 70	1 in 25
43	1 in 50	1 in 20
44	1 in 40	1 in 23
45	1 in 30	1 in 14

*The large discrepancy between the two columns can be accounted for by:

(*i*) miscarriage and still birth of Down syndrome cases after the time of amniocentesis

(*ii*) unbalanced chromosome abnormalities other than Down syndrome; some of these are more severe than Down syndrome (e.g. trisomy 18), others are less severe (e.g. sex chromosome anomalies).

Single gene anomalies

There are many disorders, both congenital and of later onset, caused by single gene defects. Most are rare (1 in 10,000 births or less), but studies in Western populations have shown that around one person in 100 suffers from one of these disorders. A few, such as the thalassaemias, sickle cell anaemia, and cystic fibrosis, have become common in specific populations and make a major contribution to morbidity (see Table V).

Autosomal disorders are those caused by defects of genes carried by chromosomes 1-22, the autosomes. These are transmitted identically by males and females. An individual inherits a copy of each gene from each parent. Autosomal dominant disorders are those which are caused by a single copy of a defective gene, its partner being normal.

TABLE V. Single gene disorders associated with particular ethnic groups or geographical areas

	Ethnic group or geographical area	Prevalence at birth	Heterozygote frequency (approximate)
Thalassaemias	Greece, Italy, Cyprus, Middle East, parts of India and SE Asia	Variable up to 1/200	1/20–1/7
Thalassaemias	China, SE Asia	Variable up to 1/200	Up to 1/7
Sickle cell anaemia	Central and West Africa, US Blacks	Up to 1/100	1/15–1/5
Cystic fibrosis	Northern Europeans	1/2000	1/22
Tay Sachs disease	Ashkenazi Jews	1/3600	1/30

Autosomal recessive conditions require both copies of a gene to be defective before they are expressed.

Defects in genes carried by the X chromosome show a special type of inheritance. A male transmits his X chromosome to all his daughters but to none of his sons. Most of these conditions are recessive, so that females carrying the defect in single dose are unaffected, but on average half their sons will be affected and half their daughters will be carriers.

It is essential before offering genetic counselling for any single gene disorder to have an accurate diagnosis, especially if the pedigree is uninformative. There are many examples of genetic disorders which superficially resemble non-genetic conditions and of similar disorders having different modes of inheritance.

Autosomal dominant disorders

The commoner examples include Huntington's chorea, neuro-fibromatosis, and the 'adult' type of polycystic kidneys. Each child of an affected parent, male or female, is at 50% risk of inheriting the condition.

As long as the condition does not reduce fertility, one finds pedigrees showing generation to generation transmission; however,

301

some autosomal dominant conditions do reduce fertility and these are maintained in the population by fresh mutations. A significant proportion of cases then have unaffected parents, and the recurrence risk for these couples is low. The affected person, even though a fresh mutation, has the normal 50% risk to his or her children.

Many autosomal dominant disorders are variable in severity, and it may be necessary to examine an at-risk family member very carefully before pronouncing him or her unaffected. Conditions of delayed onset, like Huntington's chorea or myotonic dystrophy, also present difficulties in defining the risks for individuals.

Autosomal recessive conditions

Couples at risk are not usually identified as such until they have an affected child; thereafter, the risk to further children is 1 in 4 (25%). The aim of population screening for carriers is to identify at-risk couples before the first affected child, and this is practicable for some of the autosomal recessive conditions which are common in particular ethnic groups (see Table V).

Disorders of this category are more likely to occur in the children of blood relatives. Thus it is particularly important that consanguineous partners should attend any local carrier screening programme. This will detect part of their increased risk, but much of it is for rare disorders which cannot be foreseen.

An increasing number of autosomal recessive disorders can be detected prenatally, especially those whose biochemical basis is understood, and those for which DNA markers are available (see page 308).

Risks are usually low for the offspring of an affected person, a parent of an affected child who changes partners, and for cousins, nephews and nieces.

X-linked recessive conditions

These include Duchenne muscular dystrophy, classical haemophilia and several varieties of X-linked mental retardation, including the fragile X syndrome.

A woman with two affected sons, or with an affected son and an affected brother or uncle, is a known carrier; however, allowance may need to be made in calculating carrier risks for the likelihood of mutation at different stages in the pedigree. Carrier tests, such as serum creatine kinase in Duchenne muscular dystrophy and factor

VIII levels in haemophilia, may be necessary. These and several other such tests, however, do not discriminate fully between carriers and non-carriers, and results should be interpreted carefully together with pedigree data, a job requiring expertise.

Fortunately, DNA analysis will provide more efficient tests for many of the X-linked disorders in the next few years.

Multifactorial disorders

Many common diseases of post-natal onset as well as common congenital anomalies are thought to be caused by the interaction of multiple genetic factors and environmental factors. These conditions include asthma, schizophrenia, hypertension, coronary heart disease, anencephaly, spina bifida, cleft lip, club foot and many others.

Recurrence risks in first-degree relatives (sibs or offspring) are considerably increased over the general population risk, but in absolute terms the risks are normally relatively low, in the region of 2-5%. Unlike single gene disorders, risks may increase with the number of relatives already affected. There are pitfalls in genetic counselling for these conditions, which may be avoidable by careful evaluation of the pedigree and the diagnosis. Some single gene disorders may mimic a more common multifactorial disorder, and unless the true diagnosis is made, falsely low recurrence risks may be given. Conversely, multifactorial disorders will occasionally affect several close relatives, but the risks to further children in the family will usually be lower than for a single gene pedigree.

Congenital anomalies

Significant abnormalities are found in 3% of all births. Some of these are obvious at birth, such as neural tube defects or cleft lip, but some, such as deafness or congenital heart disease, may not be diagnosed until later. Congenital anomalies usually occur singly but about 25% are multiple; of this 25%, about a third are chromosomal in origin.

The aetiological mechanisms of these malformations are approximately:

Multifactorial	50%	(mainly isolated anomalies)
Chromosomal	8%	} (usually multiple anomalies)
Single gene anomalies	3%	
Known teratogen	2%	(congenital infections, drugs, alcohol)
Unknown	37%	

Genetic counselling in this area requires a precise diagnosis, which may entail an expert clinical evaluation of the affected child, and various special investigations. Those dealing with malformed still-births and neonatal deaths must bear these needs in mind and try to make sure that all necessary diagnostic procedures have been carried out before disposal of the body.

Genetic counselling

Genetic counselling is concerned with the giving of the genetic facts and risks to the couple in a way that is understandable, so that they can realize the significance of the risks in their particular family circumstances. The ideal time for counselling is when the mother is not pregnant. Then there is time to investigate, if necessary, the parents for heterozygosity or for chromosome anomaly. The options of further pregnancy or contraception are then still open to the parents.

Many couples will identify themselves as being at risk by the birth of a child with a developmental abnormality, or by a child developing a handicapping disease in childhood. Others may think they are at risk because of some known abnormality or disease in themselves or a close relative.

The first essential for genetic counselling is an accurate diagnosis of the presenting case. The second is an accurate family history which may give clues to the mode of inheritance even if the diagnosis is obscure. From the diagnosis, the family history and knowledge of the aetiology of the condition, the risk of recurrence of the specific disease within the family can be estimated and given to the couple. In difficult family pedigrees this calls for a specialist in genetic counselling, who is not always easily available.

The significance of the risk of recurrence depends firstly on the degree of handicap of the particular disease and secondly on the ability of the family to cope with the handicapping situation. A 1 in 2 recurrence risk of polydactyly (a dominant condition) is acceptable to most parents, one of whom is also affected, but a 1 in 4 risk of a second child with a severe progressive fatal illness such as Tay-Sachs disease is daunting to most parents. Where the abnormality is so severe as inevitably to cause stillbirth or neonatal death, a 1 in 4 risk may be acceptable because there is no risk of a continuing handicapping illness.

Where the risks of recurrence are low, such as in congenital malformation because of multifactorial inheritance, or when the condition is treatable (cleft lip), the risk may be acceptable. However, parents differ greatly in their reaction to abnormality and recurrence risks, and each family has to be considered individually. There are no hard and fast rules with regard to 'high' and 'low' risks. In addition, factors such as existing family size, social circumstances and finance inevitably influence the decision.

Most genetic counsellors do not have as their primary object the reduction of incidence of genetic abnormalities in the population. A couple who take a high risk do not necessarily represent a failure of genetic counselling, as long as their decision is an informed one. All genetic counsellors are familiar with the referral from a colleague which is a thinly-veiled request to make a couple 'see sense' and have no more children, but directive counselling is generally unhelpful.

During the discussion of genetic risks, an opportunity should be given to the parents to air their fears and fantasies about the occurrence of abnormality in their offspring. Often reassurance can be given and guilt feelings allayed by open discussion and factual information.

Where prenatal diagnosis is possible for an abnormality under discussion, the consultation should cover the nature of the tests available, stage in pregnancy when they would be carried out, the reliability of the results, and the timing and method of abortion (should that be requested after an abnormal result). The couple should be helped to consider their reactions to the various possible outcomes of the procedure. Any couple should be free to opt out of prenatal testing if they decide they would rather take the risk of an affected child.

Prenatal diagnosis

Many serious disorders can now be detected in the fetus. All the available approaches call for a high degree of technical expertise. No centre should attempt prenatal diagnosis until suitable experience has been acquired, for mistakes can do a great deal of harm.

Fetal abnormalities may be detected by routine tests in pregnancies not previously known to be at risk, or the couple may have begun the pregnancy aware of a risk and requesting a particular test.

The implications of a fetal abnormality, and the couple's likely response to it should ideally always be discussed with them before a test is carried out. While it is not normally helpful to restrict testing to those couples who agree to abortion in the event of an abnormal result, those who would not contemplate abortion under any circumstances should consider carefully whether the test (particularly if it has a risk attached) would really help them.

Methods of prenatal diagnosis (Table VI) can be considered under four headings: fetal imaging, fetal tissue sampling, amniotic fluid chemistry, and maternal blood sampling.

Fetal imaging

At present this is practically synonymous with ultrasound scanning.

In general, structural malformations are not reliably detectable before 16 weeks of pregnancy. Between 16 and 20 weeks, scanning may detect anencephaly, hydrocephaly, microcephaly, encephalocele, congenital heart defects, abnormalities of the kidney and renal tract, limb shortening, spina bifida, diaphragmatic hernia, abdominal wall defects, hydrops fetalis, and large tumours or swellings. It must be stressed, however, that the reliability of these diagnoses depends both on the quality (resolution) of the equipment and the experience of the operator.

It is important to be aware that some of the above malformations may occur as part of a chromosomal syndrome, such as trisomy 13 or 18. Thus, if the option of continuing a pregnancy is being considered, with what appears to be a repairable defect, fetal karyotyping should be carried out.

Fetal tissue sampling

The most widely used technique is amniocentesis at 16-18 weeks of pregnancy. Amniotic fluid cells, which are of fetal origin, can be cultured for chromosome analysis and for biochemical assays. The

TABLE VI. Some indications for prenatal diagnosis

Method	Indication
Chromosome analysis	(*i*) Maternal age (see Table IV) (*ii*) One parent carries balanced chromosome rearrangement (*iii*) One parent has a numerical anomaly (complete or mosaic) (*iv*) Parents had previous chromosomally abnormal baby.
DNA analysis	Parents known to be at risk of transmitting single gene disorder *and* responsible genes/linked markers have been shown to be identifiable.
Ultrasound scanning	One parent suffers from, or parents known to be at risk of, a serious chromosomal abnormality which is identifiable in the fetus.
Amniotic fluid alpha fetoprotein and acetyl cholinesterase	(*i*) one or both parents with neural tube defect (*ii*) previous child with neural tube defect (*iii*) raised maternal serum alpha fetoprotein during pregnancy.
Fetal biochemistry (usually on cultured fetal cells)	Parents at risk of a specific biochemical disorder which is expressed in an accessible fetal tissue (usually, one affected child already born to the couple).

latter are applicable in families known to be at risk of specific metabolic disorders, mostly rare. DNA can be extracted from cultured amniocytes, but chorion villus sampling (see below) is usually preferred for DNA testing. Fetal blood sampling is sometimes carried out in looking for haemoglobinopathies where DNA analysis is not possible. It is also used in some situations for chromosome analysis in the late second trimester of pregnancy.

Chorion villus sampling can be carried out by either transcervical or transcutaneous aspiration at 8-10 weeks of pregnancy. As with amniocentesis, ultrasound guidance is necessary. Villi may be used for fetal chromosome analysis, some biochemical assays and DNA analysis. The risks of villus sampling are still being evaluated but, in expert hands, are probably not more than 2% for inducing abortion. The comparable risk for amniocentesis, is $\frac{1}{2}$-1%. Many couples are prepared to accept a slightly higher risk in return for an earlier result.

Amniotic fluid chemistry

The main application here is the measurement of alpha fetoprotein and acetyl cholinesterase in the diagnosis of neural tube defects. Because other conditions can be associated with a high amniotic fluid alpha fetoprotein, the interpretation of these tests requires experience and a good ultrasound scanning service.

Maternal blood sampling

Maternal blood alpha fetoprotein levels can be used as a population screening test for neural tube defects, but a raised level is less specific than a raised amniotic fluid level; in fact, only a minority of women with blood levels above the 'upper limit of normal' will have a baby with a neural tube defect; the test is merely an indication for a repeat test and further investigation by ultrasound (if possible). In parts of the world where neural tube defects are uncommon, this form of pregnancy screening is unlikely to be helpful.

Methods of concentrating fetal cells from maternal blood may in future allow non-invasive fetal tissue sampling.

DNA analysis

The diagnosis of some single gene disorders has been revolutionized in the last few years by recombinant DNA techniques which can be applied to blood samples or chorionic villi. The reader who wishes to learn about these techniques should consult a book by A. E. G. Emery.*

The number of conditions that can be diagnosed by DNA analysis is rapidly growing. An important distinction must be made between those conditions for which a gene-specific DNA probe is available, and those where the gene itself has not been identified, but a linked DNA probe is available.

In the former group, which includes sickle cell anaemia and the thalassaemias, the most prevalent group of genetic disorders world-wide, a precise and fully reliable diagnosis can be made. In the second group which (at the time of writing) includes cystic fibrosis, X-linked

---

*Emery, A.E.G. (1985) *An Introduction to DNA Analysis.* London: Churchill Livingstone.

muscular dystrophy, and Huntington's chorea, family studies usually need to be carried out before diagnosis can be offered, not all families are informative, and there may be a small but significant error rate. This is because one is using normal DNA variants ('polymorphisms') to track genes through the family.

Family planning advice

If there is no added risk to future offspring or if the risk is acceptable to the couple, contraceptive advice will not differ from that given to any other couple wishing to space or limit their family. However, if the risk is felt to be too high to embark upon a further pregnancy, then the contraceptive advice given must pay due regard to the genetic situation.

When the high risk is due to one or other parent being the carrier of a single abnormal dominant gene or a balanced chromosome anomaly, the high risk will still hold with any spouse of the affected person. Similarly, if a woman is a known carrier of an X-linked abnormal gene, she will carry the 1 in 2 risk of having an affected son with any partner. In these cases reliable contraception is essential, and sterilization of the carrier may be indicated even at a relatively young age if he or she fully understands the situation and requests sterilization. It is important to retain the reproductive ability of the unaffected partner who carries no added risk.

In the older woman, where the risk of chromosomal anomaly continues to rise, safe, reliable contraception and probably sterilization should be offered. It must be remembered that the techniques of prenatal diagnosis will become more generally available in the future. Also, further advances will make the prenatal diagnosis of a greater number of abnormalities possible.

Where both partners are carriers of the same abnormal recessive gene the risk of having a further affected child is 1 in 4. However, if a new marital partnership should be established, the risk of affected children will be eliminated unless the new spouse also carries the same abnormal gene, which is statistically unlikely. It is reasonable, therefore, for both partners to seek to retain their reproductive potential. Oral or injectable contraception is nearly always indicated, as all other reversible methods carry a higher risk of pregnancy. Should accidental pregnancy occur, the choice lies between continuing with the pregnancy, knowing throughout that there is a high risk of abnor-

309

mality, or obtaining a therapeutic abortion, if legal, even though there is a chance that the fetus would be normal.

Artificial insemination by donor

Where the male partner is the carrier of an abnormal dominant gene or of a chromosomal anomaly, or where both partners are carrying the same abnormal recessive gene, artificial insemination by donor may be an acceptable way of increasing family size without taking a high genetic risk. Very careful counselling is essential before a decision is made in this direction.

Chapter 20

Non-clinic Service Delivery

Community based distribution of contraceptives

Introduction

In many developing countries up to 80% of the population live in rural areas. In these same countries trained health personnel, such as doctors, nurses and midwives, are in short supply. The ratio of doctors to population can be as low as 1 per 10,000 to 1 per 100,000 population: for family planning programmes in these countries the greatest challenge is to reach the rural poor who live in far-flung villages widely separated by fields, mountains and rivers, and where transportation is poor or non-existent. Clinic-based, health-personnel orientated family planning services cannot be expected to reach most of these rural poor.

One solution to this dilemma has been the use of village or household points for the distribution of certain fertility regulation methods. This community based distribution (CBD) has as its objective the extension of family planning services and supplies beyond the clinics. This can bring them directly into the daily lives of the people, where they will easily be available to everyone. The extension of services through such programmes reduces the reliance on clinics and broadens service delivery. This is frequently done by employing staff who do not necessarily have previous medical training, but who have a well-organized back-up referral system.

The methods of family planning best suited for CBD programmes are condoms, spermicides and oral contraceptives. It has been recognized that these can be supplied without clinic procedures and with new, more flexible patterns of supervision.

CBD programmes must pay special attention to the programmatic requirements of using widely dispersed lay distributors (workers). These concerns include: the number and types of contraceptive methods these workers can deliver effectively; the frequency and content of their interaction with clients; methods of training and supervision suitable to the needs and educational levels of the workers; and programme evaluation which takes into consideration workers' record-keeping capacities, and the geographical dispersion of much of the field work.

Given the extensive health needs of communities, CBD projects have been responding to a growing demand to provide a broader mix of services. It has frequently been suggested that integrated health and family planning services reinforce the effectiveness of any one intervention, and increase service efficiency.

Training

The importance of developing a well-trained cadre of workers prepared to deal with the unexpected situation and with the demands of their role in far-flung communities, cannot be over-emphasized. CBD workers range from health personnel to housewives in the community. Geographical dispersion and irregular work schedules are common factors in CBD projects, and regular supervision becomes difficult. These factors all make the initial training and subsequent retraining very important.

Training of CBD workers must be based on a clear understanding of the activities of the programme and must take into account the capabilities of the worker. The training must be practical and include the problems of field situations. Training should help them cope with unexpected situations without the need to seek immediate help in every case, and also to recognize their limitations. Role playing and practice in which field situations are duplicated are essential components of training programmes.

Trainer selection is important. Field personnel who are senior to designated CBD workers, but who perform or have performed work similar to that of these workers have proved to be well suited to the teaching role: they understand field situations and can express concepts in a manner understandable to the students.

Supervision

Supervision is a key factor in successful CBD programmes. Ideally, supervisors should have had field experience in the type of field work being performed and should be accessible on a regular basis. Regular meetings between field workers and supervisors (monthly or more frequently) can serve a number of purposes, including assessment of performance.

A chain of referral must be established for all CBD programmes. Depending on the community, the referral will reach trained nurses, midwives and doctors if necessary. Referrals are required when clients prefer, and are better suited for, methods not available through CBD programmes; for example, sterilization or implants.

Supplies

The importance of maintaining a secure supply system cannot be over-emphasized. Breaks in supplies can occur owing to in-country shortages in international shipments, and national customs regulations at port of entry. Since supply breakdown can lead to loss of client confidence, wherever possible stockpiles, back-up supply sources or alternative input strategies should be available.

Evaluation

Most community-based projects operate in areas with inadequate census and vital statistics, resulting in a lack of baseline information. Many projects are also of short duration and unlikely to result in measurable changes in births averted or maternal, infant and child mortality and morbidity. In addition, in many cases, community workers are illiterate or semi-literate. All of the above make assessment of the impact of projects difficult. Much of the regular evaluation will depend on routine service statistics determining the numbers of contraceptives distributed.

Checking the clients

Screening of clients by CBD workers is carried out by having check lists or simple interviews. This screening serves health and ethical functions and may also increase project acceptance among the medical profession in the community. Screening should not be so stringent as to disqualify women unnecessarily. On the other hand screening should make easier the identification of women at risk from particular methods of contraception. The preparation of check lists (see page 66) should be based on known health risks in a given population. Existing check lists for other communities could be modified to serve local

313

needs. CBD workers should have appropriate training to master the check lists, to interpret the findings accurately, and to direct clients to appropriate alternatives.

Offering a contraceptive method mix within one programme allows the CBD worker and the client to determine which contraceptive is best suited to the client's needs, and to provide alternative methods if the contraceptive originally selected proves not to meet changing needs.

Social marketing of contraceptives

Over the past 20 years another way of getting contraceptive supplies to those who need them has evolved through the use of social marketing. This has been defined as 'the correct application of basic marketing principles to achieve a social good'. A climate can be created in a community where subsidized sale of socially desirable products such as contraceptives becomes part of the daily life of the market place.

Contraceptive social marketing (CSM) began in 1968 with the start of the Nirodh condom initiative, in which, with help from the Ford Foundation, a programme was instituted in several Indian states to supply condoms at subsidized rates to 170,000 existing retail outlets for sale at lower than usual prices to those wanting them. This programme included active advertising of the product through various media, and is still continuing successfully today.

Further programmes of CSM were initiated, another successful one being the Preethi condom programme in Sri Lanka, organized by Population Services International with help from the IPPF. This started in 1973 and was also very successful. Now there are programmes in about 30 developing countries. Existing commercial distributors, such as retail shops, pharmacies and village stores which supply the day-to-day needs of a community, are involved in the schemes. They are sold various contraceptives below commercial rates. They then sell these to clients at low prices. The sales are accompanied by radio, press and other forms of advertising.

In several countries, notably Colombia, Costa Rica, the Dominican Republic, Egypt, El Salvador and Sri Lanka, the local family planning associations have undertaken the administration and management of the social marketing programme. Excellent results, with increasing sales of condoms, oral contraceptives and spermicides, have been reported. In 1986 the Sri Lankan FPA made a reasonable profit from sales, after widespread advertising through various media and careful supervision of retail outlets. In Egypt, the FPA has brought intrauterine devices into its CSM programme as well.

The main contraceptives sold through CSM programmes are condoms, oral contraceptives and spermicides. IUDs are fitted in Egypt, as mentioned above. In this case, of course, women choosing IUDs must have them fitted by trained health workers.

The programmes do not expect to be self-supporting, but the money received from sales goes some way to off-set costs. It has been found that prices have to be low enough so that clients can afford to buy the contraceptives, but high enough to assure them that the products are of good quality. Also, the retailers, and wholesalers where they are used, must be able to make a reasonable profit. Many donor organizations help to subsidize the programmes, the main one for several years being the US Agency for International Development (AID). Social Marketing for Change (SOMARC) is active in helping to set up new programmes in a number of developing countries.

To give some idea of the scope of CSM programmes, some fairly recent figures from Bangladesh are of interest. By 1984, contraceptives were available in more than 90,000 retail outlets there, organized through 5,000 stockists and 22 wholesalers. They were supplying more than a million couples with contraceptives (7% of eligible couples in Bangladesh). In 1983 sales of condoms were almost 100 million, and two million oral contraceptive cycles and more than five million spermicidal tablets had been sold through the retail outlets. As the Social Marketing International Association said at the time, "The results accomplished in Bangladesh clearly demonstrate that basic marketing principles of research, distribution, promotion and advertising can be applied to generate a social good. This is social marketing."

As with community based distribution, there is a system for back-up advice for clients, especially those buying and using oral contraceptives. This safety-net is important, for programmes can be disrupted and adversely affected if clients have any side-effects from the contraceptives they buy, without some means of having these attended to. And, of course, users of hormonal contraceptives, whether they obtain them from clinics, CBD distributors, or retail shops, must know that there is a chain of help for any difficulties or adverse effects right back to nurses and doctors, if needed.

Promotion of contraceptive products is carried out in CSM programmes by positive advertising, imaginative poster campaigns, and

315

the use of special public relations techniques. Advertising on radio and television (where applicable), in newspapers and cinemas, and in public places is very effective. Easy-to-see displays and posters at the retail outlets are important. Public relations techniques which will attract public attention, such as the boats carrying loudspeakers and advertising posters on the rivers in Bangladesh, are very successful in drawing attention to the CSM programmes. Advertising CSM programmes not only highlights these programmes but also tends to increase interest in contraception generally in the country in question.

More and more of the contraceptive needs in many countries are being met by social marketing programmes. These programmes are contributing actively to the expansion of the use of several forms of contraception in the developing world.

IMAP Statement on Community Family Planning Services

Community Family Planning Services (CFPS) represent a comprehensive approach to delivery of family planning services through a community-based network. They offer an efficient and effective way of expanding the availability and increasing the acceptability of these services to large numbers of people in urban and rural areas.

CFPS include the distribution of contraceptives with appropriate and adequate back-up available at health centres, clinics and hospitals, accompanied by the provision of information, education and counselling through community channels. Where possible, CFPS should be integrated with other efforts to improve the quality of family and community life. They can also provide channels for broad-based community education and for provision of other services.

The effectiveness of CFPS depends on the extent to which they are able to draw on existing local resources, including commercial networks. The participation of the community itself in the design, delivery, management and evaluation of these services helps ensure that they respond to the needs and the preferences of the people they serve and increases the possibility of community self-reliance. In this respect, a community can consist of a social group, such as young people, factory or farm workers, as well as a geographical locality.

Choice of methods

The choice of methods to be distributed in the community depends on the acceptability of methods, laws prevailing in the country and the availability of back-up and referral services. Condoms and spermicides are easily distributed through local channels. Injectables, IUDs and diaphragms may be considered for inclusion in CFPS after careful assessment of available facilities, proper training of personnel and adequate supervision. CFPS workers should be familiar with the advantages and disadvantages of these as well as surgical methods of family planning and, when necessary, be able to refer clients to a facility where these methods are available.

Most CFPS channels are well suited for distribution of oral contraceptives. When distributing oral contraceptives outside the clinics, special criteria should be followed: from a medical standpoint, pills containing over 50 μg of oestrogen should be excluded; pills containing 30 μg of oestrogen are suitable for most women and should be the oral contraceptives available through local outlets. However, because of the higher incidence of break-through bleeding with these pills, it is advantageous to have available through back-up facilities pills containing 50 μg of oestrogen. Back-up may also include two different progestagens in combination with the different dosages of oestrogen.

Physical and/or pelvic examinations are not essential to the use of oral contraceptives. However, back-up facilities should be available where such examinations could be carried out.

Education and counselling

Provision of education and counselling before, during and after the adoption of a contraceptive method is an integral part of the responsibility of CFPS workers. They should be able to provide information on the possible effects on the health of the consumer of the use or non-use of different contraceptive methods, and on the options available to help users make their own choice of an appropriate method. A basic training programme for CFPS workers should be devised to cover all the above aspects, including the use of a checklist for screening clients and the maintenance of basic records for patient management and programme evaluation.

A number of policy, legal or administrative obstacles may impede the scope and the effectiveness of community family planning services. Where consistent with the protection of user safety, IPPF may work towards the removal of obstacles preventing easy and equal access to contraception.

(Adopted by the IPPF Central Council, November 1981, and amended by the Central Council, November 1982.This statement replaces earlier statements adopted in 1973, 1974, 1975, 1976 and 1978.)

Chapter 21

Statistical Methods Explained

Introduction

Epidemiological studies and statistical methods are used in the assessment of different attributes of contraception, such as effectiveness, use continuation, cost (or cost effectiveness), acceptability and safety. What follows is not intended as an introduction to statistics (a number of excellent books on that topic are already available), but an attempt in the context of these methods to discuss and define a number of concepts and terms which family planning doctors may meet in their work. This may be either when they are sifting information about the assessment of family planning methods and services, or when they are themselves involved in the collection of research data.

Any doctor planning to undertake a clinical trial or a particular study of a family planning method would be wise to seek full statistical advice before embarking on such a venture.

Theoretical and use effectiveness

The varying success of any single method of contraception has resulted in the knowledge that its effective use requires a certain minimum level of motivation on the part of contraceptive users if they are to succeed with it. Many studies have been published which show a wide variation in pregnancy rates and other unwanted side-effects associated with any method of contraception. These varying failure rates have been attributed to a number of personal, social and cultural factors relating to the contraceptive user, the person responsible for providing the method, and the user-provider relationship. It is now generally accepted that differences in the reported failure rate must be due, in part, to these non-medical and non-technical influences.

These differences in the failure rate associated with a single birth control method have led to a distinction being made between the 'theoretical effectiveness' of the method and its 'use effectiveness' (or clinical effectiveness). The theoretical effectiveness is an abstract term which describes the use of the contraceptive under ideal conditions, where it is used consistently and exactly according to instructions. This level of effectiveness can only remain as a theoretical abstract, for such ideal conditions cannot continue once the human factor is introduced. In practice, theoretical effectiveness measures the effectiveness of a contraceptive method after attempts have been made to *minimize* the human factors also involved.

The main purpose in describing the theoretical-effectiveness rate is to provide a baseline—although an imprecise one—on which the more gross variations in the use-effectiveness rate can be assessed. The use-effectiveness rate is the rate of effectiveness actually obtained by contracepting couples and is usually very different from the theoretical-effectiveness rate described above. It is clear that the 'use effectiveness' of a particular method of contraception is a more realistic, though more complex measure than its 'theoretical effectiveness'. The use-effectiveness rate acknowledges the influence of other variables; these may be sociological or psychological as well as physiological.

The gap between theoretical and use effectiveness varies among different populations. This is because the consistency of use is known to vary across social groups, across variables of a psychological nature, and even in the same individual or couple over time. It is known that fecundity varies, but so also does willingness to contracept.

If it were possible to reduce the part played by the contraceptive acceptor—i.e. reduce the human factors involved—it would be expected that the rate of use effectiveness would more closely approach the rate of theoretical effectiveness. This is already the case with sterilization. Use effectiveness of this method is more dependent on the skill of the surgeon than on the characteristics of the acceptor.

It is commonly assumed that the intrauterine device (IUD) is the only reversible contraceptive method in general use today that even remotely approaches such an ideal. The IUD appears to minimize the part played by the acceptor in that it has to be fitted and removed by a third party. (Implants are in this category also, but are not yet in widespread use.) Consistent use of the IUD is inevitable once fitting has taken place, provided it is not expelled or does not perforate, and its use does not require any reliance on memory or anticipation of need. It would seem that here is a method that brings together theoretical effectiveness and use effectiveness in a way that is not possible with the more traditional methods of contraception or their modern alternatives, the oral contraceptive and other hormonal methods. But evidence collected over the years indicates that even with this method of contraception, factors associated with the IUD user and the person directly responsible for its fitting play an important part in its successful use. Age, parity, social class, cultural or ethnic differences, as well as factors associated with the prescribing and fitting of the IUD, have all been shown to affect the reported pregnancy, expulsion and removal rates. It seems that *who* fits and receives the IUD may be as important as *which* IUD is fitted!

This attempt to include personal and social factors in the assessment of the use effectiveness of family planning methods also permits a shift in emphasis from the consequences of using specific methods to those associated with method acceptance. To be able to define the pre-existing characteristics of method users which will lead to subsequent effective use has an obvious attraction. With the increasing awareness of such characteristics, an emphasis on the selection of appropriate acceptors possessing favourable characteristics for a particular method becomes possible. This change in emphasis from the purely medical consequences of method use to the social and personal considerations of potential users highlights the importance of the relationship between the provider and the user in ways that were not considered in the early days of contraceptive development.

Incidence and prevalence rates

Incidence

This is the occurrence of a particular event among a population during a specific period of time, usually one year. In the area of contraception, the event may be the acceptance of a method, or it may be a side-effect or complication or pregnancy. The population can be defined geographically as, for example, individuals in a particular country or region. It can also be defined by any other characteristics, such as the use of a contraceptive method, sex, age, etc. As an example: all reported new cases of stroke in 1987 among women using oral contraceptives in the USA would be the incidence of stroke in 1987 among that specific population.

Prevalence

This refers to the proportion of a population having a particular condition at a specific point in time. The condition may be the use of a method of contraception or an illness; the point in time can be by a certain date (usually calculated at mid-year) or at the time the information was collected. For example, the proportion of women in India using a contraceptive method by mid-1987, would be the prevalence of that contraceptive use in 1987 in India.

The following example will show further the difference between incidence and prevalence: the proportion of women of reproductive age who obtained an IUD during 1987 in Kenya would be the incidence of acceptance of the IUD in that particular country in 1987. The proportion of women who were using an IUD by mid-1987 in Kenya would be the prevalence of IUD use in Kenya in the same year. Prevalence would include women who obtained the IUD before 1987, but only those who obtained the IUD in 1987 would be included in the estimate of incidence.

Epidemiological studies

Three main methods are used to study the consequences of contraceptive use: case-control studies, cohort studies, and retrospective cross-sectional surveys.

Case-control studies

In these studies the histories of individuals who currently have a particular condition are compared with the histories of individuals who do not show the condition, in an attempt to discover if a common predisposing factor linked to the condition can be identified. It is this 'looking back' over previous experience which has led to case-control studies sometimes being described as *retrospective* studies. In order to provide evidence that a link between the two events (the previous experience and the current condition) is present, a comparison is made by reference to a group of otherwise similar people who do not show the current condition.

If the group with the current condition being studied has a significantly higher record of the previous experience than the group who do not have the condition, this suggests that the previous experience is related in some way to the condition being studied. For

321

example, if some members of a group of women attending hospital for the treatment of pelvic inflammatory disease had previously used a particular IUD, and such IUD use is significantly higher in this group than among a group of otherwise similar women attending for some unrelated reason, then, at first sight, evidence is present that the use of that par-ticular IUD is related to the pelvic inflammatory disease. The first group of women are the 'cases' and the second group of women are the 'controls'; hence the description 'case-control studies'. The use of a control group provides a standard against which any deviation can be compared.

Cohort studies

These studies differ from case-control studies in that they 'look forward', and for this reason they are often called *prospective* studies. Again, two groups are used for comparative purposes, with one exposed to the predisposing factor to be monitored and the other not exposed. The two groups are matched as closely as possible, but with this one factor differentiating them. The two groups are then monitored — or followed longitudinally — during the succeeding period of time (which can be days, months or years) and the incidence of any observed conditions recorded. If there is a significant difference in the subsequent experience of the two groups, then the risk factor being monitored may be related to the subsequent experience. For example, if a group of women accepting oral contraception is compared with a group of similar women not using oral contraceptives, and it is found that the oral contraceptive users subsequently demonstrate a significantly higher incidence of thromboembolism than the control group, then at first sight evidence is present that taking oral contraceptives is related in some way to the thromboembolism. Cohort studies are very similar to *experimental* studies, but differ in that the persons being studied in the exposed condition group are self-selected. In an experimental study the allocation to the 'experimental' and 'control' group is undertaken at random by the experimenter or researcher.

Possible biases

In both case-control and cohort studies, a sufficient number of cases is required in order to obtain statistically significant results and avoid the possibility that the results may be explained by chance. The number of subjects required is usually much greater for cohort than for case-control studies.

When the results are not statistically significant, that does not mean that no association exists between the risk factor and the outcome. It only means that the number of cases was not sufficient to test this. In addition, it is necessary to control for different sources of bias:

1. In some studies the results may be biased because the data were not collected in the same way among the two groups being compared; for example, a personal versus a telephone interview.

2. Another bias may be that the control group was not selected properly and does not represent the general population, or is too different from the group having the predisposing factor or the condition being studied. For example, there may be large differences in the average age of the two groups.

3. There may be another factor which is related to the predisposing factor and the condition being studied which is more prevalent among one of the two groups. For example, in some studies a possible association between oral contraceptives and cervical cancer may be explained because the use of oral contraceptives may be more prevalent among individuals who are promiscuous, and promiscuity has been identified as a risk factor for cervical cancer.

4. The presence of the risk factor affects the chances that the condition being studied will be identified. If it is a disease, the chances of the diagnosis being made will be enhanced. For example: if users of oral contraceptives have more chance of having cervical smears done, it may explain the finding of a greater incidence of cervical cancer among them.

Comparing case-control and cohort studies

A comparison of case-control and cohort studies reveals that there are advantages and disadvantages for each in evaluating the risks and benefits of different contraceptive methods. These are summarized in Table VII.

Cross-sectional surveys

Surveys are conducted to collect data from individuals about themselves, about their households, or about their communities. The term 'survey' is broadly defined as a systematic method of collecting data necessary for the objectives of a particular study.

TABLE VII. Comparison of case-control and cohort studies

Case-control	Cohort
Usually quick, cheap and relatively easy to do.	Usually slow, expensive and difficult to do.
May be the only way to study rare diseases.	Usually only practicable for fairly common diseases.
Will often permit study in great depth (e.g. of sexual history) and will allow many possible aetiological factors to be considered.	Numbers usually preclude collection of highly detailed information on each subject.
By definition concerned with only a single disease.	Enables many different diseases to be studied at once.
Notoriously subject to bias in the selection of both cases and controls.	Generally less subject to bias (but not necessarily so).
Usually provides an estimate only of relative risk.	Provides information on both relative and absolute risk.
Cannot study variables which may be altered by the disease event (e.g. 'hormonal status' in breast cancer).	Can study variables which may be altered by the disease event.
May be recall problems (and bias) in measuring exposure.	Normally, no problems of recall.

From: Vessey, M.P. (1979) Design and interpretation of case-control and cohort studies. *British Journal of Family Planning*, **5**, 56–57.

The cross-sectional survey is a one-time activity and the individuals are generally interviewed. It is cross-sectional in the sense that respondents are at various stages of their life-cycles. Some, for example, are in their twenties, while others may be in their forties. In addition, the survey describes respondents in various situations, just like a snap-shot. For example, in a cross-sectional survey, some women may be found pregnant, while others are breast feeding, contracepting, or in none of these three categories. The interviews or clinical examinations, as required by the study, are done only once.

Cross-sectional surveys can be subdivided into: (1) current status; or (2) retrospective; according to the type of information obtained. For example, such information as marital status or whether a method is being used or not, refers only to the point in time when it is collected and, therefore, it is called 'current status' (i.e. status at the time the information is obtained). However, when respondents are asked about past events, such as age at marriage, date when the method was first used, or date of live-births, etc., the information is retrospective for it relates to events which occurred in the past. It is possible to analyse this retrospective information as if it comes from a longitudinal design, but the methods of collecting such data are different. Longitudinal data are relatively more accurate; retrospective reports are affected by how well a respondent remembers the information required of her, or him.

Another aspect in survey research is the study population. More specifically, whether the study aims to collect information from the entire population or to draw a sample from a particular population. The 'population' is narrowly defined as the 'study population' to imply the group to which study findings refer. Therefore, if the study refers to contraceptive users, all individuals using a method form the study population. In many cases, it is expensive and time-consuming to cover the entire study population and, therefore, a representative sample is drawn and included in the study. The information is obtained from the sample respondents, but the results can be generalized to the study population. Scientific procedures in sampling theory are adopted so that the information obtained from a sample is representative of the population under study. Sometimes, such surveys are called 'sample surveys' in order to indicate that information is obtained from a 'representative few' and not from the entire group, though findings are attributable to the entire group.

The coverage of a survey can be national, regional, district, from a rural area, or from a number of clinics in a particular geographical area. The coverage also depends on the objectives of the study.

The above information is general to all surveys. Some examples may be helpful to indicate the usefulness of this approach for the topic under discussion. A cross-sectional survey will be useful to ascertain information on the prevalence of contraceptive methods, types of methods used, reasons for non-use (among non-users), and satisfaction with the method being used (among users) in a community or a region. The usual approach would be to select a sample (generally of women in the reproductive age-range) and interview respondents with a questionnaire.

Lastly, it is important to note that interviews and questionnaires (or forms) are the usual approach for the collection of information. The questionnaires can be pre-coded, with categories already ascribed for various questions, or open-ended. An example of the former is to have a list of possible side-effects for a question on 'what side-effects did you experience when using (method)?' The latter will be of the type 'Why are you not using a contraceptive method?', which requires the response provided by the interviewee to be written as she or he tells it.

Measures of effectiveness

In order to translate clinical findings into quantifiable information on which knowledge of the benefits and risks of family planning methods is based, it is important to know something about 'events' and 'months of use' (sometimes described as 'months of observation' or 'months of exposure'). The definition and calculation of events and months of use represent the central features of all statistical procedures used to measure the effectiveness of a family planning method.

Events

The term 'event' is used to describe any experience subsequent to the commencement of a trial or study of a family planning method which is considered relevant by those setting it up. At one level, the descriptions of such events are relatively straightforward — for example, when they refer to the general incidence of unwanted pregnancy or to unacceptable changes in menstrual bleeding patterns. But the precise definition of these events often varies between researchers, depending on the degree of specificity required in research design. This often creates difficulty in comparing results across or between studies. For example, the description of unwanted pregnancies might include those resulting from the misuse of the method by the user (e.g. when the oral contraceptive is not taken as instructed and forgotten on some days) or when other events may have intervened, such as the unnoticed expulsion of an IUD before conception. Similarly, the definition of menstrual disturbances might — or might not — depend on the subsequent behaviour of the women concerned.

A *complaint* about such a disturbance might be regarded as an event in one study, while in another study such a complaint might be associated with a decision to stop using the family planning method before it is classified as an event. In most oral contraceptive studies a complaint of bleeding disturbance is usually recorded and reported in publication, whereas in most IUD studies attention is only drawn to such complaints if they lead to the removal of the IUD. If such is the case, a comparison of published reports of these 'bleeding' events among users of the two methods may be misleading and inappropriate.

Months of use

The term 'months of use' raises issues of definition (what is a month?) and of calculation (how many months?). In general, the basic unit of analysis when recording the time intervals between commencing use of a family planning method and the experience of a defined event (or the end of the study) is, by convention, a month.

This means that if a contraceptor ceases to use the method as a result of experiencing a defined event the day after commencing use of the method, one month of use will be credited. From this it can be seen that the minimum period of use is one month. Conventions have been established which permit the calculation of the total months of use by taking the commencing date as month one, and adding another month on the same day in each subsequent calendar month. This procedure provides the number of *ordinal* months.

Examples

(*a*) *Commenced taking oral contraceptives 18 February and estimated date of conception calculated as taking place on 24 December.*

18 February to 17 December = 10 months
18 December to 23 December = 1 month
11 months of use

(*b*) *IUD fitted 3 January and IUD expelled 4 January.*
months of use = 1 month

(*c*) *Commenced using diaphragm 2 June and study ended 31 July the following year with no event reported.*

2 June to 1 July (following year) = 13 months
1 July to 31 July = 1 month
14 months of use

(*d*) *Commenced using condoms 2 June and gave up owing to dislike of method 2 July.*
Months of use = 2 months

It can be seen from these calculations that a month is identified for each period of 28, 29, 30 and 31 days, depending on which calendar months are being observed. In addition, any part of a remaining month is added as an additional month. Recently, and in an attempt to be more precise, some researchers have begun to calculate each ordinal month by taking the total number of days of experience and dividing by 30 (or 31). However, the important point to notice is that similar *ordinal* months may be calculated for each contraceptor in any study irrespective of the day in the *calendar* month when recruitment took place.

Calculation of risk

There are several ways of measuring or stating the possibility of failure of a contraceptive method, and calculating associated side-effects. These include the rate, ratio, relative risk and attributable risk. These are discussed briefly below.

Rate

Rate is the measurement of the probability of occurrence of a particular event among a population. For example: the occurrence of pelvic infection among users of the IUD can be expressed in terms of the rate of pelvic infection among IUD users; in this case the event is pelvic infection and the population is users of the IUD.

Ratio

Ratio is the measurement of the frequency of occurrence of a particular event relative to the occurrence of a different type of event. For example: the maternal mortality ratio can be expressed as the number of maternal deaths per 100,000 live births; in this case one event is maternal mortality and the other event live births. In contrast, the rate of maternal mortality can be expressed as the number of maternal deaths per 100,000 women of reproductive age. In this case women of reproductive age are the concerned population.

Relative risk

Relative risk (RR) is the comparison between the incidence of a particular event among a population exposed to a risk factor and the incidence of the same event among a population not exposed to the risk factor. The RR is estimated by dividing the rate in the exposed group by the rate in the unexposed group. For example: if the incidence rate of a disease among users of a contraceptive method is 9 per 1,000 users and the rate of the same disease among individuals not using that method of contraception is 3 per 1,000, the relative risk of that disease among users of the contraceptive method compared to non-users would be 3 (9 divided by 3). The interpretation of the relative risk in this example is that the risk of developing the disease among the users of the contraceptive method is 3 times the risk of developing the disease among non-users of the method.

Attributable risk

That is the incidence or amount of an event or condition that can be attributed to the exposure to a risk factor. This is estimated by subtracting the rate of the event or condition among the unexposed group from the rate among the exposed group. So, using the same example as above, the attributable risk will be estimated by subtracting 3 from 9, and the result will mean that 6 cases of the disease out of 9 per 1,000 individuals using the method will be due to the use of the method. The attributable risk is useful for assessing the public health implications of the association between a risk factor and a disease.

Measuring effectiveness

The Pearl Index

In 1932, Pearl introduced a method of measuring effectiveness which takes into account the length of time the woman has been exposed to the risk of a defined event. Known as the Pearl Index, the calculation is expressed in terms of a rate per 100 woman-years of exposure (abbreviated as HWY). The method of calculation is as follows:

$$\text{Rate per HWY} = \frac{\text{Total number of defined events} \times 1200}{\text{Total months of use}}$$

The denominator includes the total months of use for all those using the method being studied. Using the Pearl Index it is possible to compare the relative efficiency of two or more methods even though the women are using each method for differing lengths of time.

The rate per HWY is a statistic which could erroneously give the impression that the rate given applies to 100 women who have been followed for at least one year. This would be incorrect because the calculation of the rate is based on the total months of use for all women taking part in the study, and a similar number would be recorded for 150 women who are each followed for an average of 12 months as for 300 women who were each followed for an average of six months of use.

A disadvantage of the Pearl Index is that it assumes that the monthly probability of an event remains constant over a period of time. Long-term studies have demonstrated that this assumption is incorrect. This limitation was recognized as a serious weakness of the Pearl Index when it became known that the risk of certain events varies according to the length of time a particular family-planning method is used. Nevertheless, frequent reference to the Pearl Index still appears in publications reporting the effectiveness of family-planning methods. While the Pearl Index may be useful as an initial crude measure of the risks and benefits of a particular family planning method, its limitations should be recognized.

Life-table analysis

The more advanced life-table approach, which is similar to the technique used by life insurance companies in assessing risks, permits the calculation of a rate for a specific risk (e.g. pregnancy) over a defined period of time, taking into account the presence of other competing risks (e.g. removal and expulsion of an IUD) during the same time. It also assesses the changing probability of risk for defined events over a period of time. The calculations are expressed in terms of a rate per 100 women after 'N' months or years of observation.

Gross and net rates

In life-table analysis, the calculation of risks is usually based on two approaches yielding qualitatively different rates. While both use similar definitions and data collection procedures, they should not be confused. The first is described as the *gross* event rate and refers to the risk of a defined event taking place without reference to the likelihood of any other, competing, events occurring. The second rate is described as the *net* event rate and refers to the risk of a defined event occurring bearing in mind that other, competing, events may take place before the defined event has had an opportunity to take place. (E.g. what is the risk of an unplanned pregnancy for an IUD user bearing in mind the chance that the IUD might be removed following a complaint of excess bleeding before the pregnancy can occur?).

While both *gross* and *net* rates can be calculated for different periods of time, it is clear that only the net event rate takes into consideration the risk of a variety of events. Care should be taken in checking which of the rates is being presented in publications describing the effectiveness of family planning methods. The most commonly presented statistic is the net event rate; but sometimes this is inappropriate. For example, net event rates will always be lower than their equivalent gross rates because the net rates will be taking into account the possibility of other, competing, events. If an IUD has a moderate gross pregnancy rate and a very high gross expulsion rate, then the *net* pregnancy rate will be considerably lower than the *gross* pregnancy rate simply because of the high risk of the competing event of expulsion. By publishing only the net pregnancy rate in such circumstances, a false impression could easily be given that the product is more protective against pregnancy than it really is. Most published reports provide only net event rates but, strictly speaking, this is not a proper procedure when comparing one product with another.

Conclusion

The design, data collection, analysis and interpretation of information concerned with measuring the risks and benefits of family planning methods is a complex business. Much depends on the type and specificity of the information required. A healthy dose of scepticism when examining the statistical treatment of any information is not a bad thing, but the often repeated advice of the computer programmer that 'junk in' leads to 'junk out' should not be forgotten. If information is not carefully recorded in an accurate and consistent manner, no matter how refined the statistical tool may be, the quality of the data will remain flawed.

Chapter 22

Legal Aspects of Family Planning

Introduction

Family planning has an obvious legal dimension, especially in its relationship to the provision of health care services. Laws and regulations define how these services are to be provided, by whom, for whom, where and under what conditions.

Laws and regulations at the national level about contraceptive distribution, sterilization, abortion and the use of non-doctor personnel determine the conditions under which family planning services can be made available. Other legal factors that affect the supply, demand and procurement of family planning services in any given country may be found in customs regulations, currency restrictions, quality control of manufacture, and advertising restrictions. Of course, the doctor making these services available is under a duty to provide them in a manner which conforms with acknowledged patterns of medical practice. Any deviations from accepted norms of medical practice in providing the actual service may result in the doctor's liability for negligence if, as a consequence, the health of the recipient is impaired. Thus the legal and policy requirements that affect family planning use are many and varied, and any doctor involved in this field should be familiar with those in his or her particular country. If there is some doubt, readers should contact their own family planning association, their local medical defence organization, or the International IPPF offices for advice.

The current pattern of contraceptive use has reflected a revolution in family planning practice. Estimates by the Population Information Program indicate that currently about 77 million women world-wide use the IUD, about 56 million use oral contraceptives (OCs), about 35 million couples use condoms, and smaller numbers use other reversible methods. In addition, an estimated 72 million women and 33 million men rely on voluntary sterilization, and as of 1980 it is estimated that about 70 million abortions occur annually, some 20 million of these illegal. Recent legal and policy changes have both encouraged and reflected this revolution. Laws and policies, once thought to be major barriers to family planning practice, have helped expand the availability of family planning services in a number of ways. All of these are not applicable to all countries, but form the totality of new thinking in:

- Legalizing distribution of contraceptives
- Widening the categories of workers who are allowed to supply contraceptives
- Allowing increased public information and advertising of contraceptives
- Providing services or education for young people
- Easing import requirements
- Establishing a legal basis for voluntary sterilization, and
- Liberalizing laws affecting abortion services.

These changes have made it easier to obtain safe and effective contraceptives through the private sector as well as through government services.

This chapter will survey the major legal and policy issues that affect family planning service delivery and will review the various ways these have been addressed in recent years. World-wide, there is no uniformity in the approaches taken, and in most cases there are numerous alternatives.

Contraceptive information and advertising

The basic right of individuals to the 'knowledge' and 'means' necessary to "determine freely the number and spacing" of their offspring, with its origins in the 1968 Conference on Human Rights (Tehran), was endorsed in the Plan of Action which emerged from the World Population Conference (Bucharest) in 1974 and again in Mexico City (1984). In other words, individuals have the right to contraceptive information and services, a concept that is endorsed nearly unanimously throughout the world—in fact, 96% of the world's population live in countries that do so. The constitutions of some countries actually require the government to develop family planning programmes.

Yet laws and policies of various types — criminal as well as drug regulatory — have often undercut efforts to disseminate accurate, up-to-date information about family planning. Some of these laws are based on rationales that seek to protect public morality, some are based on opposition to the idea of family planning itself. Fortunately, restrictive laws are becoming less prevalent, but they still exist. One of the vestiges of the French legal system illustrates this point. In Chad, Article 98 of Law No. 28 of 29 December 1965, which draws its inspiration from the French anti-contraception law of 31 July 1920 (no longer in force in France), makes it a *criminal* offence to disseminate 'contraceptive or anti-natalist propaganda' through speeches in public places, or by placing in 'public channels' books, written material, drawings, pictures or posters which advocate family planning.

Advertising and display of contraceptives

Law and policy may affect access to information in at least three ways. First, drug regulations often permit advertisements on the methods among the medical and pharmaceutical professions only. For instance, notices which focus on a specific brand of oral contraceptives or condoms are often not circulated to the general public. Because of this, the public may remain ignorant not only of the various alternatives available to them, but also of the risks and benefits involved.

Second, access to information on family planning may be blocked by the views of the public or private authorities that control the modes of advertising. Attempts to advertise about specific family planning methods are often rejected on the grounds that the material is too sensitive, although advertisements informing the public where family planning services in general can be acquired have been allowed. This is not the case in Mexico and Colombia, where contraceptives are openly and vigorously promoted. The use of the radio as a means of promoting contraception is permitted and encouraged in several Latin American countries. On the other hand, authorities who control broadcasting policy in the USA have been very reluctant to permit such practices, despite the fact that broadcasting codes governing them were ruled out in 1982.

Third, rules controlling the display of contraceptives often require that they be hidden away from public view. If such is the case, a form of 'self-advertisement' is precluded and the knowledge that contraceptives are available is more difficult to come by. 'No display' requirements are really only a matter of aesthetics; they serve no legitimate health purpose.

Recently, however, many countries have liberalized laws and policies governing information about contraceptives.

Contraceptive distribution

Many new schemes for contraceptive distribution have been developed over the past few years. Most of these depart from the traditional pattern of doctors providing contraceptive services. There is a discernible trend towards the use of health personnel other than doctors as providers of contraceptive services. Community-based distribution programmes (CBD) and commercial-retail sales programmes (CRS) are two of these (see page 311). The aim is to make high-quality services as widely available as possible.

Minimum standards for any distribution scheme should seek to provide the contraceptive user (consumer) with adequate information and care. At the same time, they should be designed to reduce the risk of liability to doctors and other personnel involved in the actual distribution. Both of these goals can be achieved if proper guidelines are established. The IPPF Central Medical Committee and the Law and Planned Parenthood Panel (Law Panel) suggested in 1975 that the following precautionary procedures, appropriately adapted to each national setting, be established as guidelines for distribution programmes, whether clinic or community-based:

"The distributor (*a*) should obtain from the consumer appropriate information as to the consumer's personal circumstances which may affect the competence of the consumer to give informed consent to the use of particular products or methods, and (*b*) should, in the light of the best available medical knowledge, provide appropriate information on the possible effect on the health of the consumer of the use or non-use of any particular contraceptive.

"Distributors, wherever possible, should work within a framework which offers appropriate information and service on a variety of family planning methods so that the consumer can be aware of the possible options available to him or her and so that he or she may choose whichever method he or she prefers. The distributor should provide to the consumer appropriate information on how to use the method chosen.

"The distributor should supervise, monitor and evaluate the on-going use of contraceptives by consumers and maintain a system of referral to assure that the right of the consumer to appropriate care is protected."

With these general guidelines in mind, we shall now consider laws and policies as they affect the various contraceptive methods.

Oral contraceptives

The distribution of oral contraceptives is governed in many countries by the requirement that only a doctor can prescribe them. The sale and distribution of oral contraceptives after prescription are often further limited to pharmacies under the direct supervision of a registered pharmacist or to other authorized outlets. These restrictions are usually part of the regulations applicable to all drugs in these countries.

With this traditional legal framework in mind, the IPPF Law Panel and Central Medical Committee in 1976 recommended that the following ways of interpreting the prescription requirement be used to make the wider distribution of oral contraceptives within the clinic setting easier:

The technique of 'standing orders': Under this approach the doctor in charge of the clinic issues 'standing orders' to trained non-doctor health personnel on how and when to administer oral contraceptives. This is accomplished by giving them a short list of questions they should ask the woman during screening (see page 66). If the woman answers 'no' to all the questions, the distributor is authorized to issue the oral contraceptives; if the woman answers 'yes' to any one of the questions, she will be referred to a doctor for further consultation.

The technique of signed prescriptions: At the beginning of the week, the doctor presents the non-doctor health personnel on the staff with a prescription pad of blank, signed prescriptions along with standing orders or instructions indicating which kind of women can receive oral contraceptives and under what conditions. They are then allowed to issue these under the standing orders by using the signed prescription sheets from the pad.

The technique of counter-signing prescriptions: Under this system, trained non-doctor health personnel write the prescription and the doctor counter-signs it. This technique is particularly appropriate for programmes with a large number of trained midwives and nurses but very few doctors. As with the other techniques, because the midwife or nurse can usually spend more time with the women than the doctor, they get a better response, thus enabling better care to be given.

The technique of long-term prescriptions: In addition to the above, the health manpower resources available for the distribution of oral contraceptives may be more wisely used if long-term prescriptions are given, thereby saving valuable doctor time. This technique involves prescriptions made out for 12 months or more after initial screening by the doctor. Subsequent repeats of the contraceptives are supplied without the necessity of seeing the doctor again. Once the 12 months have passed, the woman sees the doctor for a check-up and a new prescription.

Trends in oral contraceptive prescription and distribution

While the prescription requirement is widespread, in a number of countries responsibility for distribution of oral contraceptives is being shifted to non-doctor distribution in clinics and to community based non-clinic distributors (see page 311). This has meant that legal limitations like the prescription requirement, established as standards when health care was organized in a different manner than it is today, have been modified.

As examples, new laws and health regulations have been adopted in a number of countries to allow trained non-doctor health personnel to prescribe and distribute oral contraceptives. The actual provisions vary widely and are in a state of constant change, and in many countries a huge gap exists between law and practice.

Insertion of intrauterine devices

Usually, the insertion (fitting) of intrauterine devices (IUDs) is not governed by specific regulations. A few countries, though, specifically require that a doctor, or in some particular cases a gynaecologist, insert IUDs. Others permit appropriately trained health personnel to perform the insertion.

In the absence of specific regulations, the insertion procedure is generally assumed to fall within the definition of the practice of medicine and therefore is often undertaken only by doctors. There is, however, some room for flexibility here, and in some instances it is permissible for appropriately trained health personnel to perform the insertion. Where neither laws nor regulations forbid insertion by non-doctors, it is legally permissible to use such personnel by delegating the function to them. The doctrine of custom and usage permits delegation of medical tasks as long as the doctor maintains supervision. The doctor, however, remains legally responsible for the action of the trained health personnel.

Contraceptive safety

Most countries require that hormonal contraceptives meet some national safety and quality standards. A number of developing countries base these standards on those that have been established in developed countries. Some countries require a certificate of free sale which essentially certifies that the drug being imported is sold in the exporting country. Some require that either the Food and Drug Administration (USA), the Committee on Safety of Medicines (UK) or the Board of Drugs (Sweden) approve the drug for use. This requirement is sometimes specified in the Ministry of Health regulations, but often it is an unwritten *de facto* policy.

Import and manufacture of contraceptives

Many countries have rules that affect the importation of contraceptives. In countries where contraceptives are not manufactured the rules affect the availability of contraceptive methods. Import rules exist for various reasons: to raise revenue, to conserve foreign exchange, or to protect local manufacturers, as well as for safety reasons. Some countries, realizing that price is a factor in wide-spread contraceptive use, have either lowered or dropped tariffs. The import duties vary widely. For example, Bangladesh, Egypt and Tunisia allow contraceptives to enter duty free, while Uganda imposes a 50% duty. In Colombia, tariffs range from 26% to 45%. Import duties have been removed from contraceptives in South Korea, Sri Lanka, and Thailand. In French overseas territories, the import and manufacture of contraceptives has been authorized. In Ireland the manufacture and import of contraceptives requires a licence from the Ministry of Health.

Voluntary sterilization (surgical contraception)

Voluntary sterilization (surgical contraception) has become one of the world's most widely used methods of family planning. An estimated 105 million couples of reproductive age have made voluntary sterilization their method of choice. The IPPF Panel of Experts on Sterilization suggested that the following principles should govern the general approach to voluntary sterilization:

(*a*) Each individual (as a matter of human rights) has the freedom of choice to control his or her fertility. Indeed, freedom of choice in this area is guaranteed by many national constitutions.

(*b*) Where there is no law forbidding voluntary sterilization, it is legally permissible to perform the procedure.

(*c*) Under normal circumstances, consent voluntarily given legitimizes a medical operation.

Since voluntary sterilization for contraceptive purposes is a relatively new procedure, most countries do not have laws which specifically regulate sterilization. In the large number of countries without any statutory law specifically against sterilization, the operation is apparently legal, even though it may not be common medical practice.

The trend throughout much of the world has been to reduce or remove restrictions on voluntary sterilization and to clarify its legality. However, in some countries, confusion still exists as to the legal status of voluntary sterilization. At present, laws and policies can be placed into four basic categories:

Countries where voluntary sterilization for family planning is specifically permitted by special provisions of law — either statutes, ministry regulations, or presidential decrees (24 countries containing 13.5% of the world's population).

Countries where voluntary sterilization is legal because there is no law that can be interpreted as prohibiting it. The largest number of countries fall into this category (52 countries containing 59% of the world's population).

Countries that have not clarified the legality of voluntary sterilization. This category includes some civil-law countries — those with legal codes based on continental European practice — including most French-speaking African countries and some countries of Europe and Latin America. In these countries criminal code provisions banning intentional bodily injury have been interpreted as applying to voluntary sterilization for family planning even though the person voluntarily consents. In these countries prosecutions of doctors performing voluntary sterilizations are virtually unknown. These include 29 countries containing 14.5% of the world's population.

Countries where voluntary sterilization for family planning purposes is illegal under statute, ministry regulations, or decree (29 countries containing 11.9% of the world's population).

As with other laws affecting family planning, practices and law sometimes differ. For example, voluntary sterilization procedures are generally available in Belgium and France even though legal doctrine has until recently considered them clearly illegal. In Japan, voluntary sterilization for contraception is readily available even though the law authorizes sterilization only for eugenic and therapeutic purposes. In a number of countries where statutes do not specifically address sterilization, government agencies offer voluntary sterilization, thus making it clear that the procedures are legal.

Consent

Since voluntary sterilization is generally irreversible, the primary responsibility of those who provide sterilization services is to ensure that the individual gives mature, informed, unpressured consent to the operation, is legally adult and legally and socially competent to give that consent. To this end those providing sterilization have a responsibility to ensure that the individual seeking the operation receives and understands information about the procedure.

Some governments, in an effort to prevent coercion or abuse of voluntary sterilization, have established individual informed consent procedures. In some cases there are rules for spousal, parental or guardian consent. They have also set age, parity and other requirements on who may obtain voluntary sterilization.

Turkey, in an effort to prevent coercion, established a penalty of two to five years' imprisonment for anyone who performs sterilization without the consent of the person involved. The age of consent in some European countries is 25 years. In other countries, consent for voluntary sterilization is the age of majority, usually 18 or 21. Some developing countries have set the age at 30 or 35, but Singapore allows voluntary sterilization on request for those over 21. India has set different age requirements for men and women — 25 for men and 20-45 for women (age is linked with parity in some programmes, so the age of consent varies). Some countries also have parity requirements. Egypt requires that a couple have three children, one must be male, and Bangladesh requires that a couple have two children and the youngest must be over one year old.

Parental or guardian consent is required for minors, incompetents, or the mentally ill in certain countries.

In counselling the prospective recipients of voluntary sterilization the provider should include a discussion of the procedure's irreversibility, availability of alternative reversible methods of contraception, advisability of the procedure as a contraceptive method, the description of the techniques used in the procedure itself, and the long- and short-term benefits and risks to health. It should be made clear to the individual that, at present, sterilization should be considered a permanent procedure. On the other hand, it should be stressed that the operation does not necessarily guarantee the prevention of pregnancy in every case, particularly during the immediate post-sterilization stage for males. In the case of male sterilization, the individual should be provided with some contraceptive measures for at least 12 ejaculations.

It is also advisable to secure in writing the voluntary informed consent of a legally competent, fully informed person who wishes to be sterilized. This is necessary for two reasons: (1) to ensure that the person being sterilized fully understands and consents to the procedure and the consequences which attend it, including possible failure; and (2) to protect the doctor and/or the institution where sterilization is performed from any liability which might attach if consent were not acquired. The voluntary informed consent also removes the possibility of viewing sterilization as falling within the criminal law prohibitions on, for example, mayhem or mutilation. None of the above, however, will insulate a doctor from liability for an operation which is performed negligently. This is in keeping with the accepted rules governing surgical procedures.

Care should also be taken to ensure that a marriage partner, or a third party, does not encourage an individual to accept sterilization against his or her will. Conversely, where the individual being sterilized has given informed consent, under most legal systems it is not legally necessary to obtain the consent of the other spouse for the purpose of protecting the doctor or the institution concerned. However, the non-consenting spouse may have a right of action against the person being sterilized, based on the general principles of marriage or family law in a given country. For example, sterilization without either the knowledge or consent of the other spouse, or against his or her expressed wish, may be grounds for divorce or separation in some countries. It is therefore advisable, but not legally mandatory, to get the signatures of both spouses where possible. However, the spousal consent policy should not be used in such a way as to deny the procedure to individuals who want it and can give informed consent.

Abortion services

Since 1967 the abortion laws in no fewer than 40 countries have been altered. In all but two of these, the grounds for abortion have been expanded. At present nearly two-thirds of the world's population lives in countries where laws permit abortion on a wide variety of grounds. In five out of the six most populous countries of the world, abortion is widely available — China, India, Japan, the USA and the USSR. The trend towards liberalization is clear, though in recent years pressure has been growing to restrict this move. Not surprisingly, as the IPPF Ad Hoc Expert Panel on Abortion which met in Bellagio in 1978 observed, current abortion laws take a variety of forms, impose a variety of restrictions, and differ considerably in their content. They differ in the degree and extent to which they permit women to select abortion as a method of fertility regulation. Nevertheless, certain general provisions and legislative patterns emerge in respect of the following indications:

1. *Risk to the life of the woman (the life indication).*

2. *Risk to the woman's health (both physical and mental health) from continuation of pregnancy, meaning risk beyond that normally associated with pregnancy (the health indication).*

To avoid problems over the definition of the word 'health', the Panel concluded that where countries have subscribed to World Health Organization principles it would be appropriate to use the WHO definition of health in interpreting their abortion laws: "Health is the state of complete physical, mental and social well-being and not merely the absence of disease or infirmity".

3. *Some degree of likely physical or mental impairment of the child if born (the fetal indication).*

4. *Pregnancy by rape or incest or other specified sexual crimes (the juridical indication).*

5. *The effect of childbirth upon the health and welfare of the woman and her existing children and family (the social, socio-medical or socio-economic indication).*

6. *Jeopardy to the social position of the woman or her family (the family indication).*

7. *Failure of a routinely employed contraceptive means (the contraceptive indication).*

This type of provision is unusual. The law in India (1971) was one of the first to contain a provision that permits the interruption of the pregnancy where there was a contraceptive failure.

8. *On request, usually during the first trimester.*

Legal requirements governing the provision of abortion care

The following kinds of requirements, usually found in more liberal laws, are among those that govern the provision of abortion care:

Requirements as to who should perform abortions

The requirements in this respect range from those that have no regulations at all about who may undertake abortion procedures, to those that require they be performed only by registered medical practitioners, or that medical practitioners have additional special qualifications, e.g. a specialty in gynaecology. A number of contending arguments emerge from legislation which confines the procedure to the few. It is not easy to oppose concentrating abortion procedures exclusively in the hands of the most qualified doctors. Protection of the health of women is an interest of the highest individual and social priority.

The argument in favour of ensuring high standards is compelling, especially since adverse reactions to routine procedures may in principle arise in any individual case. Nevertheless, the argument can be overstated, and its emphasis upon excellence has sometimes been found to affect the widespread availability of abortion services. When laws or regulations require performance of abortion by only the most highly skilled, many fewer procedures are legally undertaken than if the law permitted performance by others who are adequately trained. The doctors who oversee childbirth itself, which in most countries usually presents a greater hazard to women's health than early pregnancy termination, are not generally governed by special legal requirements or qualification.

It has been suggested that the person providing general health care to the community should be the person responsible for the provision of abortion services. If the care is provided by a registered medical practitioner, no special qualifications should be required for all other comparable procedures.

In both developed and developing regions of the world properly trained midwives, public health nurses and comparable health and auxiliary personnel perform many medical and surgical procedures and are also able to conduct procedures safely early in pregnancy under adequate supervision. An advantage of their involvement is their ability to provide equal or higher quality of pre- and post-abortion care and counselling than a busy doctor can offer, thereby securing better and perhaps more confidential care. They already play an important role in fertility regulation, including menstrual regulation, to which the earliest abortion is analogous. Further, as research produces non-surgical abortifacients with controllable side-effects, and as the doctor's involvement in their employment can therefore be reduced, effective management can be projected along more extended lines of delegation.

Doctors delegate many procedures, for which they remain medically responsible, to their staffs. They train, advise, supervise and are at hand, of course, in the event of emergency, but do not attend in person. Legally restricting medical services to the most scarce and costly personnel may prejudice service to the community. It is important to point out that, to date, the only country to specifically authorize non-doctors to perform surgical abortion is China.

Requirements as to where care should be provided

Some laws either restrict the provision of abortion services to specified institutions or leave the choice of place to the discretion of the health professions.

The argument that has favoured detailed supervision is that it promotes a high quality of care, and reduces or accommodates emergencies. Similarly, strict supervision may be required in late, surgical abortions when a viable fetus may be produced. The argument on the other side is that sometimes such regulations can greatly reduce the availability of safe abortions.

Requirements as to when care should be provided

While legislation cannot itself guarantee a supply of resources for abortion services, it can be designed to make such services more easily available to all, and to protect the health of the woman by encouraging the earliest possible abortion.

344

Another approach taken by some countries is to make it progressively harder to obtain abortions sought after the first trimester. For example, the permissible indications for abortion are often narrowed or the approval of a second doctor is required after the first trimester. Requirements that may cause delay should not be incorporated in abortion legislation.

Legality of treatment of incomplete abortion

Abortion laws are often the most stoutly defended yet least enforced on national statute books. Their symbolic role in defence of the defenceless has a powerful emotive appeal. Instances of enforcement, however, are notoriously unsuccessful. Police do not normally tend to move to enforce legislation that is obviously obsolete or out of accord with public opinion, nor do they normally proceed against a woman who performs an abortion on herself even in countries where women inducing their own abortion are liable to prosecution. Nonetheless, where the law is restrictive, women are often deterred from seeking proper treatment for incomplete abortion, and health workers are often hesitant to proceed with treatment, because they think it is illegal. The treatment of incomplete abortion is legal despite the provisions of restrictive abortion laws. Indeed, it is a duty under the law of most countries. Since such treatment is governed in the same way as other medical procedures, it does not usually fall within the rules of the abortion law. Only the legal principles of necessity and consent govern the treatment of incomplete abortion, as they do other medical procedures. Further, where such treatment is denied, the person who denies it would, in most cases, be open to charges of violation of the rules of medical ethics and possibly those relating to negligence in the delivery of health care.

Requirements as to the provision of contraceptives

Some laws, such as in Finland, specifically require the provision of contraceptive advice and services to women in the post-abortion phase. Iceland suggests that the woman's partner also be given contraceptive advice. The law states that: "Where the woman is married or cohabiting, the man shall, if possible, likewise be given instructions regarding contraception".

Social justice considerations require that the poor be afforded equal rights to health care with those who are not poor, including the right to safe medical procedures to terminate pregnancy. By encouraging contraceptive practice the programme extends beyond the mere enactment of abortion legislation; indeed such legislation is not the end of the programme, it is the beginning. Abortion in some countries is part of an overall fertility regulation programme that gives priority to family life education and instruction in contraceptive methods.

In this spirit, the 1975 Icelandic enactment is appropriately called the Law on Counselling and Education Concerning Sex and Childbirth and on the Termination of Pregnancy and Sterilization. Similarly, the 1973 South Korean law regulating abortion and other matters of maternal health is called the Maternal and Child Health Law.

Other matters affecting providers

When indications exist upon which medical opinion would consider abortion necessary or justified, doctors and health facilities are obliged to consider abortion as a legitimate medical option. Qualified practitioners and health facilities should therefore be made aware that they may be in some legal peril if they do not conform, or at least consider an abortion procedure as a therapeutic option. Many doctors and health facilities are anxious about their involvement in abortion for reasons of self-protection; this is usually because they are unsure about their legal position.

They should be made aware, however, that in adopting this attitude, they risk legal liability. In rejecting medical treatment on non-medical grounds, qualified practitioners and health facilities may be sued for negligence (that is, for falling below the medical standard of care), and if the pregnant woman's health is damaged through continued pregnancy and/or giving birth, they may be liable for negligence. If death follows a non-medically grounded refusal of abortion, furthermore, malpractice liability in manslaughter by criminal negligence could arise.

The only exception to this is where conscientious objection is permitted under the law. Even so, providers must ensure that the woman who has met the legal requirement for an abortion is referred to those individuals who can provide it.

Menstrual regulation

The way in which the law affects menstrual regulation (MR) depends on how the law defines the crime of abortion. Some laws make attempted abortion a crime whether or not the woman is pregnant, others implicitly require the existence of a pregnancy as an element of the criminal offence.

The majority of Commonwealth countries still have laws reflecting the restrictive legislation passed initially in England in 1861 or in India in 1860. Similarly, the French Penal Code abortion provisions, although liberalized in France, still apply in the majority of former French colonies. In 1979 in the UK it was agreed that menstrual regulation could be carried out under the provisions of the 1967 Abortion Act. Both of the 19th century British and French statutes made an attempt at abortion a felony, irrespective of whether the presence of pregnancy is proved or not. However, in other legal systems, such as those that apply in much of South America, proof of pregnancy is a prerequisite for a successful abortion prosecution. In this situation, it might well be easier to defend the performance of menstrual regulation, as a legal procedure on women who have sought help soon after missing a period and before pregnancy could be verified clinically.

No test cases on menstrual regulation *per se*, as opposed to proof of pregnancy, are known to have been brought or reported. There was, however, a recent experience in England which is relevant. An English gynaecologist performed an MR procedure after a missed period but before a diagnosis of pregnancy could be made. After an anti-abortion group complained, an investigation was held and a report submitted to the Director of Public Prosecutions (DPP). The doctor ceased doing the procedure when the DPP informed him that MR "might be illegal". (If MR were not subject to the Abortion Act of 1967, it might have been prohibited by the 1861 law described above.) After considering the matter, the DPP took the view that Section 1 of the Abortion Act 1967 "affords protection to doctors using menstrual aspiration in the circumstances described in the article . . . ".*

---

* MR is a speculative treatment which can be performed before a pregnancy can be verified. For this reason, some are performed at this stage. It is therefore argued by some that the position taken by the DPP is too simplistic, that MR should not be subject to the Abortion Act of 1967, but rather be treated as other gynaecological procedures which are not the subject of special legislation.

In the absence of any other precedent, doctors and others will have to depend on legal advice they may be given concerning the application of the abortion law to menstrual regulation in their respective countries. However, the trend seems to be to treat menstrual regulation, for the purposes of terminating pregnancy, as falling within the provisions of already existing abortion laws and regulations. Although there is still some doubt whether these should apply or not, MR practice in many countries has developed in spite of apparent legal problems.

Undoubtedly, further evolution and definition of the legal status of the new option of menstrual regulation will take place in the future. For the present, in instances where there is doubt about the effect of restrictive abortion laws on MR, it is probably safe to say that MR may be performed legally in those countries which require proof of pregnancy as an element of the crime. Certainly, as indicated above, where abortion is available for a variety of reasons, particularly where it is available on request, the technique can be used as long as providers conform with other requirements of the abortion law.

Sexually transmitted diseases

Worldwide, there is considerable legislative interest in the control and treatment of sexually transmitted diseases (STDs). Legislation, in addition to establishing prophylactic and therapeutic measures, also seeks to regulate STD in the areas of: penal matters, prostitution, pre-marital and prenatal examinations, sperm donors, blood donors and wet nurses.

The law in many countries requires any person who is aware or believes he or she is suffering from an STD to seek treatment and to disclose names of partners who might be similarly affected and need treatment. In some countries, notification of health authorities is required. While most can be kept anonymous to encourage individuals to seek treatment, some countries require the name of the person to be given. A number of countries require pre-marital and prenatal examinations as a way to control STDs. In some countries the intentional transmission of an STD (sometimes through negligent behaviour) is a criminal offence.

In response to a growing incidence of STD, especially in youth, some countries have enacted or changed laws to allow access to confidential treatment for a wider range of the population. This has taken place in three forms: (1) enabling all minors, irrespective of age, to seek treatment; (2) enabling minors of a certain age to seek out treatment independently; and (3) requiring that parental consent is necessary before a minor may seek out treatment.

After an STD is diagnosed, legislation in some countries places responsibility on the parents (guardians) and/or the doctor to ensure that the treatment is carried out.

AIDS and HIV infection

The legislative response to what has been described as the pandemic of the acquired immune deficiency syndrome (AIDS), and infection by the human immunodeficiency virus (HIV), has been quite unprecedented, at least in many of the industrialized countries. As of mid-1987 some 40 countries (as well as virtually all sub-national jurisdictions in Australia, Canada and the USA) had introduced some form of legislation on AIDS; no less than 550 bills on the subject were introduced in the USA State legislatures between January and the end of August 1987.

A significant number of these bills called for mandatory testing of applicants for marriage licences. At least three USA States have now enacted such laws, the clear intent of which is to endeavour to prevent perinatal transmission of HIV — it is now established that between 30% and 50% of sero-positive (i.e. HIV-infected) pregnant women will transmit the infection to their offspring either before, during or shortly after childbirth. In two USA States, applicants for marriage licences are now required to receive information on AIDS and the availability of testing facilities. There have also been calls for the mandatory testing of pregnant women, but available information suggests that only one country has so far adopted such a measure. Elsewhere, the voluntary testing of pregnant women belonging to high-risk groups is encouraged, generally by guidelines rather than by statute.

Fully reliable evidence of transmission of HIV by breast milk is very limited, but at least one country now requires the testing of milk donors. It is of course evident that HIV can be transmitted by semen, and legal or administrative measures have been adopted in a number of countries to ensure that donated semen for artificial insemination by donor is free of HIV antibodies (see page 237).

Although not directed to family planning, other AIDS legislation may be significant in some jurisdictions. Testing of prostitutes for HIV has been instituted in a few countries. AIDS is now classified as a sexually transmitted disease in some countries, and restrictions on the advertising and availability of condoms have been liberalized in at least two European countries because their use is considered to reduce the risk of STD, including AIDS.

Perhaps most important have been the campaigns—often legislatively mandated—to educate sexually active persons (and others) about the disease and its modes of transmission and about the critical role that condoms can play at present in limiting its spread. Such campaigns may have a beneficial side-effect, namely the promotion not only of 'safer sex', but also of safer and more responsible sexual lifestyles and, hopefully, parenthood.

Compensation, incentives and disincentives

Some 40 governments reinforce population or family planning policies by rewarding those who follow the policies and by levying charges or penalties on those who do not. The benefits are usually provided from national funds rather than from any external funding source. In some countries, incentives are used to encourage higher fertility rather than decrease it.

In family planning programmes, the incentive type of reinforcement can take at least five different forms: (1) payments or bonuses to health personnel who provide family planning services; (2) compensation, in cash or in kind, to acceptors of specific family planning methods; (3) long-term economic or social benefits for families under a specified size; (4) economic opportunities for communities or businesses that meet or exceed national goals; and (5) loss of benefits or outright penalties for those who do not follow policies.

Payments to providers or recruiters are sometimes a feature of incentive programmes. These range from a set fee for an IUD insertion or a sterilization procedure to higher stipends for family planning workers who meet acceptor targets. A major ethical concern, however, is whether payments specifically for permanent methods lead providers to pressure users who would really prefer a reversible method.

Policies which authorize a direct one-time payment to individual acceptors are almost entirely confined to Asia. Most relate to voluntary sterilization. In most cases, payments cover lost wages, transportation, and other costs of operation. This type of reimbursement has been shown to increase the number of acceptors, especially of voluntary sterilization. However, in the case of payments to providers, excessive promotion of any one method rather than an emphasis on informing individual choice may sway people who might regret the decision later and discontinue the method they were talked into using.

The objective of long-term incentive programmes is to create a strong motivation to limit family size by providing important long-term advantages. This long-term approach is used most extensively in China and other countries of South-East Asia. In China, where the government is promoting the goal of the one-child family, benefits are the largest and most varied.

Community incentives represent another approach to increased family planning practice. These are intended to create a sense of social responsibility within a group and to reduce the central government's administrative involvement. One drawback for programmes which rely on peer pressure is that without proper education or a strong belief in the ultimate goals of the programme, resentment and opposition often arise.

Some countries use disincentive programmes. They include a monthly charge for each child after the second one, a threat to the children's education and work, an increase in delivery and crèche charges for each succeeding child, and less tax deductions for further children.

The issues raised by incentive and disincentive programmes are important ethically, administratively and politically. Ethically, arguments range from the view that they infringe on individual freedom of choice and action in determining family size, to the view that they actually increase choices, especially for the poor, by relieving them of responsibility greater than the family can handle. In some countries, the argument that what is good for society as a whole may have to take precedence over the rights of individuals has currency. The potential tension between the right of individuals to choose the size of their families and the interest of governments to limit population growth, thereby protecting the welfare of current and future generations, is at the core of the ethical debate.

In recognition of the potential problems and ethical issues, some donor governments and international agencies have prepared specific guidelines for any payments related to voluntary sterilization.

The administrative pitfalls of the incentive/disincentive programme range from the abuse of the system to the possibility of it becoming extremely expensive for programmes which offer financial incentives. Moreover, the delivery and monitoring of an incentive/disincentive programme that may be easy in the city may be hard and expensive to implement in the rural areas.

Politically, incentives and disincentives have been most acceptable and successful where public opinion supports policy goals to which they are related. Where it does not, friction and resistance to the programme will cause difficulties in implementation and this will only serve to fuel political resistance to the programme. While incentive and disincentive programmes are in use in various countries, it is still considered better to have good family planning programmes with a strong educational component.

The use of trained health and auxiliary personnel

Over the past few years numerous studies have shown that, when properly trained and supervised, health and auxiliary personnel are capable of assuming a wide variety of family planning duties, including screening women for and prescribing oral contraceptives, inserting intrauterine devices, and providing differing forms of follow-up care.

In family planning the trend appears to be in the direction of expanding the roles of these personnel. Whether or not non-doctor personnel can legally provide family planning services is determined by laws governing the practice of medicine in general, the prescription of drugs and devices, and laws dealing specifically with family planning methods.

Some medical practice statutes tend to define the practice of medicine in a way that precludes the use of non-doctors in family planning except as providers of information. These statutes are now being criticized for their excessive rigidity. In a broader context of health care, it is probable that thousands of non-doctors throughout the world perform duties which legally would be considered medical practice although they are not always protected by law. Midwives and nurses are regarded as part of a 'caring' not 'curing' profession. They are able to carry out technical procedures on instruction, but in many countries are not allowed decision-making authority, and lack the ability to play an independent role in fertility regulation.

Pharmaceutical laws place legal requirements on the distribution of medication including certain contraceptives, through the doctors' prescription and pharmacy sale requirements. In general, these laws tend to protect the general public from indiscriminate use of potent drugs, self-medication, or administration by untrained personnel. In the case of contraceptives, however, these statutes used to be one of the single most effective limitations on the role of non-doctors. However, some countries have begun to re-evaluate their health care systems and to revise the laws regulating them, to allow a more active involvement of non-doctor personnel. Much initial effort has been made to demonstrate that non-doctors, when properly trained, provide suitable health care services. There are various approaches which enable the individual doctor or clinic to use non-doctor personnel more fully within the traditional legal setting of medical practice (see page 336).

Family planning services for adolescents

Laws relating to providing family planning services to adolescents vary greatly. In many countries, by virtue of laws or policies on public morality, it is essentially illegal to provide family planning information and services to adolescents. These laws and regulations apply to married and unmarried adolescents alike in some countries. In others, the law does not specify whether such activities are legal or illegal, yet custom prohibits the practice.

Where it is legal to supply family planning information and services to unmarried adolescents, parental consent may be required. This practice may prevent adolescents seeking family planning advice. However, it may be valuable for parents to offer constructive support at this time, although many sexually active adolescents would prefer not to involve their parents. A few countries permit adolescents themselves to consent to receiving family planning advice and services.

There are basically two ways in which adolescents receive information about contraception. One is through a formal programme such as used at school, and the other is informally. In countries where most adolescents are in school it is easier to disseminate information. However, in the developing world where only 36% (Latin America), 22% (North Africa and the Middle East), 20% (South Asia) or 6.9% (Africa) are in a secondary school programme, other approaches must be used. Numerous laws regulating the type of information reaching the general public may inhibit or forbid dissemination of sexual health information. Malta's regulations treat information on reproduction as immoral. Indonesian law makes specific mention of adolescents under 17 in forbidding the dissemination of contraceptive information. However, the government provides 'family life education' to adolescents. In the

Philippines, 'instruction and information on family planning and responsible parenthood' must be given before a marriage licence may be issued.

Parental concern about the type of information made available to adolescents on sex and family health has resulted in these subjects being excluded from some population education programmes. Reluctance to include sex education in school curricula is beginning to change in some of the developed countries, particularly since the advent of AIDS. In a survey carried out in the USA in 1982, 82% of adults supported sex education in the school system. Latin American countries, however, have some of the most restrictive laws and policies on reproductive health education. In Argentina, sex education which includes information on contraception is considered a criminal offence, particularly if it takes the form of 'propaganda'. The Argentine decree prohibits any "dissemination of information on fertility regulation to the public". Much of the same attitude still exists in many Francophone countries in Africa where remnants of the 1920s French anti-contraception legislation still affect the legal rule.

In a general analysis, two somewhat contradictory features exist. First, though countries may favour family planning as a reproductive health strategy and seek to inform adults, they resist instructing the young. And second, where religious precepts are threatened, the political rather than the legal process is used to stifle its acceptance. For example, in many Latin American countries instruction on 'responsible parenthood' is acceptable as long as it conforms to the doctrinal approach of the Catholic Church. Where contraceptives are available to adolescents, it is usually to married adolescents. This adds another dimension to the problem.

The IPPF policy on the subject is as follows: (*a*) Fertility regulation information and services should be freely available on request to all young married people irrespective of parity or length of marriage. (*b*) Priority should be given to "programmes which aid in the removal of barriers to the availability of sex education and fertility-related services to youth, including information and counselling on sexually transmitted diseases and other matters of concern to youth". (*c*) "Wherever pre-marital conception is a social and clinical problem, family planning services should be available for the unmarried".

INDEX

355